K

Ethical Patient Care

Ethical Patient Care

A Casebook for Geriatric Health Care Teams

EDITED BY

Mathy D. Mezey, R.N., Ed.D.
Christine K. Cassel, M.D.
Melissa M. Bottrell, M.P.H., Ph.D.(c)
Kathryn Hyer, Dr.P.A., M.P.P.
Judith L. Howe, Ph.D.
Terry T. Fulmer, R.N., Ph.D.

The Johns Hopkins University Press
BALTIMORE AND LONDON

The Johns Hopkins University Press
2715 North Charles Street
Baltimore, Maryland 21218-4363
www.press.jhu.edu

Library of Congress Cataloging-in-Publication Data

Ethical patient care: a casebook for geriatric health care teams /
edited by Mathy D. Mezey ... [et al.].
    p.   cm.
Includes bibliographical references and index.
ISBN 0-8018-6770-3 (pbk. : alk. paper)
    1. Geriatricians—Professional ethics. 2. Geriatrics. 3. Medical
ethics. I. Mezey, Mathy Doval.
[DNLM: 1. Health Services for the Aged. 2. Ethics, Medical.
3. Patient Care Team. 4. Terminal Care. WT 31 E84 2002]
RC952.5E85 2001
174′.2—dc21   2001000335

A catalog record for this book is available from the British Library.

    The Case for Megateams   295
    Judith L. Howe, Jeremy Boal, Kirsten Ek, and Christine K. Cassel

17 Emerging Ethical Issues in Geriatric Team Care   317
    Peter J. Whitehouse

    Glossary, compiled by Chandhana Paka   *333*
    Index   *343*

Jeremy Boal, M.D., Assistant Professor of Medicine and Geriatrics, Mount Sinai School of Medicine, New York

Melissa M. Bottrell, M.P.H., Ph.D.(c), Project Director, Division of Nursing, New York University, New York

Russell Burck, Ph.D., Associate Professor of Religion, Health, and Human Values; and Director, Program in Ethics and Ethics Consultation Service, Rush–Presbyterian–St. Luke's Medical Center, Chicago

Christine K. Cassel, M.D., Director, Geriatrics Research, Education, and Clinical Center (GRECC), Bronx Veterans Affairs Medical Center; and Professor and Chairman, Brookdale Department of Geriatrics and Adult Development, Mount Sinai School of Medicine, New York

Joann Castle, M.A., Project Manager Emeritus, Henry Ford Health System, Detriot, Michigan

Eileen R. Chichin, R.N., Ph.D., Codirector, Center on Ethics, Jewish Home and Hospital, New York

Phillip G. Clark, Sc.D., Professor and Director, Program in Gerontology and Rhode Island Geriatric Education Center, University of Rhode Island, Kingston

Theresa J. K. Drinka, M.S.S.W., Ph.D., Consultant and President, River's Edge Consulting, Waupaca, Wisconsin

Nancy Neveloff Dubler, LL.B., Professor and Director, Division of Bioethics, Montefiore Medical Center, Bronx, New York

Carmel B. Dyer, M.D., Associate Professor of Medicine, Baylor College of Medicine and Director of the Baylor College of Medicine Geriatrics Program at the Harris County Hospital District, Houston

Kirsten Ek, B.A., Writer, Brookdale Department of Geriatrics and Adult Development, Mount Sinai School of Medicine, New York

Catherine Eng, M.D., Medical Director, On Lok Senior Health Services, San Francisco

Terry T. Fulmer, R.N., Ph.D., FAAN, Professor and Director, Muriel and Virginia Pless Center for Nursing Research; and Codirector, the John A. Hartford Foundation Institute for Geriatric Nursing, Division of Nursing, New York University, New York

Judith L. Howe, Ph.D., Assistant Professor and Associate Director for Education, Geriatrics Research, Education, and Clinical Center (GRECC), Bronx Veterans Affairs Medical Center, Bronx, New York; Codirector, New York Consortium of Geriatric Education Centers, Brookdale Department of Geriatrics and Adult Development, Mount Sinai School of Medicine, New York

Kathryn Hyer, Dr.P.A., M.P.P., Coprincipal Investigator, GITT Resource Center; Director, USF Training Academy on Aging; faculty in Departments of Gerontology and Health Policy and Management, and Clinical Instructor, Department of Internal Medicine, University of South Florida, Tampa

Rosalie A. Kane, M.S.W., Ph.D., Professor, Division of Health Services Research, Policy, and Administration, University of Minnesota School of Public Health, Minneapolis

Susan Kornblatt, M.A., Project Director, Geriatric Interdisciplinary Team Treaining (GITT) Program On Lok Senior Health Services, San Francisco

Ernestine Kotthoff-Burrell, M.S., R.N., C.S., Project Director, School of Nursing, University of Colorado Health Sciences Center, Denver

Stanley Lapidos, M.S., Project Coordinator, Rush GITT Program, Rush–Presbyterian–St. Luke's Medical Center, Chicago

Laurence B. McCullough, Ph.D., Professor of Medicine and Medical Ethics, Center for Medical Ethics and Health Policy, Baylor College of Medicine, Houston

Mathy D. Mezey, R.N., Ed.D., FAAN, Director, the John A. Hartford Foundation Institute for Geriatric Nursing, and Independence Foundation Professor of Nursing Education, Division of Nursing, New York University, New York

Trang Nguyen, M.D., Assistant Professor of Medicine, Baylor College of Medicine, Houston

Ellen Olson, M.D., Chief, Extended Care and Geriatric Programs, and Associate Director for Clinical Programs, Geriatrics Research, Education, and Clinical Center (GRECC), Bronx Veterans Affairs Medical Center, New York; and Associate Professor, Brookdale Department of Geriatrics and Adult Development, Mount Sinai School of Medicine, New York

Kate O'Malley, R.N., M.S., G.N.P., Inter-regional Director of Cancer Control, American Cancer Society, Oakland, California

Chandhana Paka, B.A.(c), Research Assistant, Division of Nursing, New York University, New York

Linda Farber Post, J.D., B.S.N., M.A., Bioethics Consultant and Assistant Professor, Division of Bioethics, Montefiore Medical Center, Albert Einstein College of Medicine, Bronx, New York

Jill A. Rhymes, M.D., Assistant Professor of Medicine, Geriatrics and Extended Care Service, Veterans Affairs Medical Center; and Huffington Center on Aging, Baylor College of Medicine, Houston

Bruce Robinson, M.D., M.P.H., Professor of Geriatrics, University of South Florida College of Medicine, Sarasota

Lori A. Roscoe, Ph.D., Assistant Professor, Office of Curriculum and Medical Education, College of Medicine, University of South Florida, Tampa

Steven K. Rothschild, M.D., Associate Professor, Department of Family Medicine, Rush–Presbyterian–St. Luke's Medical Center, Chicago

Eileen Silverman, L.S.W., Supervisor, Adult Protective Services Division, Texas Department of Protective and Regulatory Services, Houston, Texas

Nancy L. Smith, Ph.D., A.P.R.N., C.S., Associate Professor, School of Nursing and Dental Hygiene, University of Hawaii at Manoa, Honolulu

Thomas A. Teasdale, Dr.P.H., Assistant Professor of Medicine and Statistician, Geriatrics and Extended Care Service, Veterans Affairs Medical Center; and Huffington Center on Aging, Baylor College of Medicine, Houston

Peter J. Whitehouse, M.D., Ph.D., Professor of Neurology, Integrative Studies, Case Western Reserve University, Cleveland

Nancy L. Wilson, L.M.S.W., Associate Professor of Medicine, Huffington Center on Aging, Baylor College of Medicine, Houston

The face of the U.S. population, and indeed, the world, is changing rapidly. Not only are Americans becoming more racially and ethnically diverse, but also the population is aging. Successes in enhancing the health and longevity of the population have been achieved through public health advances and improved medical care, as well as through higher levels of education, better diets, and safer housing and workplaces. These unprecedented successes ensure that a larger proportion of Americans will have the opportunity to grow old and to spend a substantial portion of their later years independent and in good health. There is considerable evidence that these population trends are continuing and that the limits of longevity have not yet been reached, even in countries with the longest-lived citizens. There is also strong and growing evidence that rates of disability are declining, even among the oldest groups. Despite this unexpected good news, increased population longevity means growing numbers of older persons who are experiencing substantial burdens of health and social problems. These problems are complex, interrelated, and difficult to disentangle and manage.

For half a century, professionals focusing on the care of older persons have argued that the knowledge and skills of multiple disciplines are required to address the multifaceted problems associated with chronic illness and the many losses experienced in later years. More recently, a cornerstone of geriatric clinical practice and education in the health professions has been the use of multidisciplinary teams working together to address the complex problems of older patients and to provide integrated care. Barriers to achieving this ideal have been substantial, and both organizational and financial disincentives are daunting. Nonetheless, efforts to develop and maintain interdisciplinary teams for improving geriatric care have continued across the United States and abroad. These teams have involved an assortment of professional disciplines in an array of service-delivery systems, depending on a variety of funding mechanisms.

Appreciating the obvious logic of interdisciplinary team approaches for geriatric patients, but also noting the rather underwhelming success (or survival) of such teams, the John A. Hartford Foundation launched an innovative program to stimulate the development of interdisciplinary teams and to better understand factors contributing to success, as well as the barriers challenging those successes. Much has been learned in this effort, as the projects struggled with the real-life issues of developing and maintaining teams, along with the everyday concerns involved in caring for geriatric patients. In particular, the teams struggled with ethical issues and moral dilemmas raised by efforts to develop innovative programs in changing health care systems; to care for patients with multiple problems in the context of their families and other care providers; to integrate the knowledge, skills, and cultures of various professionals; and to negotiate transitions among settings.

This book results from an effort to share insights and strategies developed as a part of the geriatric interdisciplinary team training project and to involve a larger audience in consideration of the many ethical issues surrounding team-based care specifically and geriatric care more generally. The book succeeds nobly in illustrating the complexity of the problems and the importance of careful consideration of ethical issues, cultural mores, and professional values. It also suggests effective strategies for addressing ethical conflicts and difficult decisions. The use of real-life experience and case studies adds flesh and feeling to the skeletal structure of theoretical systems and ethical constructs.

The authors very effectively "speak from the trenches," at each turn demonstrating their grounding in the real world as they apply ethical principles and philosophical values to the everyday problems and conflicts arising in interdisciplinary team care. This book is a valuable resource for practitioners considering team-based care, for professionals providing care to patients with multiple problems, and for ethicists and philosophers concerned with providing ethical guidance to caregivers, families, and health professionals.

Terrie Wetle, Ph.D.
Associate Dean of Medicine for
Public Health and Public Policy
Brown Medical School

Effective and collaborative teamwork by physicians, nurses, social workers, and other health professionals is a core resource for the care of older adults; interdisciplinary care is the hallmark of good geriatric care. No one health discipline has all of the knowledge needed to deal with multiple complex chronic illnesses. No one discipline can establish effective continuity of care across multiple locations ranging from the patient's home, to acute care hospitals, to rehabilitation and long-term care institutions. No one discipline can cost-effectively focus resources on functional outcomes to assure that older patients maximize their independence in activities essential for independent living.

Few if any geriatricians or geriatric nurse practitioners function well without a team. Many community physicians who care for older patients also routinely collaborate with other professionals in a team. But, "teams" take many different forms. Some comprise practitioners who work in a multiple-specialty group practice or long-term care settings. Others are "virtual teams," bringing professional expertise and collaboration to bear depending on the complexity of a specific patient's needs. What creates a team is agreement on the organization and priorities for services around a common goal—the patient's care plan.

Working in teams is not a skill that comes naturally to everyone. "Teaming"—cross-training and learning about how teams function—is rarely an explicit part of the curriculum of programs preparing health care professionals. Health professionals, even those in geriatrics, rarely train together in teams, understand team function, or appreciate the range of expertise and skills of other health professions. In 1995 the John A. Hartford Foundation launched a major initiative to stimulate models of interdisciplinary team training in geriatrics in settings ranging from tertiary academic health centers to community health care networks. The goal of this $12 million Geriatric Interdisciplinary Team Training (GITT) Program was to substantially enhance the understanding of factors critical to the success of interdisciplinary geriatric care by strengthening the training of interdisciplinary geriatric team members. Thirteen universities and health care systems around the country and a resource center experimented with creating models of team training. Since the project's inception, more than eighteen hundred health care professions students and practicing professionals have participated in GITT educational programs and documented the outcomes of GITT effectiveness. Curriculum and insights into developing these programs are available from the New York University Resource Center (www.gitt.org).

In the process of implementing GITT, some participating faculty interests coalesced around ethics. Clinical ethics has long embraced interdisciplinary teams as a model for mediating and resolving ethical issues in health care, sometimes constituted as an "ethics committee." Geriatrics is rich with important and difficult ethical issues in managing individual patients and interactions between patients, family members, and health care providers. GITT faculty developed case studies and teaching materials for teams encountering ethical issues in the process of providing patient care. As we shared materials, the idea for this book emerged. Quite simply, we realized we had a rich body of material that could be of great use to people in teaching programs working with interdisciplinary teams in medical ethics or geriatrics or both.

We were encouraged by the response from Wendy Harris at the Johns Hopkins University Press. Ms. Harris was supportive throughout, and she pressed us to focus and strive for cases and analyses that were sharp, incisive, and new.

This book represents the determined efforts of many people. Of course, the authors of the cases and the chapters were important colleagues. Not only were they essential to getting the job done but also we learned from each other and created lasting friendships in the process. In addition to their authorship activities, Kathryn Hyer and Judith Howe took on strong editorial and organizational leadership roles. Melissa Bottrell's intellectual incisiveness, organizational and editing skills, and gentle but persistent pressure to meet deadlines helped moved the project from concept to reality. Finally, we owe special gratitude to the John A. Hartford Foundation of New York, and particularly to foundation staff who provided inspiration and friendship as well as funding: Corinne Rieder, Donna Regenstreif, Laura Robbins, and Christopher Langston.

We hope that the reader senses our excitement with the new intellectual territory we discovered in developing this book. The insights that we gained have added immeasurably to the quality of our practice. We hope you will find the book valuable, perhaps even in surprising ways. We expect it will be useful for training programs for physicians, nurses, social workers, and other health professionals, especially those expecting to care for older patients and most especially those specifically focusing on a career in geriatrics. We also expect people involved in bioethics teaching and in organizational development research and scholarship to find here new insights that they may not find in the traditional textbooks in those fields. Those in the world of practice, where ongoing continuing education is a major commitment, will find real-world lessons here. We welcome communications from individuals who find this book useful and invite you to share with us comments about the book's strengths and weaknesses and ideas that you have for improvement.

PART I

Introduction

CHAPTER 1

An Introduction to Bioethics as It Relates to Teams and Geriatrics

Christine K. Cassel, M.D.,
Mathy D. Mezey, R.N., Ed.D., and
Melissa M. Bottrell, M.P.H., Ph.D.(c)

Patients and health care providers are confronted daily by an ever-growing number of options for the diagnosis and management of disease. Health care management becomes more difficult when the patient is older and therefore is more likely to be subject to multiple interacting illnesses and conditions. The multifaceted nature of geriatric care and the complex ethical dilemmas that can arise when patients become more functionally and cognitively dependent make providing appropriate and ethical care for older adults more challenging.

Over the past thirty years, interdisciplinary teams have been suggested as an effective approach to enhance care for people with multiple and chronic health care needs. An extensive body of literature describes the processes and positive outcomes associated with care delivered by these teams. Recently, managed care has triggered a renewed interest in teams as health care providers and institutions respond to new modes and locations of practice and changing reimbursement structures.

Nowhere in health care has the team concept taken greater hold than in geriatrics. Geriatric teams are now standard practice in geriatric assessment and rehabilitation and are mandatory in nursing homes receiving Medicare or Medicaid reimbursement. A growing body of literature documents the association between improved outcomes for older patients and care management by interdisciplinary teams (Rubenstein et al. 1984; Applebaum and Austin 1990). When a frail, cognitively impaired older resident has no family, the nursing home team often takes the place of family members in addressing the resident's everyday and long-term needs and care goals.

Teamwork implies improved communication between care providers such that teams are valued for their ability to avoid conflicts among providers, patients, and family members that if unaddressed would lead to ethical confrontations about patient care. Yet despite its known benefits, team care management may create ethical dilemmas by the very nature of team dynamics. Poorly functioning teams, perhaps because of disciplinary cultures and values that create barriers to communication, can distort ethical analysis. Even in seemingly well-functioning teams, the voice of the patient may be lost among health care providers who, acting collaboratively, have institutionalized their analytic and decision-making patterns. Teams organized for the express purpose of reducing costs can become a mechanism to convince the patient to select a "fiscally sound" treatment that may not represent the patient's interests or preferences.

In this chapter we describe the complex needs of geriatric patients and the role of teams in facilitating their care. We discuss ethical concepts that ground the analytic framework for ethical decision making and introduce ethical issues that can both inform and intrude when geriatric teams care for elderly patients and their families. We also discuss our choice of Jonsen, Siegler, and Winslade's (1998) framework as the basis for analysis and discussion of the ethical dilemmas confronting teams presented in the remaining chapters.

Overview of Geriatrics

The increasing number of people in our society living upwards of thirty years as older adults—from the age of 65 and into the mid- and late nineties—challenges health care providers with an extraordinary panoply of health care conditions. Normal age-related changes couple with diseases that manifest in later life. Dementia strikes a minority but nonetheless large subset of older people (25–50 percent prevalence in people 85 and over) (American Psychiatric Association 1997). Family and other age cohort members that used to assist with or be present for decision making and recovery die or move away, making them unavailable. Thus, older adult patients, and especially very old patients, challenge the communication, informational, and teaching skills of physicians, nurses, social workers, and others who are drawn into the elder's care.

With people age 65 and older expected to make up 33 percent of the world's population by 2050 (Population Division, Department of Economic and Social Affairs 1998), most nations' health care systems are confronted by previously unthinkable problems. Anticipating that at age 65 people will live an additional twenty years or more, the focus of care needs to shift to health promotion, disease prevention, and the control of disease sequelae that hamper independent functioning. On the other hand, older people with acute illness, recurrent and progressive chronic illness, and severe functional and mental frailty will continue to require care, preferably at home or in community settings, but also in acute care and long-term care institutions.

Most elders prefer to receive care at home. It is estimated that 65–70 percent of all home health patients are 65 years of age and older (Martin 2000). In 1995 Medicare-certified home care agencies made more than 252 million home visits to approximately 1.5 million Medicare beneficiaries (Mitty and Mezey 1998). Some 41.2 percent of these were for licensed nursing visits, while another 48.2 percent were home health aide visits (Health Care Financing Administration 1999).

Older patients with chronic diseases experiencing complications or acute exacerbation of existing illnesses occupy many medical and surgical hospital beds. Older people are admitted to hospitals approximately three times more often than the overall population, and 42 percent of all acute care hospital days are for people aged 65 and over. The level of complexity of elderly patients is evidenced by their average length of stay of 6.5 hospital days, as opposed to 4.3 days for younger patients. In 1996 the number of days of care of discharged hospitalized patients over 75 years of age was about twice that of those 65–74 years of age and five times that of the population 45–64 years old (U.S. Census Bureau 1998).

Nursing homes are a necessary option for the small but substantial portion of people 65 and over who, because of severe functional and cognitive impairments (inability to perform at least three activities of daily living [ADLs] and many instrumental activities of daily living [IADLs]), are unable to live independently. In 1997 nearly 1.6 million residents were cared for in more than 17,000 nursing homes in the United States (Gabrel 2000). More than 78 percent of residents were aged 75 and older, of whom more than 40 percent had bladder or bowel incontinence. Approximately 48 percent of all nursing home residents were thought to have a dementing illness (Krauss and Altman 1996).

Approximately eighteen hundred agencies provide hospice care to terminally ill patients of all ages in free-standing hospices, at home, and in hospitals and nursing homes (Haupt 1998). Only about 20 percent of dying patients are referred to hospice; referred patients typically receive between seventeen and twenty-one days of hospice services prior to death (Lamnari 2000).

Managed care is starting to address the care of frail older adults. Until recently managed care companies with Medicare risk contracts sought to enroll only the "well elderly." A few mature capitated model programs for the frail elderly exist: the Program of All-Inclusive Care of the Elderly (PACE) demonstration projects (Eng et al. 1997), social HMOs (Newcomer, Harrington, and Kane 2000), and nurse practitioner–physician collaboration models such as the nurse-run nursing home–based EverCare model (Kane and Huck 2000), and For Health. The PACE and SHMO models enroll both frail and well elderly persons.

Overview of Teams

A comprehensive history of teams is beyond the scope of this text (for an in-depth discussion, see Pfeiffer 1998). Brill (1976, p 14) defines teamwork as: "work which is done by a group of people who possess individual expertise, who are responsible for making individual decisions, who hold a common purpose, and who meet together to communicate, share and consolidate knowledge from which plans are made, future decisions are influenced and action determined." Several aspects of Brill's definition are worth noting. Physicians, nurses, social workers, and therapists come to the team experience with strong discipline-specific skills, perspectives, experiences, and propensities (Pfeiffer 1998). Effective interdisciplinary team members have confidence in the unique body of knowledge and skills that they bring to patient care needs. The communication and negotiation that are hallmarks of a mature team are best done by seasoned professionals who have sufficient confidence in their own skills to welcome the complementary skills of the other team members.

Second, while team members are responsible to one another, they are also responsible for individual decision making. Parsimonious resource use supports the concept of "task-specific roles" for different team members; each member takes on those tasks that they do best and that are within the purview of their discipline. But for a team to function effectively, all the members must be supportive of the team's common purpose.

Third, Brill's definition strongly underscores that team members have a stake in the outcome of their deliberations. A health care team is a group of professionals with a common goal. Explicating a clearly defined purpose and goal of care is often the most difficult but also the most useful aspect of team deliberation. While at minimum the purpose is to fulfill the care obligations to the patient, clarifying the scope and content of that obligation and the subsequent actions is a key task of teamwork. Similarly, participants on a team have joint accountability for the short- and long-term consequences of the advice given to the patient and family and of the mutually supported decisions.

Brill's definition fails to capture the leadership component of successful teamwork, yet leadership issues can create internal conflict. Historically, clinicians of different disciplines worked together to provide patient care and ensure positive patient outcomes. In such "informal teams" the physician was the de facto team leader, but communication between members about care decisions was generally open and unfettered. Organizational structures typically recognized the physician as the formal leader; this was sometimes necessary for legal purposes to mark accountability and liability for treatment decisions. But effective teams recognize, use, and try to develop leadership skills among team members. Shifting leadership is an important task in the development of formal teams (Purtilo et al. 1998); it positions the discipline with the most to offer the patient *at the time* such that other disciplines assume a supportive role.

Creating a formal team is a process with discrete steps that evolves over time (Pfeiffer 1998; Tsukuda 1998). Often-quoted stages of team development are forming, storming, norming, and performing (Tuckman 1965). *Forming* involves developing a sense of trust among members and establishing the methods by which the team will operate. This stage spills over into the *storming* phase which is characterized by resisting the team's "rules" and testing whoever happens to be in the leadership role at the time. Each phase allows time for team members to understand and appreciate the roles and contributions of their colleagues and to reflect on their own roles. *Norming* occurs when a set of common goals and values are incorporated or internalized by all the team members. The final stage, *performing,* occurs when team members come to see themselves as a mutually supportive group whose members provide constructive feedback. The experience of the Interdisciplinary Team Training Program in Geriatrics (Panneton et al. 1982) and the John A. Hartford Geriatric Interdisciplinary Team Training Program (Siegler et al. 1998), among others, has shown that team skills can be successfully taught to health profession students and practicing professionals.

There can, however, be a dark side to teamwork (see Chapters 10 and 11). Groupthink can obscure the goals of care or interrupt adequate appreciation and encompassing of patient or family goals. Lack of leadership and the "maintenance roles" of group work can cause dissension and delay decision making. Role dilemma and strain appear to be associated, in part, with the time required for team participation (e.g., preparation and meeting attendance) and lack of administrative support. Yet despite the hazards of teamwork, the benefits of team care, especially for older patients, continue to make inroads in a variety of health care settings.

Interdisciplinary teams are particularly useful for patients who require the attention of multiple disciplines, that is, patients described as having "wicked problems" (Drinka and Clark 2000). Teams are needed when patient problems are both complex and nonroutine (ibid.) due to the multitude of options and unpredictable patient responses to treatment. A team can help the patient and family to identify the benefit, burden, and consequences of various treatment options.

Knaus et al. (1986) documented the association between good communication among physicians and nurses and reduced mortality and morbidity for patients in intensive care. Physicians are coming to recognize the implications of poor communication between themselves and nurses in acute care and other settings. Other studies have confirmed the benefits of teams in caring for patients with chronic health problems and those requiring rehabilitation (Diller 1990; Keith 1991), hospice (Eng 1993), and Alzheimer disease services (Snyder 2001).

In geriatrics, improved outcomes were found for patients cared for in geriatric assessment units as compared to other units throughout the hospital (Rubenstein et al. 1984). More recently, interdisciplinary team care has improved outcomes for older patients and their family members in a primary geriatric care setting (Applebaum and Austin 1990). Perhaps the most important function of a team is the ability of team members to hear the patient's wishes from multiple perspectives and to clarify patient and family concerns.

Managed care organizations evaluate outcomes relative to episodes of illness rather than episodes of care. When evaluating an episode of illness, the desired outcome of disease management—for example, congestive heart failure—is not the hospital length of stay but rather the overall annual cost of care and the functional and quality-of-life outcomes. Focus on the episode of illness has accelerated movement toward more formalized interdisciplinary teams to both improve care and contain costs. Caring for such patients, however, can also uncover if not create a variety of ethical dilemmas that teams must resolve.

Overview of Bioethics

Moral issues have always been part of health care practice, even at the time of Hippocrates. But with the advent of modern science and technology, moral issues now occupy center stage and are more complex. Bioethics, an interdisciplinary field involving philosophers, theologians, lawyers, social scientists, and clinicians, has grown as an independent scholarly discipline, especially since the 1980s. The field examines issues as diverse as recombinant DNA research and genetic engineering, public health concerns such as the international AIDS epidemic, and economic issues such as fair allocation of limited financial resources for health care. Cultural relativism is a concern of bioethics because different nations and different ethnic groups within nations may have different health priorities and values from the mainstream society. For example, the U.S. Constitution and legal system emphasize the protection of the individual and the right to self-determination far more than do many other cultures and legal systems. Bioethics research contributes to the framing and analysis of ethical problems and perspectives on the moral or legal resolution of social issues and describes ethical aspects of the health care attitudes and choices of patients, families, and clinicians.

Clinical work in bioethics has generally involved ethics consultation or ethics committees. Ethics consultation is now common in American hospitals and, to some degree, in nursing homes. An ethicist is an expert in the fundamental literature of bioethics and in law related to health care. Called to consult in cases when difficult moral dilemmas arise, the ethicist becomes a member of the clinical team caring for a patient. Rarely does an ethicist make a final decision in a difficult situation; rather, he or she provides a combination of helpful information, mediation, and facilitation of the group process toward resolution of confusion or disagreement.

An ethics committee is an interdisciplinary group of staff that often includes a lay person or community representative. Mandatory in hospitals and a growing presence in nursing homes, these committees may be charged with developing institutional policies for informed consent, resuscitation, and genetic diagnosis and disclosure in order to establish consistent practice within the institution. Ethics committees may advise clinicians on individual cases as they occur. Ethics committees may also educate staff about ways of evaluating and resolving ethical dilemmas and about new medical technologies and laws that might have implications for clinical practice.

Ethical Decision Making

An ethical dilemma is a situation in which two or more important competing values conflict, yet one must be chosen. Moral behavior may be defined by widely accepted codes of social behavior or by the duties of citizenship. But even within the philosophical literature, ethics—"the moral evaluation of human behavior"—does not have a single agreed-upon framework or set of principles with which to resolve ethical dilemmas. Some argue from a "principled" standpoint that difficult decisions should be analyzed against the template of those widely agreed-upon rules. For example, "Thou shall not kill," a widely accepted moral rule, could influence one to oppose physician-assisted suicide or abortion. On the other hand, a priority of respect for individual autonomy might result in a clinician's decision to help a terminally ill patient end his life or to help a woman terminate an unwanted pregnancy. Rule-based ethics can nevertheless end in conflict between different rules and the surrounding process of setting priorities between the rules. These priorities are in some instances reasoned to be absolute. For example, some religious frameworks may argue that the proscription against killing trumps the right to self-determination.

Other philosophers suggest that ethical rules should be relative to situation. Despite calls to rule-based reasoning, *situational ethics*—sometimes referred to as "casuistry"—is what most clinical bioethics discussions become in practice. Its widespread use is attributed to a number of factors, perhaps the strongest being the absence of a single dominant religious framework in the United States (even though religious beliefs often strongly influence standpoints in medical ethics). Precisely because of the diversity of beliefs and cultures in the United States, the Constitution explicitly protects and strengthens the rights of individuals to make their own decisions. Thus, bioethical conflicts that arise often require analysis and setting of priorities between different values, taking into account moral beliefs, ethical principles, and the rights of the individuals involved. For this reason, mediation skills are central to the effectiveness of an ethics consultant or committee. The process of understanding and giving voice to the beliefs, fears, concerns, and questions of all relevant parties (patient, family, and clinicians) is often as important as the final decision that resolves an ethical conflict or dilemma.

In addition to rules and situational ethics, two related schools of ethical analysis—*consequentialist* and *utilitarian*—focus on the likely outcome of a decision and how the greatest good can be accomplished. A strict consequentialist analysis examines a decision's specific consequences for the people involved. A utilitarian analysis will examine what is best overall—or, as it is often phrased, the greatest good for the greatest number.

Modern medicine has brought ethics into health care in an explicit way. Philosophers, legal scholars, and religious experts often participate in teams' clinical decision making and are familiar with the language and culture of clinical medicine. Many clinicians, in turn, study ethics and are knowledgeable about the language and analytic framework of philosophical ethics and the basic legal background of important medical decisions. These clinical ethicists may also join an interdisciplinary team, even if they are not caregivers for the patient under discussion.

Out of this rich interdisciplinary discourse have come several practical approaches to clinical bioethical problem solving. One of these approaches, often referred to as *preventive ethics* (McCullough et al. 1995; see also Chapters 5 and 7 in this volume) tries to anticipate and prevent ethical dilemmas and conflicts from arising. A paradigm example of preventive ethics is advance directives. Patients express their preferences concerning life-sustaining treatment in the event of a critical or life-threatening illness, in advance of that illness occurring and the potential incapacity that may accompany it. Another approach to preventive ethics is to improve communication about a patient's values and treatment goals throughout the course of a primary care relationship or an episode of serious illness. This kind of "values" history taking not only yields easier and more open communication but gives the clinician a measure of confidence about treatment decisions if the patient permanently or temporarily loses the capacity to speak for himself.

In another approach, Russell Burck (Chapter 3) uses the language of defining "the good, or the not so good" when dealing with ethical dilemmas. "The good" may be an individual personal good or a broader social good, such as reducing the risk of communicable disease or ensuring universal access to health care.

Burck's definition strives to evaluate the good based not on abstract concepts but on answers to the following types of questions:

- What are the right actions? Which actions are more right and not as right? What principle or standpoint is being used to analyze this question?
- What is the responsibility in this situation, and who bears that responsibility?
- What is the proper use of power?
- What is the appropriate relationship of means and ends in this specific situation?

Central to many ethical dilemmas, especially in the care of older adults, is the determination of decision-making capacity. Much of American bioethics rests on the right of individuals to decide for themselves, derived from almost a century of case law (see *In re Schloendorff v. Society of New York Hospital* 1914). How do we know whether an individual has sufficient ability to understand his or her situation so as to make an independent decision? If the person does not, then the responsibility moves to the care providers to make a decision based either on *substituted judgment* (what that patient would have decided for himself) or on a *best interest* standard (if we don't know enough to make a substituted judgment determination).

Determinations of capacity are frequently based on psychiatric research, yet many in psychiatry will assert that they are not well trained in capacity determination. Capacity determination may be only a legalistic concept or perhaps a legalistic fiction in some situations. For example, patients with short-term memory impairment may be able to understand the benefits of a proposed treatment and express their values. If they don't remember the next morning when the operating room gurney arrives, is the consent invalid? Many elderly people may be mildly demented or simply a little "eccentric," making decisions that do not appear to have any sense in the context of what we know about their future and the actual risk involved. A patient may refuse to be evaluated for coronary artery disease, for example, because to her an electrocardiogram suggests a myocardial infarction, while coronary artery surgery appears safe. This decision would strike us as "irrational," yet even an individual who is not diagnosed as psychotic might make that decision. Is she therefore "crazy"? If a patient with a known diagnosis of schizophrenia or other psychotic disorder made such a decision, he would be assumed to not be in his right mind and the legal system would override his decision or appoint a guardian. What do we do in the gray area between the obviously psychotic patient and the "eccentric" patient?

Finally, surrogate decision making becomes very complex. Many states, on the assumption that family members act in the best interest of relatives, stipulate a legal hierarchy by which the entitlement to make proxy decisions occurs. For example, in the case of an elderly man, the decision may first go to the wife, second to the adult children, third to the siblings, and so on. The issue of surrogacy raises questions about the nature of families, possible conflicts of interest in the event of an inheritance, and the presumption of family solidarity and good spirit. While most families probably do speak in the best interest of their loved one, making such decisions may stir up deep-seated emotional conflicts or raise questions of financial gain. The clinician must ascertain if the surrogate speaks from a perspective of substituted judgment, the best interest of the patient, or the best interest of the family overall.

Other values that are often used to frame the analysis of ethical dilemmas are virtues, rights, and justice. A *virtues focus* tends to center on the care provider. What would the virtuous nurse, physician, or other health professional do in this situation? The question appeals not to abstract ethical rules or moral principles, but to the idea of a moral or virtuous person and what that person might do. Interestingly enough, this kind of analysis can allow for a ground-up approach to determining the right action. It may alternatively allow for a situational or consequentialist approach in which the resolution emerges from the impact on people who are confronted with making that decision—a combination of patient, family and health care provider.

A *rights-based analysis* usually focuses more on the patient and asks whether a person has certain rights that ought to be respected regardless of the values or cultural beliefs of others. For example, if a patient has, a "right to life" or, alternatively, a "right to die," appropriate responses to a clinical situation will differ depending on the right appealed to and the ability of the right to trump other considerations, such as "do no harm." Interestingly, the rights approach may often end up looking very much like an autonomy-based approach in which the base priority is the value of actions as determined by the individual patient. As we continue to develop methods to communicate with individuals with various dementias and redefine and enhance our definitions of decision-making capacity, we are in essence redefining concepts of individual personhood (see Chapter 17), which may have implications for rights-based analyses.

A *justice-based perspective* is often contrasted with the rights-based, or individual autonomy, perspective. Justice involves the notion of fairness to a group of people, often those who are disadvantaged socially, economically, or by our health care system. Justice issues may concern distribution of scarce resources, such as organs for transplantation, or broader financial allocations. For example, one could argue that a younger person should get preferential access to a liver that is available for transplantation because that person may benefit more—for example, through a likelihood of more productive years of work—than an older person may. Organ transplantation is one area of health care in which age-based rationing is widely accepted within the United States. In situations where organ transplantation is highly dependent on the ability to pay privately for such services, then the ability to pay may trump any sense of fairness or justice related to age or other criteria.

Other issues of justice occur in the general area of health care expenditures. A frequently articulated concern is that the American health care system favors elderly people unduly because the federally financed Medicare program provides universal health insurance for those over 65. Given the large and growing number of uninsured people in the United States, this sense of favoritism leads to questions of justice and intergenerational equity. Countries that provide universal health insurance regardless of age do not have this kind of justice problem. They do, however, have to deal with problems of how best to distribute the scarce resources among the population covered. Such arguments in the United States concern whether new services ought to be covered by federally funded programs like Medicare. Oregon's attempt to rationally decide, based on a cost-benefits standard, which treatments it would and would not provide for its Medicaid beneficiaries is one example of a policy attempt to deal with such issues. The distribution of funding for acute high-technology interventions versus home care and hands-on care by nurses, nurse aides, and personal care attendants also creates issues of justice.

As more and more patients need care in circumstances where providers have a financial incentive to either withhold care or to manage finite resources over a broader population, the ethical issues associated with the cost of caring for the functionally dependent geriatric patient moves analysis of the ethical issues from the individual to the institutional context (see Chapters 14–17). How institutions manage resources—both financial and structural—can create a variety of ethical dilemmas for providers attempting to meet the medical and psychosocial needs of older adults. Such justice issues become even more complex when considered within the context of society's responsibility to the older adult and the older adult's responsibility to society, particularly when the older adult is cared for by a health care team.

Ethics and Teams

Team ethics has its own complexities. As we will see throughout this book, the members of the team need to develop cohesiveness and a sense of group identity. Even an effectively functioning team may be at risk for overlooking or avoiding difficult issues due to unspoken pressures to maintain collegiality and agreement. A team also bears a different kind of responsibility from an individual. McCullough (see Chapter 5) calls this the "co-fiduciary responsibility of teams." While caregivers need to consider their individual fiduciary relationship to the patient, the team needs to understand its collective fiduciary relationship to the patient and assure that that responsibility is acknowledged and addressed.

Not uncommonly, issues are brought to an ethics consultant or an ethics committee not because they are actual ethical dilemmas, but because the team members are uncomfortable dealing with them. Suppose a patient with metastatic cancer is unresponsive to treatment but acknowledges that death is near; she wants only pain treatment. Her case may be presented to an ethics consultant because the clinicians involved are uncomfortable confronting death and mortality. They may have failed to adequately communicate with the patient and may feel that her request for dying comfort care is tantamount to requesting euthanasia. In this situation there is no real ethical dilemma because there is no real choice. Rather, it is the result of a communication failure among team members and between the team and the patient.

A geriatric team offers an important advantage in resolving ethical dilemmas in that it creates a forum for persons with different perspectives to ensure that a decision is thoroughly discussed and that all points of view are taken into account. Even since ethics committees were spawned by the Karen Ann Quinlan case in 1976 (*In re Quinlan* 1976), a significant literature studying the processes of ethics committees has sparked debate about their effectiveness in making good decisions (Andereck 1992; McDaniel 1998; West and Gibson 1992).

Some issues raised in the debate about ethics committees apply equally to the consideration of interdisciplinary teams as venues for the resolution of ethical issues. Sometimes the process of reflecting as a group on the issues and values itself gives rise to a better sense of the right course. In addition, new information from different team members sometimes emerges that makes the solution or path clear. On the other hand, the downside to teams confronting ethical conflicts is groupthink. Every group has its own dynamics, with member leaders and nonleaders. Strong individuals may dominate the committee process, inhibiting a full hearing of diverse opinions. Strong personalities can be so persuasive that fundamental disagreements are ignored or moral objections inappropriately addressed. Members may feel that their decision must be right since they don't want to talk about it any more.

Compromise is an important part of the group process and sometimes may lead to the best resolution of a disagreement. At other times, however, it may not—sometimes there really is a right and a wrong answer, and a compromise may not be in the best interests of the individual patient. Still, for the sake of smooth process, a group may reach such a compromise. This problem raises the general issue of whether the patient and family should be members of the team.

The existence of a team itself may raise ethical issues in the delivery of health care. These issues rarely surface directly as ethical dilemmas, but they nevertheless can have enormous ramifications for patient care. For example, questions may arise about appropriate disclosure to the patient of the team's existence and its role in decision making. How does the team incorporate the patient's voice in its decisions? How does it choose or reject members of the team? The confidentiality of information and potential conflicts of interest of individual team members or of the team itself are also important issues. Elderly patients may be concerned that decisions that go beyond what they might normally consider health care—for example, about whether they have the capacity to live at home—may be made without their input.

Issues related to the role of interdisciplinary teams in raising and resolving ethical dilemmas can be divided into four categories. The first category comprises issues that relate to the team's obligation to ensure the centrality of the specific patient or family, especially with respect to the providers' obligation to the best interests of the patient.

The second category relates to functioning among *members* of the team: Who should be on the team? What is the role of the patient or family? Do different health professionals have different standing on the team? by virtue of their profession? by their proximity or responsibility to the patient? For example, does the view of the nurse practitioner who is the primary care provider hold more weight than that of the occupational therapist who has only seen the patient a few times? Similarly, issues related to team care generally, irrespective of patient care, emerge: How does the team weigh the value of information? How does power get shared? What are the group's rules for discussion and weighing information? To some degree, this category encompasses primarily process issues: How sensitive and sophisticated is the team in creating plans of care and in surfacing ethical conflicts? How and under what circumstances does the team seek ethics consultation and input? How does a team relate to an existing ethics committee? How is such ethical expertise evaluated and documented?

The third category includes issues that have implications for ethical decision making across institutions or between institutions and the community. How do the team members relate individually and as a team to the overall health care management structure? Increasingly complex and competitive health care systems make open communication among providers and different health care systems difficult. A team may inhibit discussion of complex ethical dilemmas because providers are managing multiple roles on the team, maintaining their ethical responsibility to the patients and balancing their legal and financial responsibilities to organizations. Providers from different disciplines may experience discomfort discussing ethical issues in a group where power, education, and access to the patient are uneven—an issue that particularly surfaces in nursing homes and in home care.

The fourth category consists of ethical dilemmas that arise because professionals represent both their clinical training and the institution or organization that employs them. The obligations of a group of professionals who are caring for an elderly patient, for example, are weighed against their obligations as representatives of institutions and organizations or mechanisms that finance health care. These multiple roles and the potential conflicts of interest are not only important for ethical analysis but may have a negative influence on group processing of information and ultimately team performance.

Evaluative Criteria and a Framework for Ethical Analysis

A variety of structures are available to frame ethical analysis of clinical care issues for geriatric patients, including Lo's *clinical ethics* approach (Lo 1995), McCullough and Jones's *preventive ethics* approach (Purtilo et al. 1998), and Purtilo's *five-step process of ethical decision making* (Purtilo 1993). While each structure is valid and useful for examination of ethical dilemmas in clinical cases, we chose the case analysis process used by Jonsen, Siegler, and Winslade (1998) because it is the only one to focus explicitly on the identification and analysis of the contextual factors—implicitly geriatrics and team care—that enhance or intrude on ethical decision making. But to enhance the process's teaching value for ethical analysis, we have slightly modified the case analysis template to more clearly indicate the order of steps to be taken in analyzing and resolving ethical disputes.

Jonsen, Siegler, and Winslade (1998) organize information gathering and case analysis through four different aspects: medical indications, patient preferences, quality of life, and contextual features. The modified structure used in this book more broadly indicates the environment in which team care exists and the range of ethical issues—from patient centered to organization centered—addressed in each chapter. Each case is thus analyzed through a series of steps that require teams to: (1) gather the clinical information; (2) identify patient and family preferences; (3) evaluate quality-of-life issues; (4) consider contextual issues (especially team-related issues); (5) resolve the ethical issues and create a plan of care; (6) implement the plan; and (7) evaluate the plan after it is implemented. While Jonsen, Siegler, and Winslade include family preferences within the topic of contextual issues, our structure includes family preferences within the topic of patient preferences, to more appropriately recognize the multifaceted aspects of individual health care decision making and the variety of decision-making structures used by patients and families from diverse cultural and ethnic backgrounds. We also added Steps 5, 6, and 7 to encourage providers not just to ruminate over the various ethical issues but also to construct and implement a plan of action. (See Table 1.1.)

The chapters in this book focus the bulk of their analysis on Steps 2, 3, and 4. Infused into these steps are discussions stemming from various evaluative criteria, including virtues, consequences, rights, or justice and equality. But the chapters discuss only those ethical issues that specifically apply to the case(s) presented and use only evaluative criteria that most appropriately apply to the discussion. Students and teachers looking for suggestions as to how to use the modified Jonsen, Siegler, Winslade structure should refer to Chapter 2, which clearly highlights the special circumstances and conundrums posed when an interdisciplinary team manages health care.

TABLE 1.1
Template for Case Analysis

1. Gather the Clinical Information
   a. What is the patient's medical problem? history? diagnosis? prognosis?
   b. Is the problem acute? chronic? critical? emergent? reversible?
   c. What are the goals of the treatment and care?
   d. What are the probabilities of success?
   e. What are the plans in case of therapeutic failure?
   f. In sum, will medical and nursing care benefit the patient and harm be avoided?
2. Identify Patient and Family Preferences
   a. What has the patient expressed about preferences for treatment?
   b. Has the patient been informed of benefits and risks, understood, and given consent?
   c. Is the patient mentally capable and legally competent? What is evidence of incapacity?
   d. Has the patient expressed prior preferences (e.g., advance directives)?
   e. How does the patient want to include family or friends in the decision-making process?
   f. If the patient is incapacitated, who is the appropriate surrogate? Is the surrogate using appropriate standards?
   g. Is the patient unwilling or unable to cooperate with medical treatment? If so, why?
   h. Are there family issues that might influence treatment decisions?
   i. In sum, is the patient's right to choose being respected to the extent possible in ethics and law?
3. Evaluate Quality-of-Life Issues
   a. What are the prospects, with or without treatment, for the patient to return to a normal life?
   b. What biases might prejudice provider evaluations of the patient's quality of life (i.e., is the patient or family's definition of quality of life or the provider's definition used)?
   c. What physical, mental, and social deficits is the patient likely to experience if treatment succeeds?
   d. Is the patient's present or future condition such that, if it continues, he or she might judge life undesirable?
   e. Is there any plan and rationale to forgo treatment?
   f. What are the plans for comfort and palliative care?
4. Consider Contextual Factors
   a. Are there provider (physician, nurse, etc.) issues that might influence treatment decisions?
   b. Are there financial and economic factors?
   c. Are there religious or cultural factors?
   d. Is there any justification for breaching confidentiality?
   e. Are there resource allocation problems?
   f. What are the legal implications of treatment decisions?
   g. Is clinical research or teaching involved?
   h. Is there any provider or institutional conflict of interest?
5. Resolve the Ethical Issues and Create the Plan
6. Implement the Plan
7. Evaluate the Plan

TEACHING RESOURCES

Beauchamp, T. L., and J. F. Childress, 1994. Respect for autonomy. In *Principles of biomedical ethics, 4th ed.* New York: Oxford University Press.

Gervais, K. G., R. Priester, D. E. Vawter, K. K. Otte, and M. M. Solberg, 1999. *Ethical challenges in managed care: A casebook.* Washington, D.C.: Georgetown University Press.

Glaser, J. W., and R. P. Hamel, 1997. *Three realms of managed care: societal, institutional, individual.* Kansas City: Sheed and Ward.

Johnson, T. F. 1999. *Handbook on ethical issues in aging.* Westport, Conn.: Greenwood Press.

Lo, B. 1995. *Resolving ethical dilemmas: A guide for clinicians.* Baltimore: Williams and Wilkins.

Mezey, M., J. Teresi, G. Ramsey, E. Mitty, and T. Bobrowitz, 2000. Decision-making capacity to execute a health care proxy: Development and testing of guidelines. *Journal of the American Geriatrics Society* 48(2):179–87.

REFERENCES

American Psychiatric Association. 1997. *Practice guidelines for the treatment of patients with Alzheimer's disease and other dementias of late life.* http://www.psych.org/clin_res /pg_dementia_2.html#d [2000, August 1].

Andereck, W. S. 1992. Development of a hospital ethics committee: Lessons from five years of case consultations. *Cambridge Quarterly of Healthcare Ethics* 1(1):41–50.

Applebaum, R., and C. Austin. 1990. *Long term care case management: Design and evaluation.* New York: Springer.

Brill, N. 1976. *Teamwork: Working together in the human services.* Philadelphia: Lippincott.

Diller, L. 1990. Fostering the interdisciplinary team, fostering research in a society in transition. *Archives of Physical Medicine and Rehabilitation* 71:275–78.

Drinka, T. J. K., and P. G. Clark. 2000. *Health care teamwork: Interdisciplinary practice and teaching.* Westport, Conn.: Auburn House.

Eng, C., J. Pedulla, G. P. Eleazer, R. McCann, and N. Fox. 1997. Program of all-inclusive care for the elderly (PACE): An innovative model of integrated geriatric care and financing. *Journal of the American Geriatrics Society* 45(2):223–32.

Eng, M. A. 1993. The hospice interdisciplinary team: A synergistic approach to the care of dying patients and their families. *Holistic Nurse Practitioner* 7:49–56.

Gabrel, C. S. 2000. An overview of nursing homes and their current residents: Data from the 1997 National Nursing Home Survey. *Advance Data from Vital and Health Statistics,* vol. 311. Hyattsville, Md.: National Center for Health Statistics.

Haupt, B. J. 1998. Characteristics of hospice care users: Data from the 1996 National Home and Hospice Care Survey. *Advance Data from Vital and Health Statistics,* vol. 299. Hyattsville, Md.: National Center for Health Statistics.

Health Care Financing Administration, eds. 1999. Medicare and Medicaid Statistical Supplement, 1999. *Health Care Financing Review.* Baltimore: U.S. Department of Health and Human Services.

In re Schloendorff v. Society of New York Hospital. 1914. 211 N.Y. 125; 105 N.E. 92.

In re Quinlan. 1976. 70 N.J. 10, 355 A.2d 647.

Jonsen, A. R., M. Siegler, and W. J. Winslade. 1998. *Clinical Ethics, 4th ed.* New York: McGraw-Hill.

Kane, R. L., and S. Huck. 2000. The implementation of the EverCare demonstration project. *Journal of the American Geriatrics Society* 48(2):218–23.

Keith, R. A. 1991. The comprehensive treatment team in rehabilitation. *Archives of Physical Medicine and Rehabilitation* 72:269–74.

Knaus, W. A., E. A. Draper, D. P. Wagner, and J. E. Zimmerman. 1986. An evaluation of outcome from intensive care in major medical centers. *Annals of Internal Medicine* 104(3):410–18.

Krauss, N. A., and B. M. Altman. 1996. *Characteristics of Nursing Home Residents, 1996.* http://www.meps.ahcpr.gov/papers/99-0006/99-0006.htm [2000, August 2].

Lamnari, A. 2000. Hospice. In M. M. Mezey, B. J. Berkman, C. M. Callahan, T. T. Fulmer, E. L. Mitty, G. J. Paveza, E. L. Siegler, N. E. Strumpf, and M. M. Bottrell, *The encyclopedia of elder care.* New York: Springer.

Lo, B. 1995. *Resolving ethical dilemmas: A guide for clinicians.* Baltimore: Williams and Wilkins.

Martin, K. S. 2000. Home health care. In M. M. Mezey, B. J. Berkman, C. M. Callahan, T. T. Fulmer, E. L. Mitty, G. J. Paveza, E. L. Siegler, N. E. Strumpf, and M. M. Bottrell, *The encyclopedia of elder care.* New York: Springer.

McCullough, L. B., N. L. Wilson, J. A. Rhymes, and T. A. Teasdale. 1995. Managing the conceptual and ethical dimensions of long term care decision making: A preventive ethics approach. In L. B. McCullough and N. L. Wilson, eds., *Long-term care decisions: Ethical and conceptual dimensions.* Baltimore: Johns Hopkins University Press.

McDaniel, C. 1998. Hospital ethics committees and nurses' participation. *Journal of Nurse Administration* 28(9):47–51.

Mitty, E., and M. Mezey. 1998. Integrating advanced practice nurses in home care: Recommendations for a teaching home care program. *Nursing and Health Care Perspectives* 19(6):264–70.

Newcomer, R., C. Harrington, and R. Kane. 2000. Implementing the second generation social health maintenance organization. *Journal of the American Geriatrics Society* 48(7):829–34.

Panneton, P. E., K. P. Moritsugu, and A. M. Miller. 1982. Training health professionals in the care of the elderly. *Journal of the American Geriatrics Society* 30(2):144–49.

Pfeiffer, E. 1998. Why teams? In M. Siegler, K. Hyer, T. Fulmer, and M. Mezey, eds., *Geriatric interdisciplinary team training.* New York: Springer.

Population Division, Department of Economic and Social Affairs. 1998. *United Nations 1998 revision of the world population estimates and projections.* New York: United Nations.

Purtilo, R. 1993. *Ethical dimensions in the health professions.* 2d ed. Philadelphia: W. B. Saunders.

Purtilo, R., B. W. Shaw, and R. Arnold. 1998. Obligations of surgeons to non-physician team members and trainees. In L. McCullough, J. W. Jones, and B. A. Brody, eds., *Surgical ethics.* New York: Oxford University Press.

Rubenstein, L. W., K. R. Josephson, G. D. Wieland, P. A. English, J. A. Sayre, et al. 1984. Effectiveness of a geriatric evaluation unit: A randomized clinical trial. *New England Journal of Medicine* 311:1664–70.

Siegler, E. L., K. Hyer, T. T. Fulmer, and M. D. Mezey. 1998. *Geriatric interdisciplinary team training.* New York: Springer.

Snyder, L. 2001. Care of patients with Alzheimer's disease and their families. *Clinics in Geriatric Medicine* 17(2):319–35.

Tsukuda, R. A. 1998. A perspective on health care teams and team training. In E. L. Siegler, K. Hyer, T. T. Fulmer, and M. D. Mezey, eds., *Geriatric Interdisciplinary Team Training.* New York: Springer.

Tuckman, B. W. 1965. Developmental sequences in small groups. *Psychological Bulletin* 63: 384–99.

U.S. Census Bureau. 1998. *Statistical abstracts of the United States.* http://www.census.gov/prod/www/statistical-abstract-us.html [2000, August 1].

West, M. B., and J. M. Gibson. 1992. Facilitating medical ethics case review: What ethics committees can learn from mediation and facilitation techniques. *Cambridge Quarterly of Healthcare Ethics* 1(1):63–74.

CHAPTER 2

Using This Book as a Teaching Tool

Kathryn Hyer, Dr.P.A., M.P.P., and
Judith L. Howe, Ph.D.

This book is intended to help students and clinicians who are working with frail older adults and their families enhance both their ethical decision-making skills and their team-facilitation skills. It draws on the teaching and clinical experience of faculty who participated in a national, multisite initiative funded by the John A. Hartford Foundation of New York City (Siegler et al. 1998). Beginning in 1995, the Geriatric Interdisciplinary Team Training (GITT) Program encouraged leading academic health centers and elder service providers to develop models of team training for medical residents in primary care, advanced practice nurses, master's-level social workers, and other clinicians. While developing ethical cases for teaching students, the faculty recognized that no cases merged ethics skills and team skills in practical ways that addressed the needs of clinicians on the team, elderly patients, and their families. We believe that the ethics cases presented in this book help fill this void.

Our goal has been to produce a practical text that teaches clinicians and trainees a process to analyze ethical issues that clinicians working in teams commonly face. We teach team skills together with ethical skills because in geriatric settings, after the ethical deliberations and discussions are finished, clinicians, patients, and their families (i.e., the team) must come to consensus on an appropriate course of action. The team outcome, generally an interdisciplinary care plan, should specify who does what by when. Just as clinicians need to gain skill in analyzing the ethical context of the cases presented throughout this book, they also need basic process and management tools for facilitating group discussions and decision making. Each chapter in this book reflects actual clinicians' experiences and includes intellectual musings and emotional responses to everyday ethical dilemmas, as well as a description of the process that the health care team used to resolve an ethical issue. We have included details to replicate the uncertainties and pressures clinicians face in practice, but we have altered the patients' and clinicians' identities to protect confidentiality.

Throughout the book, cases are presented both as ethics cases and as team processes. This chapter offers ways to reinforce discussion on both dimensions. While these rich ethics cases can be used exclusively for ethical discussions, we encourage a fuller discussion of the ethical complexities that arise from providing care in a team. Few trainees will appreciate the complexity of the team without explicit discussion about team process, communication techniques, conflict resolution approaches, and power differentials. Since cases require class discussion, we also include recommendations on how to lead a case discussion and how to encourage learners to come to class prepared to discuss the case.

The learning objectives for the book are:

1. to apply a team-based framework to approaching the range of ethical dilemmas facing interdisciplinary geriatric health care teams;

2. to recognize the differences and commonalties among various disciplines on a team and predict how those differences may impact team process and on patient outcomes;

3. to identify the range of settings and circumstances in which teams operate along the continuum of geriatric care;

4. to explain the benefits to the patient and the family of participating and working with a group of clinicians; and

5. to apply team skills in facilitating ethical discussions to enhance communication, resolve conflicts, create team norms, identify the challenges of interdisciplinary teamwork, and avoid "groupthink."

In this chapter, we present ways to enhance ethical discussions on teams within the framework proposed by Jonsen, Siegler, and Winslade (1998), which we have adapted to accommodate a team's need to process the ethical discussion. The rationale and ethical context for the seven steps are described in more detail in Chapter 1, but clinicians should always agree to (1) gather the clinical information; (2) identify patient and family preferences; (3) evaluate quality-of-life issues; (4) consider contextual issues (especially team-related issues); (5) resolve the ethical issues and create a plan of care; (6) implement the plan, and (7) evaluate the plan. For the ethical analysis, four different types of information are gathered and processed within the team meeting: medical indications, patient preferences, quality of life, and contextual features. Each case is thus analyzed through a series of steps that reinforces ethical consideration in fact gathering, elicits the preferences of the patient and family and the clinicians treating the patient, and processes the information in a way that focuses the group on a common task—agreement about the course of action. The final steps in the template encourage the team to realize that consensus about the plan is only part of their job.

We encourage the instructor to treat the class discussion as a team meeting. Reminding learners about their responsibility to prepare for case discussions will help them practice making a clinical summary of relevant facts and using their process skills before their peers. In clinical settings, trainees will be expected to come prepared to team meetings. Ultimately, instructors must recognize that as they teach this case-based approach, they are modeling the very team skills that they hope students will learn. By establishing the ground rules for discussions, making clarifying statements, encouraging participation from quiet observers, and quelling loquacious or domineering individuals, instructors are modeling and reinforcing the very facilitation skills that the learners need to acquire to effectively process a team discussion.

Organization of the Book

In order to describe a range of ethical dilemmas facing teams of providers and to highlight differences in values, preferences, and socialization to the elderly among different disciplines, this book presents a variety of "cases from the field." These case presentations enhance the use of the book as a teaching tool as they provide real-world examples that are livelier, more relevant, and less intimidating than a lecture on ethics. The authors are seasoned clinicians, educators, and gerontologists who selected the cases based on their experiences in caring for older adults. The cases reflect care that was provided to elders in a variety of settings—in the community, at home, in hospitals, and in nursing homes. Each case involves an ethical conundrum faced by an interdisciplinary team of health professionals who are providing care to an older adult and who may disagree on what needs to be done.

The part headings highlight types of bioethical dilemmas faced by professionals working on teams that care for older adults and their families. Part II underscores differences in discipline-specific socialization and how those forces impact the group processing of ethical issues. A team is composed of individuals who bring diverse personal and professional identities to their clinical practice. The personal identity formed by one's age, gender, culture, values, personal style, professional identity, disciplinary socialization, and expertise, along with one's professional knowledge and experience in health care settings, combine to create the unique skills, knowledge, and attitudes of each team member. But teams rarely acknowledge these differences in members' knowledge, values, and attitudes. The cases in this part demonstrate the power of professional socialization and the damage that ignoring it creates in producing unacknowledged team conflicts and unsatisfying team decision making.

Part III emphasizes the team's obligation to make choices that ensure the centrality of the specific patient or family. How teams involve patients as team members is a critical issue. The voices, power, and importance of the patient and family unfold in countless obvious and subtle ways. The ability of a team to hear the patient, to honor the patient's cultural preferences and values, and to abide by the patient's wishes are core components of ethical dilemmas, particularly as frail patients lose cognitive capacity. Patient autonomy, when it collides with the team's recommendations, requires clarification of patient motives and capacity but also submission to the patient's rights.

Part IV considers the implications for ethical decision making across institutions or between an institution and the community. Since legal and regulatory standards change as the locus of care shifts, this part highlights what happens when well-established teams of providers have to coordinate care with other teams. Both the ethical analysis and the resolution of issues are complicated when teams work across settings. Creating team norms of trust, confidentiality, and open communication is more difficult in a competitive environment with scarce resources.

Part V articulates the ethical dilemmas that arise because professionals represent both their professional training and the organization or institution that employs them. The chapters in this part weigh the obligations of groups of professionals caring for elderly patients against their obligations as representatives of institutions and health insurance companies. The implications of multiple roles and potential conflicts of interest are addressed both in the ethical analysis and in the group processing of information.

Implications of the Demographic Imperative

The coeditors compiled this book because health care professionals need to recognize the global demographic imperative of a rapidly increasing older population and its implications for themselves. The baby boomers have already turned fifty, and by 2020 more than 20 percent of the U.S. population will be over 65 years of age. By 2020 families and providers will be caring for the large numbers of older adults who will increasingly be living to more advanced ages. While many elders will be healthy and vigorous, a significant number will require assistance because of multiple chronic conditions and the associated disabilities leading to functional impairment.

The demographic revolution has more implications than simply the number of elders who will need health care services for chronic *conditions*. The color and ethnicity of aging in America is also changing. The Census Bureau projects that by 2015 some 21 percent of all elders will be non-Caucasian (U.S. Census Bureau 2000). Training clinicians to recognize the influence of culture on care and family expectations about elders' needs is a particular emphasis in the case examined by Smith and colleagues (Chapter 5). There the team was torn about advocating for a Hawaiian elder's needs and the family needs in a primary care geriatrics clinic. Other cases in the book also reflect the diversity of America's elders and reinforce the need for each clinician to acknowledge her or his own culture and values and the strong influence these personal aspects have in shaping expectations about care.

The Changing Locus of Care

In only one decade, home care has grown tenfold, from $2 billion (3 percent of the Medicare budget) in 1988 to $20 billion (9 percent of the Medicare budget) in 1998, although it has recently become the target of budget cuts (National Association for Home Care 2000). Despite these cuts, home services will continue to grow because home is the preferred setting of care for most elders and the costs are still less than in other settings. Our cases reflect the shifting locus of care to the home, which is the setting in Dyer and colleagues' chapter (Chapter 9) and in two of the cases presented in Howe and colleagues (Chapter 16); it also factors into the dilemma examined in Dubler and colleagues (Chapter 10). Dubler and colleagues emphasize the ethical issues that a hospital-based discharge planning team encounters when a patient prefers a questionable home care plan over other options that might better meet his medical and social needs. Other cases highlight the ethical issues facing a team as a patient's autonomy and the caregiver's responsibilities collide. In the case from Dyer and colleagues, a hospital team must reconcile its plan with an adult protective services team that has a different mission and a different set of operating norms. In the Howe and colleagues case of Mrs. Rodriguez, the patient's desire to die in her home must be reconciled with the team's assumption that Mrs. Rodriguez does not have the capacity to make that decision.

In Howe and colleagues's second case, in which Mr. Stokes requires hospice at home, the reader gains insight into the challenge of managing noncurative medical and support services for a terminally ill patient in the home under a capitated budget. Hospice services, like home care, have been increasing in number of providers and requests for service. While 71 percent of hospice patients have a diagnosis of cancer, this case discusses a patient with a debilitating stroke, an important and noteworthy condition appropriate for hospice services. The need to begin discussions about prognosis and palliative care (rather than curative care) is another theme that this case highlights; such discussions should be encouraged among health profession students and clinicians.

The cases also highlight the disconnects that occur in transitions between emergency rooms, inpatient units, home care services, and hospice care at home. They highlight the ethical dilemmas stemming from different legal obligations to provide service in different settings. Questionable family caregiving further complicates the cases. The cases allow a rich discussion of patient autonomy, teams, and the different rules and obligations of clinicians who provide care from within the various components of the acute long-term care system. They also highlight the problems that patients face when they are shuffled among providers and when no one team takes the responsibility to coordinate the transitions among and between providers.

Finally, the chapters discuss emerging ethical issues that have implications for teams, such as the trend toward more frequent movement from setting to setting along the care continuum, and privacy concerns around access to electronic records and from electronically created virtual teams. In a provocative chapter about the future (Chapter 17), Whitehouse addresses the privacy implications and the new forms of teams that technology makes possible. As has already been proven, new technology, virtual teams, and telemedicine raise further issues of accountability across health care settings and the need to keep teams patient-focused.

Nursing Home Teams

The majority of cases presented in the book involve the most vulnerable elders in the long-term care system—nursing home residents. Because the typical nursing home resident has complex problems, the federal nursing home reforms enacted in 1987 (OBRA 87) required nursing homes to conduct comprehensive assessments by multidisciplinary teams and since then, teams have routinely worked in nursing homes. Our cases reflect the ethical and team issues in monitoring and adjusting care for frail elders, who frequently have limited cognitive capacity. Balancing the rights of these patients, family concerns, and the rights of other residents is an ongoing challenge. We hope that the insights of these clinicians and the cases prove helpful for those working in nursing homes.

Managed Care

The book also focuses on the dilemmas facing health care teams because of changes in reimbursement systems. Ideally, managed care changes the incentives of the health care plan that is responsible for paying and arranging for services and shifts care from treatment to prevention and early intervention. Multiple providers have incentives to coordinate services and to be certain that treatments are not at cross-purposes. These incentives are especially important to frail elders, who frequently are vulnerable to multiple providers prescribing medications and treatments without full knowledge of those already in place. But many fear that managed care reduces the willingness of providers to pay for expensive services and encourages them to deny appropriate treatments

We present a number of dilemmas facing teams in managed care programs, including some of the newer organizational settings. Howe and colleagues' hospice case (Chapter 16), involves managing a patient who needs a great deal of personal care, well beyond the usual hospice budget. Kornblatt and colleagues' case (Chapter 8) focuses on the problem of managing a difficult patient who demands costly services under the On Lok / Program of All-Inclusive Care for the Elderly (PACE) model of care. PACE is a managed care program designed to keep frail elders living in the community through a series of primary care, adult day care, rehabilitation, and preventive services. In this case, the patient demanded services in a way that raised ethical and reimbursement quandaries and that also had important implications for the fiscal solvency of the program.

Difficult fiscal tradeoffs are also the theme in Castle's discussion (Chapter 14) of incentives between and among the different parts of an integrated system of care. Who has the interests of the patient at heart? Finally, Hyer and colleagues (Chapter 15) highlight the ethical dilemmas facing practitioners who receive compensation from multiple sources, an increasingly common practice. This case also discusses the incentives of a new capitated nursing home reimbursement model that operates as a Medicare replacement program in some nursing homes.

Benefits of Interdisciplinary Teams

Demonstrating the value of interdisciplinary geriatric assessment began in 1984, when Rubenstein and colleagues (1984), in a randomized control trial, demonstrated decreased mortality, more accurate diagnosis, improved function, and decreased rates of nursing home placement for elders who were evaluated and treated by an interdisciplinary geriatric team. Later studies (Baggs et al. 1992; Stuck et al. 1993) confirmed the value of interdisciplinary teams and care planning for geriatric patients.

Teamwork is a "special form of interaction and interdependence between health care providers who merge different but complementary skills in the service of patients and in the solution of their health problems" (Tsukuda 1998). The circumstance of multiple clinicians caring for geriatric patients and interacting with their families produces a team of caregivers and provides the context for group or team processing of clinical care. But team care can also provide the opportunity for group discussion of patient and family preferences and the often-related analysis of ethical dilemmas. Thus team care enhances ethical analysis beyond the ability of a sole practitioner who must wrestle with ethical issues and arrive at a conclusion alone.

We believe that clinicians do recognize the importance of discussing values and options with patient and family. But because of demands on their time and the immediate needs of the next patient, clinicians often put off ethical discussions with geriatric patients, rationalizing that with no emergency, no event forces an immediate decision. The goal of this book is to promote explicit ethical discussions with patients during routine care. Geriatric ethical issues generally unfold over a long time and arise along the continuum of care from hospitals and nursing homes to homes and community-based settings. Thus, time can be a partner in helping families and patients discuss choices and can also help clinicians shift to a "preventive ethics" framework (McCullough et al. 1995; Doukas and McCullough 1996).

Moreover, we do not believe ethical discussions should occur only with physicians. All clinicians have a responsibility to help patients, families, and their fellow clinicians understand their treatment protocol and the implications of the care they provide. Clinicians must balance their own values, their discipline-specific training, and their relationship with the patient in the context of the treatment. Yet few clinicians from any of the many disciplines routinely working with elders regularly engage patients and their families in ongoing discussions about choices, values, and priorities. We expect this book to help change that dynamic.

Teams also have an added ethical context: How does one balance the disparate and sometimes competing interests of patients, families, and clinicians? What are the implications for patients if clinicians disagree about the appropriate course of action? Can the clinicians still work a joint caseload together? Are there preferred ways to process ethical discussions and decisions in which the group of clinicians must abide by the conclusions? Why is the ethical decision-making process in teams more complicated? Is it merely that, by virtue of numbers, the interaction of values, information, and relationships is complicated? What are the dangers of a group in discussing patients' interests? How does the group guard against groupthink and keep fresh and focused on patients as unique individuals? Or does something inherent in team process require clinicians on a team to practice ethical decision making differently?

Uses of This Book

This book is suitable for use in the classroom for trainees in a variety of health professions, including medicine, nursing, social work, pharmacy, nursing home administration, case management, and the rehabilitation therapies. While every case presented here includes the physician, nurse, and patient, many cases include other clinical professionals as well. Field instructors and preceptors in these disciplines can also use this book for strengthening the ethical analysis and teamwork skills of their students.

Practicing professionals and teams are likely to find the book useful for strengthening individuals' or teams' teamwork skills in a clinical setting. We especially recommend the case-based format for practicing clinicians. In facilitating discussions, each case can be a jumping-off point for comparing ethical and team issues with current cases and problems.

Finally, the book can be used in continuing education programs, such as those in geriatric education centers, which offer workshops on team building and teamwork. Cases may also be selected as part of a grand rounds, highlighting the complex nature of decision making.

The Value of the Cases for Learners

Each chapter includes a case description, a case analysis, questions to provoke further discussion, and in some cases, a list of teaching resources. The book also contains a glossary of terms. The core of each chapter is a template for analysis of the ethical issues (Jonsen, Siegler, and Winslade 1998). This template provides consistency across chapters and a problem-solving framework for learners' analysis of their own "cases from the field," including medical indications, patient preferences, quality of life, contextual features, and plan of action.

Clinicians are familiar with the case-based approach: the teaching case replaces the lecture as the vehicle for learning, and the case, the situation, and the people described become the basis for discussion and exchange of ideas. As the clinical, ethical, and family actions based on actual events unfold in a case, trainees naturally ask how they might have prevented adverse outcomes. The careful study and analysis by learners before the discussion enables trainees to practice their analytic and process skills on actual or realistic problems under the guidance of their teacher. By studying cases, learners begin to assume the role of practicing professionals long before they graduate.

At a minimum, simulated team discussion about ethical dilemmas should allow learners to gain an understanding of what needs to be done after the meeting and how it can be accomplished. At its best, the case discussion will explore values and unrecognized assumptions that hinder the processing of ethical discussion for some clinicians. Since there are no "right answers" to the cases, the case discussions provide learners with issues, problems, choices, and information. As such, they will help learners to become comfortable with the question "What would you do if you were a clinician at the team meeting described in the case?"

Each case presented in this book is unique, yet important learning themes are consistent across all of them. Learners need to understand the specific context, locus of care, competency of the patient, agreement among family members, and disease process as dimensions critical for establishing a care plan. Additionally, learners need to understand how those aspects interact with ethical dilemmas and team discussion. How long the team members have worked together, how well they work with each other, and the respect they have for each other also warrant discussion. Not all teams in this book are long established; nor do their members always operate with high levels of mutual respect. A new physician unsettles the team in the case from Smith and colleagues (Chapter 5). In the chapter by Dubler and colleagues (Chapter 10), a physician working on a team requests an ethics consultation to stop the delaying tactics being used by the social worker to thwart a discharge plan that she believes to be unsafe.

The cases should also help learners to discern the larger environmental and organizational issues that influence and affect decision making. The reimbursement and legal risks for the institution that employs the clinician are important considerations in processing a decision. Equally important is the need to place the ethical dilemma in a broader social perspective, understanding that the process of resolving it may have important and long-lasting implications for the other team members both personally and professionally.

Through cases, trainees can learn how to clarify and resolve ethical issues and practice the process used to arrive at the solution. Learners need to realize their formal and informal role on the team, both in helping clarify an ethical dilemma and in helping the team achieve agreement. The ultimate contribution of any team member is to help the group achieve consensus and then monitor the actions agreed to.

The Facilitator's Role

While cases allow learners to examine the multiple facets of a situation, case-based learning—especially case-based learning focused on teaching team skills—requires a skilled facilitator.

The facilitator in a case discussion allows clinicians to observe, learn, and practice the skills that are essential for team resolution of ethical issues. In case presentations, we encourage the instructor to play a facilitation and leadership role during the ethical discussion. We recommend that the instructor use at least some class time to simulate a team meeting and model the skills of leading the team meeting, processing discussions, and listening effectiveness. For those classes we would recommend the following:

- Create an agenda for the case discussion.
- Assign the role of recorder.
- Assign a timekeeper.
- Move through the agenda one item at a time.
- Keep the class or team focused on the discussion.
- Establish an appropriate pace.

To help learners practice communication and appropriate decision-making methods, we recommend the instructor model the following skills:

- Active listening. This is the chance to gain agreement that what you heard was what the speaker meant. Use phrases like "Is that what you said?" By checking and using active listening, the facilitator reminds learners that listening is hard and that, as a team, all participants need to improve communication.
- Encourage all members to participate fully. Solicit information from quiet members, or ask each member state his or her view. Remind participants that silence is not agreement.
- Seek out differences of opinion. Help participants recognize that disagreements are natural. Through open discussion the group obtains more information and opinions that members can use to reach a decision.
- Balance participation whenever possible. Elicit new opinions with questions like "Does anyone else have something to contribute?"
- Probe with questions like "How did you arrive at that judgment?"
- Continuously check for agreement and understanding. Check to see if everyone understands the decision and can explain why it was the best.

The Learner's Role: Preparing for the Discussion

Adults learn through a continuous cycle of acquiring information, applying principles, and adjusting based on the reaction. Active learning—learning by applying ideas and testing—is the hallmark of case-based discussion. But learners, like clinicians, need to be prepared prior to a discussion. Just as clinicians will expect the learner to assume a specified role in the health care setting after graduation, the instructor needs to help the student prepare for a case presentation. The following general questions are offered to ensure that learners come prepared to discuss the case (in addition to specific questions assigned by the teacher):

- What decision does the team believe needs to be made?
- What is the patient's perspective? Does it differ from the family's perspective?
- Is there disagreement among the clinicians on the approach that needs to be taken? If so, what accounts for this disagreement?
- What key questions must be addressed or points resolved to reach a decision? Is there a disagreement about facts or consequences? Would any additional information help clarify the issue(s)?
- Are all possible alternative actions identified? What are the consequences of the alternatives?
- What would the learner do, given his or her clinical expertise and values? Why?

Since the cases reflect actual patients and families or are composites, instructors can use them to highlight the obvious ethical dilemmas. But we also encourage instructors to discuss the subtle ethical issues inherent in most clinical settings.

Role playing is a powerful learning strategy, guaranteed to motivate and animate most students, although it also makes many students uncomfortable. Role playing is useful when instructors want to emphasize the team skills and highlight the different approaches that disciplines bring to the clinical setting. To simulate conflict and practice communication techniques, active listening and role playing can be valuable learning tools. Issues involving value conflicts, moral choices, and timeless human dilemmas in the students' world are most effective for role-playing exercises, but role playing need not be so personal.

Since role playing can be uncomfortable for some learners, instructors should:

- Offer learners some choice in how much to participate. If learners are very hesitant, offer extra time to coach them and assuage their fears. Be supportive and remind them that they will be expected to participate in teams when they finish training.
- Allow learners time to prepare themselves for the role they will play and to understand the ethical and team issues involved.
- Define the roles clearly, based on the information in the case. If you are assigning a discipline-specific role to learners, try to assign the role they are studying. It is difficult to display the knowledge, skills, and attitudes of other disciplines, and part of the team process is contribution to the discussion.
- Assign team members the formal roles of leader, timer, and note keeper.
- Ask the class to be official observers of the meeting. They will be asked to comment on the team process, including how well the leader solicited information from all members, resolved the conflicts, and developed the action agenda.
- Allow time for debriefing. The learners need time to recognize the issues, and the actors need time to talk about how they felt and what they learned.

All individual health professionals strive to coordinate care; individual clinicians expect to create the best outcomes for the patient. But a group process is very different from an individual decision-making process, and few clinicians receive training on how to work together effectively as a team. Proven teams skills such as structuring meetings through agendas, establishing timetables, and keeping notes are obvious management tools. Yet few clinicians are taught these skills in a formal way.

Practicing team skills, either alone or in concert with examining the principles and processes of ethical deliberation, provides a valuable opportunity for learners to enhance their understanding of the variety of conundrums clinicians face as they struggle to balance the needs of the older adults and their families within a rapidly changing health care system.

TEACHING RESOURCES

Barnes, L. B., C. Roland Christensen, and A. J. Hansen, eds. 1994. *Teaching and the Case Method,* 3rd ed. Cambridge, Mass.: Harvard Business School Press.

Brown, G. F., and G. D. Chamberlin. 1996. Attitudes toward quality, costs, and physician centrality in healthcare teams. *Journal of Interprofessional Care* 10:63–72.

Drinka, T. 1996. Applying learning from self-directed work teams in business to curriculum development for geriatric interdisciplinary teams. *Educational Gerontology* 22:433–50.

Fagin, C. M. 1992. Collaboration between nurses and physicians: No longer a choice. *Academic Medicine* 67:295–303.

Fulmer, T., and K. Hyer. 1998. Evaluating GITT. In E. L. Siegler, K. Hyer, T. Fulmer, and M. Mezey, eds., *Geriatric interdisciplinary team training.* New York: Springer.

Heinemann, G. D., M. H. Schmitt, M. P. Farrell, and S. A. Brallier. 1999. Developments of the attitudes toward health care teams scale. *Evaluation and the Health Care Professions* 22: 123–42.

Howe, J. L., K. Hyer, D. J. Mellor, D. Lindeman, and M. Luptak. 2001. Educational approaches for preparing social work students for interdisciplinary teamwork on geriatric health care teams. *Social Work in Health Care* 32(4):19–42.

Hyer, K. 1998. The John A. Hartford Foundation geriatric interdisciplinary team training program. In E.L. Siegler, K. Hyer, T. Fulmer, and M. Mezey, eds., *Geriatric Interdisciplinary team training.* New York: Springer.

Katzenbach, J. R., and D. K. Smith. 1993. *The wisdom of teams: Creating the high performance organization.* Boston: Harvard Business School Press.

Lynn, Laurence E., Jr. 1999. *Teaching and learning with cases: A guidebook.* New York: Chatham House.

Ryan, D. P. 1996. A history of teamwork in mental health and its implications for teamwork training in gerontology. *Educational Gerontology* 22:411–31.

Scholtes, P. R., B. L. Joiner, and B. J. Streibel. 1996. *The team handbook,* 2nd ed. Madison, Wisc.: Oriel.

West, M. A, C. S. Borrill, and K. L. Unsworth. 1998. Team effectiveness in organizations. In C. L. Cooper and I. T. Robertson, eds. *International Review of Industrial and Organizational Psychology* 13:1–48.

REFERENCES

Baggs, J. G., S. A. Ryan, C. E. Phelps, J. F. Richeson, and J. E. Johnson. 1992. The association between interdisciplinary collaboration and patient outcome in a medical intensive care unit. *Heart and Lung* 21(1):18–24.

Doukas, D. J., and L. B. McCullough. 1996. A preventive ethics approach to counseling patients about clinical futility in the primary care setting. *Archives of Family Medicine* 5:89–92.

Jonsen, A. R., M. Siegler, and W. J. Winslade. 1998. *Clinical ethics,* 4th ed. New York: McGraw-Hill.

McCullough, L. B., N. L. Wilson, J. A. Rhymes, and T. A. Teasdale. 1995. Managing the conceptual and ethical dimensions of long term care decision making: A preventive ethics approach. In L. B. McCullough and N. L. Wilson, eds., *Long-term care decisions: Ethical and conceptual dimensions*. Baltimore: Johns Hopkins University Press.

National Association for Home Care. (1999). *Basic statistics about hospice*. http://www.nahc.org /Consumer/hpcstats.html.

Rubenstein, L. W., K. R. Josephson, G. D. Wieland, P. A. English, J. A. Sayre, et al. 1984. Effectiveness of a geriatric evaluation unit: A randomized clinical trial. *New England Journal of Medicine* 311:1664–70.

Siegler, E. L., K. Hyer, T. T. Fulmer, and M. D. Mezey. 1998. *Geriatric interdisciplinary team training*. New York: Springer.

Stuck, A. E., A. L. Siu, G. D. Wieland, J. Adams, and L. Z. Rubenstein. 1993. Comprehensive geriatric assessment: A meta-analysis of controlled trials. *Lancet* 342(8878):1032–36.

Tsukuda, R. A. 1998. A perspective on health care teams and team training. In E. L. Siegler, K. Hyer, T. T. Fulmer, and M. D. Mezey, eds., *Geriatric interdisciplinary team training*. New York: Springer.

U.S. Census Bureau. 2000. *Projections of the resident population by age, sex, race and hispanic origin, 1999–2100*. http://www.census.gov/population/www/projections/natdet-D1A.html [August 9].

PART II

Professionals

CHAPTER 3

Ethics and Cultures of Care

Russell Burck, Ph.D., and Stanley Lapidos, M.S.

Does culture make a difference in patient care? Isn't a patient a patient, no matter what the culture? Our answer is that culture does make a difference. And in this chapter, we ask: If cultures of care make a difference in the team care of the elderly, do they make any ethical difference? What are the ethical commitments, strengths, and weaknesses of particular professional cultures of elder care and of the larger culture of care that draws their contributions together?

Cultures of care transmit their ethical solutions and perspectives to their members and to new generations. But ongoing reflection on caregiving and new situations continually requires new analyses of ethical responsibility toward patients, in general and in particular. Accordingly, cultures of care teach not only established solutions but also methods of ethical analysis for practical decision making, and they assess the challenges and obstacles to ethical decision making.

Cultures are created explicitly at least as much as implicitly. This chapter states our explicit proposals for the principles and guideposts of creating a culture of care. Our concern here is to work toward the creation of a patient-centered, quality-driven, team-based culture of care for geriatric patients. Creating an ethical model of interdisciplinary teaching and training based on mutual respect, knowledge and trust will in turn influence the practical replication of a culture of care devoted to the same principles. We proceed by first defining *culture* and stating how we use the term in this chapter; then articulating principles concerning the ethical aspects of the cultures that provide team health care to elderly persons; then analyzing a case; and finally drawing some conclusions from the case.

Culture

Segall and colleagues (1990, 26) define *culture* as "the totality of whatever all persons learn from all other persons." Culture is the various matters that are developed and handed down by learning and tradition, rather than transmitted biologically. Thus, a culture of health care for the elderly is whatever the persons in particular disciplines learn from others whose life or work influences those disciplines. Cultures of health care are the mental (Senge 1994) or "explanatory models" (Kleinman, Eisenberg, and Good 1978, 252) that guide those who foster and seek to maintain health, help the sick recover, support the dying, and care for the people involved.

Another meaning of *culture* is more amorphous, like *climate* or *atmosphere*, as in *corporate culture*. A phrase like *the culture of team care* refers to attitudes and norms that are established and passed on throughout an organization, but it also suggests properties that are more difficult to name.

Hill, Fortenberry, and Stein (1990) lead us to expect to encounter, in any given situation, at least one culture of the patient, or patient and family, and a number of cultures of the health care professionals. They identify eight "distinctive cultural systems": ethnicity/nationality, race, age, gender, family, vocation, religion, disability. Each of these systems has "distinguishing cultural content categories that mediate among individuals in contemporary American society" (1072). Consequently, "patient cultures and practitioner cultures" differ "in conceptualization and preferred action." Cultural systems "offer alternative, perhaps competing, strategies for group identification, affiliation, and membership." Hence, parallels between membership in a provider culture and membership in a homogeneous tribe are justified. Provider identity and tribal identity both involve tight, sometimes unquestioning allegiances as well as clashes between and among different groups.

Moreover, cultural systems are "to some extent voluntary and arbitrary in boundary structure and content" (1072). Some people, though sick or injured, are able to reject membership in the patient cultural system, and still others fight it. The arbitrariness of sickness or injury influences whether a person is an active member of the patient culture. Membership in the patient culture is time limited, except for routine care and chronic illnesses.

Providers, for their part, enter health care professions as volunteers. But admission to the professions varies according to a person's abilities, the availability of places to study, admissions committees, financial resources, and even the marketplace. Unlike the patient culture, membership in a provider culture lasts as long as a provider chooses or membership is not revoked. Thus, cultures of providers are more enduring. Interdisciplinary or multidisciplinary groups of providers often think of themselves as *the* members of the health care team, and without including patients and families.

At the level of attitude and behavior, Hill and colleagues note, cultural systems explain "more ... attitudinal and behavioral variance than other systems." At the personal level, "each distinctive culture is a potential identity system that changes along predictable lines with changes in the social, historical, physical, geographic, or technological realms of human life. 'What is me, and what is not me?' is a question each person asks over and over again" (1072).

Thus, culture is pervasive and relatively stable, but it is also dynamic. It functions consciously but also preconsciously and unconsciously. Hence, conscious efforts to change culture are likely to set off unanticipated reverberations and to require continual monitoring.

Basic Assumptions

1. Team health care of elderly persons occurs within many cultures.

Families constitute a culture of care, developing their own understandings of care and passing them from generation to generation. Provider cultures, for their part, transmit instructions and assumptions about how care should be provided and who should receive it. These cultures in turn influence a larger culture of care that includes clinicians, patients, and families. This culture is influenced by the ageist bias that exists in the American culture.

Specific cultures of care often agree in general about what constitutes the good for a particular patient. At the same time, provider cultures have their own specific perspectives on this good and their own ideas of what the various disciplines contribute to it. Within a team, as a result, teamwork and ethical reflection upon it impose external and internal tasks on the members. Much of the external ethical task of teamwork in health care, including elder care, is to negotiate among the general and specific perspectives on the good. Much of the internal task for team members concerns the personal-professional adjustments that they have to make as they negotiate agreements and disagreements with other team members.

2. Each of the cultures that influence team health care of the elderly has its own view of its responsibility toward the patient and of the patient's responsibility for her- or himself.

Y. H. Poortinga has defined *culture* as "shared constraints that limit the behavior repertoire available to members of a certain sociocultural group in a way different from individuals belonging to some other group" (1990, 6). Poortinga's view parallels Hill and colleagues' references to "strategies" that assemble health care professionals around a common core, establish their professional identity and appropriate behavior, and distinguish their professions from others. Consequently, many of the issues of teamwork concern the interaction between the "shared constraints" of the individual disciplines and the focus of all disciplines on the patient's well-being.

But some cultures of care constrain not only members of their own group but also members of other groups. Medicine and nursing, for example, constrain the behavioral repertoire available to health care professionals who are not physicians or nurses. At the same time, the cultures of these other professionals impose fewer reciprocal constraints on medicine and probably nursing. If they so choose or are permitted, doctors or nurses can do many of the things that other disciplines do. Nevertheless, representatives of individual professions frequently have little understanding of the tasks, much less the ethical commitments, of other health care professionals or of the services that they provide to elderly persons.

One way that cultures of health care constrain their members' behavior is through ethical codes or guidelines. Codes open a window to a discipline's view of human suffering, perhaps of human flourishing, and of the discipline's responsibility to help relieve suffering and foster flourishing. They "establish norms that can protect individual patients. They articulate organizational policies and official standards of conduct, and show how the organized profession frames issues" (Rodwin 1992, 707).

Nevertheless, the limits of written ethical codes are more impressive than their value. Some practitioners ignore codes altogether. Some use them rigidly, tacitly delegating their personal moral responsibility to a code and its writers, rather than using the code as a "guide to action" (Mill 1998, 191) and reflection. Some use codes in an advisory manner, in which case they may not take them seriously enough. Some use them in a self-serving manner. Rodwin notes that "some historians suggest that the AMA has used its code to 'discredit interlopers,' to boost the profession's prestige, to stave off attacks, and to discourage external regulation. . . . Codes may have helped the medical profession to reduce external competition, to promote an oligopoly status, and to protect prominent physicians against challenges" (707). He notes that the AMA "was unable to hold physicians accountable" on fee-splitting and that later it "weakened its code to placate its members" (733).

Concerning team care, Levine and Zuckerman (1999, 148) claim that codes' ethical commitments to individual patients produce negative presumptions about families. Similarly, Smith, Hiatt, and Berwick (1999, 143) hold that major ethical codes "can divide a world of health care that badly needs unity in its work." All of these uses and misuses of ethical codes are examples of ways that ethics can be an instrument of harm.

Smith, Hiatt, and Berwick are leaders of the Tavistock Group, which developed "A Shared Statement of Ethical Principles for Those Who Shape and Give Health Care." In the *Annals of Internal Medicine,* the American College of Physicians–American Society of Internal Medicine (ACP-ASIM) published a working draft of the "Shared Statement." The preamble states, "The purpose of this statement of ethical principles is to heighten awareness of the need for principles to guide all who are involved in the delivery of health care. The principles offered here focus health care delivery systems on the service of individuals and the good of society as a whole and can offer a foundation for new and enhanced levels of cooperation among all involved" (Smith, Hiatt, and Berwick, 1999, 145).

3. Each clinician inhabits several different cultures of care.

Providers' baseline culture of care, which they never leave, is that of the whole society's interest in its members' well-being. Their second culture of care is that of the common identity and shared constraints of their specific profession. Their third culture of care grows unavoidably, de facto, from their encounters with patients' needs—the larger interdisciplinary culture of care.

The second culture of care—that of a particular discipline—is more recognizable than either of the other two. Ethical reflection on teamwork can help clinicians generate a shared interdisciplinary culture of care and negotiate conflicting commitments among the various specific disciplinary cultures of care and broader social cultures.

Further shaping the societal, the professional, and the shared interdisciplinary culture is a powerful culture that measures success in terms of financial rather than patient-driven considerations.

4. Within the team care of elderly persons, the cultures of care that instruct patient, family, and professional caregivers about how to provide health care to elderly persons are a major source of conflict.

An implication of Hill and colleagues' perspective is that all health care consists of intercultural encounters and processes. Within the patient-family nexus, issues of care conflict with other life tasks and agendas. Among professional members of interdisciplinary teams, their identities within their particular disciplines are a major source of conflict. Providers' cultures are generally more focused on the patient's needs. Consequently they can be very ethnocentric, unempathic, and demanding toward family, patient, or both. Both teamwork and the ethics of teamwork involve major efforts to balance the claims of the various cultures of care about the needs of the patient. Therefore, clashes among clinicians about health care of elders are not primarily differences of opinion or personality but are clashes among and between cultures.

5. Ethics asks about the good.

Ethics asks two basic questions that can sound like a mantra: What is the good and the not so good? How do we know? In this light, a culture of care is about a discipline's understanding of the good, its ability to enhance the good, or its ability to relieve or reduce harm.

We now ask, "What is the good when we are thinking about team care, about the cultures of care that health care professionals represent, and about the development of a larger culture of team care of elderly persons?"

The question "What is the good?" can be restated in other language that is useful when we are thinking about ethics:

- What is the good or not so good?
- What is right, or wrong, or not so right?
- What is our responsibility?
- What is the proper use of our power?
- What is the appropriate relationship of means to ends?

In this chapter, our test of the good is "the most humane and encompassing solutions to the problems at hand" (Burck 1996, 245). This statement fits two claims: (1) the patient and the family are the center of the health care team, and (2) everybody counts, not just the patient and her family.

6. As a field, ethics is composed of at least two cultures.

Each of the two questions of ethics is the center of a subculture of ethics. The question about the good is the core of what we call the *culture of established solutions*. This culture keeps and hands down the solutions to many common problems that people concerned about the good have developed.

Established solutions become customs or habits in the classic sense of the etymology of *ethical* (*Webster's* 1981). In health care, customs are called policies, procedures, or standards of care. The culture of established solutions often provides technically correct recommendations for a situation. These solutions have to be tested against standards of the greatest good. The greatest-good standard is not just a personal preference but is subject to robust public dialogue. But individuals may pioneer and champion uncustomary standards that others come to accept.

The power of the culture of established solutions is that it gathers and disseminates information about agreement among ethicists and others concerned about ethics and avoids having to reinvent the wheel all the time. It is weakest when it misunderstands itself as the whole culture of ethics. When that happens, it applies litmus tests of right and wrong, good and not so good, that may not fit a particular situation well, blind its users to salient issues, and even lead to evil actions.

The culture of established solutions is often dominant within ethics. A solution, once developed, is often applicable in many other situations. Further, if an existing solution can be applied, it is more efficient to do so than to create and test new solutions. The work of ethics can be very difficult. For example, people often begin their ethical work on a case by asking, "What should we do?" They frequently emphasize the action, not the ethical reasoning behind the action. The availability of established solutions can short-circuit reflection in favor of action.

The second question, "How do we know?" Or, "How do we determine what the good is?" is at the core of the *culture of method*. The culture of method actually develops or creates the solutions that later become established. When ethics is working well, the culture of method is always present behind the scenes, carefully checking the work of the culture of established solutions. When established solutions do not obviously fit a situation and ethical novelty seems to be called for, the culture of method reviews these situations and the proposed new solutions. This culture recognizes when established solutions will and will not work in a particular situation.

The key characteristic of the culture of method is that it is not committed to any particular established solution. Rather, it is committed to the best specific good or benefit that can be achieved in a situation: "What is the best that we can do for every person and institution that has a stake in this situation?" It seeks to find "the most humane and encompassing solutions" to the problems at hand. The strengths of this culture are that it (1) recognizes that established solutions may not be adequate when fresh ethical issues arise and (2) when one does arise, it reviews the issues freshly and in all the necessary detail. The weakness is that it can reinvent the wheel and waste time.

Taken together, the two questions of ethics, "What is the good and the not so good? How do we know?" are the north star that guides us when we are lost in details of particular ethical problems. We can easily get lost just considering ethics. We do get lost when we are considering responsibilities to patients. So in the ethics of team care for elders, getting lost becomes even easier. The two questions of ethics help us get our bearings again.

The culture of ethics states its conclusions about a proposed solution in terms like *permissible, impermissible, ethically preferable, stringently obligatory,* or *absolutely prohibited.* Some people benefit from visualizing a continuum that runs from absolute ethical obligation to absolute ethical prohibition (Figure 3.1). When asking about the ethics of a case, we ask what we are obligated to do, what we are prohibited from doing, what is permissible, and within what is permissible, what is preferable. That is, we ask, Where does this possible solution lie on the continuum?

Obligation	Permissibility	Prohibition
Absolute Stringent	More Less	Stringent Absolute
	Preferable Preferable	

FIGURE 3.1 The continuum

Source: Burck 1996, 243. NCP 11: 244, 1996. Reprinted with permission
American Society for Parenteral and Enteral Nutrition.

Principles

Principles are statements that determine where we begin our work and that provide it with an organizing structure. During our work we check our principles to see whether we have been true to our original and originating guidelines. Nevertheless, principles are not ironclad, permanent, or inflexible. We must also ask whether our principles are adequate to our task.

Principle 1. All health care occurs in teams.

All health care is team care. No provider can take care of all of a patient's needs alone. The provider will require the help of other professionals or of family members.

Principle 2. The patient and the family are the team's central members.

Providers often think that they constitute the entire health care team. At the center of the team, however, are the geriatric patient and the family.

Principle 3. Externally, a team is real work with real people. Internally, a team is a perspective on the patient-provider relationship.

Among professionals, work in teams can be difficult. Including patients and their families on a team can be a difficult conceptual or internal leap. Part of the team's internal task is to determine how to define team membership. One approach is additive: it begins with the essential members of the team and adds others only as the situation requires. A limitation of this approach is that it can overlook disciplines that could really contribute to the patient's well-being. Another approach is subtractive: it considers a wide range of potential team members and subtracts the ones that are not needed at the moment. But it keeps them in mind, in case they are needed later. We lean toward the subtractive approach.

Principle 4. All health care is the expression of ethical commitments to people.

The ethics of team health care of the elderly is not an add-on or an occasional feature of caregiving. It is intrinsic yet often almost invisible. The task of health care ethics in general, and in the care of elderly persons, is to normalize ethics.

Implicit in the two questions of ethics is the idea that health care ethics is not just, or even primarily, about dilemmas and problems. It is about the commitments of the respective cultures of health care and their practitioners to people's well-being. Commitments come first (Burck 1996, 243); dilemmas and problems come later. Hence, attention to health care ethics is about the normality, the pervasiveness, of ethics in health care, and indeed in all of human experience. Ethics is not an add-on. It is intrinsic and ubiquitous.

Principle 5. The ethics of team health care of elderly persons is about doing the good for the health of these patients through teamwork.

Through teamwork, providers address their patients' suffering and foster their flourishing. Flourishing is the preferred translation of Aristotle's term *eudaimonia*, often translated as "happiness" (Rasmussen 1999, 1–2). The goal is concretely to do as much good and as little harm as the situation allows. A culture of health care represents the perspective of a discipline on human suffering and on the causes of that suffering, and it asks what that discipline can do to restore human flourishing. Over generations, a culture of care passes on what the discipline can contribute toward human flourishing and toward relieving suffering. Through teamwork, over time, the beneficial aspects of specific disciplines can, we believe, change the context of care providers by disciplines and by the team. In the following case of Lois Mason, we consider medicine, nursing, chaplaincy, and hospital ethics.

Case Description

In this section, we present a case about an older patient; explore what various cultures of care say about team care of patients; explore two different, sometimes clashing, sometimes synergistic cultures of ethics; review the case in light of the culture of method; and test the case and the principles that we have named against one another. We shall also refer to our experience using this case to teach ethics in the Geriatric Interdisciplinary Team Training Program at Rush–Presbyterian–St. Luke's Medical Center.

Lois Mason was a 72-year-old insulin-dependent diabetic woman with end-stage renal disease. Several days after being discharged from the hospital, she presented in uremic coma after her home health aide found her unconscious.

She was put on peritoneal dialysis (PD) at home, but on several occasions she accidentally pulled out her PD catheter, and the renal service was running out of sites on which to reestablish it. During this hospitalization, while her coma was lightening but before she was fully alert, she got up, fell, and once again pulled out her catheter. The renal service was able to reestablish it only with difficulty. The service recommended that Ms. Mason be discharged to a nursing home, preferably one that had a dialysis center. They also recommended that she be switched from PD to hemodialysis (HD).

The attending physician had known Ms. Mason for some time and he knew that she had already unsuccessfully tried both of the options being proposed by the renal service. He called the hospital's ethics consultation service, and with the ethics consultant, he sought a team meeting that would include the renal service and the family. The renal service's reply to the invitation was friendly, but it said that it did not see any need to attend a meeting. It had already said what it would say, which was something like, "We're very close to the end of our ability to help Ms. Mason with PD. Put her on HD; make it easy for her to get to a center."

Remembering that Ms. Mason had had a number of falls both at home and in the hospital, her hospital nurse wondered whether her mental status would clear adequately for her to become competent to take part in decisions. Further, as a nurse, she had responsibilities to ensure that Ms. Mason was discharged to a stable and sufficiently supportive environment.

At this moment the team consisted of the patient, the attending physician, the renal service, the primary nurse, and the ethics consultant, who was also a chaplain. The attending physician expected that the family would become part of the team, but they had not yet been heard from.

No social worker was involved in this case. The chaplain-ethicist performed some of the functions that a social worker would perform, such as speaking with Ms. Mason and noting how she responded to questions about switching to HD and moving to a nursing home.

A disadvantage of having a chaplain perform the functions of a social worker is that in his hospital, acute care chaplains do not visit patients' homes, but a social worker could or could arrange such a visit. Still, a team-oriented chaplain could have asked for input about the home and what it would be like for Ms. Mason to live there. A social worker might also have been better able to imagine Ms. Mason's home, if he or she had prior experience with the care of chronic patients in their homes.

Who Should Be at a Team Meeting?

The renal service's negative response immediately raised a question about the forces that constitute teamwork. Who has to be at a meeting? Some observers might say that the renal service's decision not to be at the meeting compromised teamwork. The attending physician's request that the renal service participate could express (1) a greater awareness that the patient is the center of gravity in this case and (2) his need for more teamwork with the renal service than interaction through the chart provided.

What Should a Discipline's Recommendations Include?

When this case was presented in our Geriatric Interdisciplinary Team Training (GITT) Program at Rush–Presbyterian–St. Luke's Medical Center and Rush University, some participants said that the renal service's recommendations had important ethical implications (referring to ethics as a normal part of health care). Switching the patient from peritoneal dialysis to hemodialysis might have met the goals of medicine better, they said, but it raised questions about respect for Ms. Mason's autonomy. Some readers might wonder whether there were any advantages for the nephrologists in having a patient on HD rather than on PD. Some GITT participants heard considerable ethical force in the renal service's recommendations; that force made them uncomfortable. But internal medicine physicians noted that the renal service's recommendation to switch to HD was understandably urgent: establishing an HD shunt takes time.

Further, some GITT participants maintained that an ethics consultation should have been called to consider the recommendation of moving Ms. Mason. They believed that the renal service exceeded its responsibilities in recommending nursing home placement, because it seemed to fall outside the service's focal competence. Such comments indicate the variety of perspectives on ethics that pervade health care discussions.

That ethics is a normal part of health care can be seen in the disagreement between the renal service and the attending physician about medicine's responsibility to Ms. Mason. Differing ethical commitments (Burck 1996, 243) delineated the ethical dialogue among the professional members of Ms. Mason's health care team. At the center of the team, Ms. Mason was unable to express her idea of the good. Her attending physician said that she had previously spoken her point of view, and he stated it for her, until she could speak for herself or her family could speak for her. Her family had not yet been contacted about its idea of the good in this situation. The attending physician's concept of the good was about the patient's health as well as her self-determination. The renal service's concept of the good was about her health. The nurse's concept of the good was about the patient's self-determination, mental status, and safety. The chaplain-ethicist's concept of the good concerned (1) Ms. Mason's health, as represented in the best recommendations for treatment; her story and her own goals; and the hope that education would enable her to choose the best care for herself; (2) the family and its ability to support Ms. Mason; (3) the providers' commitments and concerns.

Where these cultures clashed was in their attention to other goods. Where they agreed and where they differed are summarized in Table 3.1.

The chaplain-ethicist noted that Ms. Mason was quite firm about refusing HD. She did not want to move to a nursing home. She liked living in the condo that she shared with her sons, who were in their late twenties. The building had a doorman at the entrance who could monitor the people whom she would buzz into the condo. The chaplain also learned that the sons were planning to move to another location and take their mother with them. Ms. Mason did not indicate whether this move concerned her, but the chaplain, the nurse, and the attending physician were concerned.

The chaplain-ethicist noted that over several days, Ms. Mason's answers became clearer and that she always adamantly refused the recommendations. He did not determine her decisional capacity, but he communicated his impressions to the attending physician and to the nurse. The attending physician noted the observations, and the nurse disagreed with them.

The chaplain-ethicist asked what her days were like at home. Both she and her children told him that she was alone from about 6 A.M. until noon or 1 P.M., that her sons worked at least an hour away from home, that they provided some help for her PD and shopped, and that they returned at about 8 P.M. During the afternoon, a homemaker was present for four hours five days a week.

TABLE 3.1
Culture of Care, Particular Goods, Shared Good, Contested Good

Culture of care	Particular "good(s)" that this culture represents	Good that these cultures share	Good over which these cultures clash
Attending physician	Patient-physician cooperation Physician's advocacy for Ms. Mason when she cannot be her own advocate		
Renal service	Removing barriers to Ms. Mason's well-being		
Nurse	Patient self-determination Protection of the patient, if incompetent choices threaten or harm her Discharge to safe environment Determining whether the patient is capable of taking good enough care of her peritoneal dialysis	Ms. Mason's well-being	What will serve Ms. Mason's well-being
Chaplain-ethicist	Spirituality in everyday life Learning the patient's story and version of her situation Patient self-determination Education of the patient in the hope that she'll choose best treatment Ability of the family to care for Ms. Mason Providers' needs		

He learned that she had worked in a high-tech field and that her sons had graduate degrees in a closely related field. In his conversations with Ms. Mason's daughter, Gail, he learned that she was the oldest of the three, she worked nights, and she was going to college.

In accordance with the attending physician's request, he also coordinated the family-physician conference with the renal service, the attending physician, and nursing.

At this point, the professional members of the team had not developed their idea of the good. Two technically correct established solutions were competing for dominance: supporting her self-determination and protecting her well-being.

Case Analysis

The chapters in this book review cases from the point of view of Jonsen, Siegler, and Winslade's *Clinical Ethics* (1998). The Jonsen, Siegler, and Winslade (JSW) model works best if it speaks to a question, such as: "The renal service recommended that Ms. Mason be placed on hemodialysis and that she move to a nursing home. Is this recommendation ethical?"

We revise this question into a "trial statement" or "maxim" (Kant 1983, 30) about ethical responsibility. A trial statement is a proposal about moral responsibility in a particular context. As a proposal for action, no trial statement can be unethical. The culture of method examines trial statements and asks what ethical commitment lies behind a trial statement. Our trial statement will be the renal service's recommendation: "The best ethical course is to place Ms. Mason on hemodialysis and to have her move to a nursing home." We shall test this proposal against the four main categories into which JSW organize information for clinical ethical analysis.

We must also know how to determine when we are finished with our ethical analysis. John Rawls (1971, 20–21) spoke of *reflective equilibrium* as a provisional end of the process of ethical analysis. One indicator that we have done our job is that we have reviewed all the categories in the JSW model and any others that are pertinent for understanding this case. Despite the tugs of intuition and urgency, we methodically review each category in detail. That way, the desire for efficiency does not cause us to inadvertently exclude information. For some categories, we can say, "This category does not contribute to our analysis of this case."

JSW's first category is labeled medical indications, but we focus on their goals of medicine. Their next category, patient preferences, can be construed narrowly and concretely, as if it did not incorporate the patient's narrative. Therefore we enlarge it to patient perspectives.

JSW recommend that, wherever possible, we make decisions within the first two quadrants, which we call goals of medicine and patient perspectives (Figure 3.2). Their third category is quality of life (QOL) (JSW, ch. 3), which has three and only three possible meanings: goals of medicine, patient perspectives, and observer bias. The fundamental goal of medicine, JSW say, is to improve QOL. So understood, QOL is consistent with the goals of medicine and patient perspectives. Even if health care cannot improve Ms. Mason's QOL,

Goals of medicine	Patient perspectives
Quality of life	Contextual features

FIGURE 3.2

practitioners may be able to maintain it, slow its decline, or raise its nadir. JSW also state three "objective criteria of QOL"—restricted, minimal, and below minimal—to which we add baseline. These criteria are not observer bias, because they can be observed and described. Ms. Mason's baseline is restricted, owing to her difficulty ambulating, her being on PD, her isolation, and her depression.

JSW's fourth category is contextual features (JSW, ch. 4), which is rich in ethical issues concerning team care: particular concerns of family members, clinicians, institutional issues, costs, questions of research, and the like. This category asks for more information from the case.

As we move into contextual features, we have not yet reached reflective equilibrium. The established solutions in the first three categories only bring our ethical analysis back to our original standoff. Practitioners within medicine disagree about the patient's management (goals of medicine); the patient disagrees with the renal service (patient perspectives); her nurse disagrees with the attending physician and doubts that the patient's PD permits her to have decisional capacity (QOL). But the patient also disagrees with the family about how well she is being taken care of at home; and the family members disagree with one another about their respective responsibilities for their mother (contextual features). Among the clinicians, the disagreements follow the fault lines of their ethical commitments to the patient.

Functioning technically, using established solutions, an ethicist would say that it was too early to tell whether the renal service's recommendation was ethically permissible. Neither of their recommendations appears to have been ethically permissible, because Ms. Mason had already entertained and rejected them. Nevertheless, the disadvantages of PD made further efforts to explore her objections to HD ethically mandatory.

Functioning methodologically, the ethicist would review the proposed solutions: "Is switching her to HD now ethically permissible? No. Is moving her to a nursing home now ethically permissible? No. Her self-determination speaks against both options." But these answers would not get us closer to whatever good is possible in the situation.

Using the Ethics Consultation to Search for a Novel Solution

The attending physician already knew the established solutions and rejected them. He asked the ethics consultant to join the team in seeking ways to keep

Ms. Mason from having to reenter the hospital. The ethics consultant brainstormed the question "What is the best ethical solution for Ms. Mason?" The shape of the good that would emerge at the end of the process would have to incorporate the intentions and goals of the patient, the family, and the various providers as well as possible.

The culture of method now brought in the core of the team: the patient and her family. The attending physician requested a family-physician conference.

For Gail, the oldest of the siblings, a family-physician conference or an ethics consultation would be satisfactory only if it mets her needs and not just those of her mother and brothers. When she was called, Gail immediately insisted that her brothers, Tom and Mike, be at the conference, because "they need to be bearing more of the load." A technical "Ms. Mason has the right to choose or refuse" solution thus failed to meet Gail's concern about the appropriate distribution of burdens among the siblings in the care of their mother. Gail was assured that her brothers would attend, but they did not, so the meeting was rescheduled.

Before the second meeting, the clinicians and the family considered whether it was ethical to meet without Ms. Mason. In our GITT meetings at Rush, some physician participants would immediately say, "No, she has to be included." Usually, they changed their minds when a social worker, occupational therapist, or chaplain suggested the family had issues to discuss without her being present, before including her. Both responses represent the culture of established solutions.

Gail, Tom, and Mike wanted to meet without their mother and then with her. That approach would give them the opportunity to sort things out, in case they needed to say anything that might offend or wound her, and still include her later.

The first family meeting included Gail, Tom, Mike, the attending physician, the nurse, and the chaplain-ethicist. At the family meeting, the family worked productively on ways to help their mother more. The family did not discuss switching her to HD or moving her to a nursing home. The implication was that they were willing to help her stay at home with them.

The chaplain-ethicist asked what had changed, pointing out that Ms. Mason had been on dialysis for several years, had not been hospitalized in that time, and now had been in the hospital twice in short order. Instantly Gail said, "Oh, I can answer that. She's mad at me because I don't come to see her as much." Gail was going to school, so she did not have as much time as she had previously had to stop by and see her mother. The suggestion was made that, if she was indeed neglecting her PD in order to get her family's attention, something should be done to address this question, so that she did not inadvertently kill herself.

The family, physician, nurse, and ethicist reassembled in Ms. Mason's room. Here again there was a thorough discussion of ways that the family could be more helpful, and all the family members agreed about how they could help more and what wished-for steps were not feasible. Then Gail asked, "Momma, are you not taking care of yourself because you're mad at us?" Instantly Ms. Mason answered, "Well, you don't come see me anymore." Gail said, "Momma, you know that I'm going to school and can't come around as often. But if I come to see you once a week, will you take care of yourself?" Ms. Mason said yes.

Further discussion addressed issues of Ms. Mason's depression and the chaplain-ethicist's concern that she needed more activities to keep her occupied. All of these solutions related to Rawls's concept of reflective equilibrium. They were asking, in effect, "What can go wrong with this plan?"

With these solutions, the team members felt that reflective equilibrium had been reached. Ms. Mason was discharged on PD, was able to improve her participation in her care, and did not return to the hospital.

This analysis discloses an unexpected meaning inherent in contextual features: "Everybody counts," not just the patient, and not just the patient and the doctor. The patient counts most, but there are clearly situations in which others are so important that solutions must take their problems into account. In turn this discovery leads to a new statement of a standard against which to test trial statements: the most humane and encompassing solution(s) to the problem(s) at hand. This standard is not perfectionist. It is also not about compromise. There may be winners and losers in the decision. But those who use it seek to achieve the highest good possible, to understand the losers' view, and to achieve their goals as best as the situation allows.

Disagreements among clinicians are not personal differences but reflect the cultures of their respective disciplines. In Ms. Mason's case, from a cultural perspective, we can readily understand the disagreement between the attending physician and the consulting service, the nurse and the attending physician, and the nurse and the chaplain-ethics consultant. Each represents a culture that says: This is the way we do things. The responsibilities of each culture are well rationalized: We do things this way, because they're good for the patient. The tones of intercultural misunderstanding are easy to hear.

Intercultural misunderstanding is rooted in, among other things, clashes between customs. Such clashes are profound, because they involve understandings of responsibility and loyalty and thus commitments. A companion to customs is expectations about what behavior is fitting. With expectations comes judgment. So our consideration of cultures of care leads us to expect that team members will appeal to customs. Through clashes between customs we encounter intercultural misunderstanding, interdisciplinary clashes, and tones of judgment.

Among Ms. Mason's adult offspring, the disagreement followed the fault lines about their own life plans. It referred to scarcity and individuation: She needs more attention; they are close to their limits. The siblings accepted responsibility for their mother, but they also had responsibility for themselves.

An additional culture clash came between the providers and the family. Whatever differences existed among the providers' cultures of care, they all had one theme in common: Ms. Mason's well-being. But this theme collided with family members' responsibility to take care of themselves and not just of their loved one. To the extent that the patient/family is the core of the health care team, then a culture clash between providers and patient/family can occur at any time. In fact, the wonder is that this culture clash does not occur more often, because health care providers understandably limit their responsibility to fostering the patient's recovery and potential for flourishing, whereas the patient and family are responsible for their own flourishing and for their own contribution to the patient's well-being.

Issues about finances did not play an explicit role in this case, but it is hard to imagine that they were far from the surface. Certainly, Ms. Mason's well-being was at the top of the physician's agenda, but his agenda also appropriately included efficient use of his HMO's resources. In this case there was no tension between the patient's well-being and cost savings, but in some decisions about team care of the elderly, cost savings are part of the culture.

The Principle of Proportionate Care

Another way that we test whether we have arrived at the most humane and encompassing solution is to ask, "What can go wrong with this plan?" Have we reached Rawls's reflective equilibrium? To answer this question, we turn to the principle of proportionate care. The responsibility of the health care team is to determine the treatment and the ancillary actions that are most likely to provide the best balance of benefits over burdens for the patient (Jonsen, Siegler, and Winslade, 1998).

If the agreed-upon solution fits one or more of the definitions of "the good," why did the renal service's recommendation seem to insist on another course of action, namely, switching the patient to HD and moving her to a nursing home? The answer is that the service was exercising its responsibility under the principle of proportionate care—recommending the treatment most likely to confer the greatest balance of benefits than burdens upon the patient. This principle describes the fiduciary responsibility of the physician and of the entire team toward the patient. The recommendation of HD and a nursing home does not yet include the patient's assessment of the benefits and burdens of the treatment. The negotiation with the patient starts from there.

We are now ready to summarize Ms. Mason's case on the basis of JSW in Table 3.2.

The Team, Ethics, and the Culture of Care

We have sought to state principles and guideposts for creating a larger culture of care that will draw together the contributions of the various specific professional cultures. One issue that such a culture must address is whether it considers the patient a member of the health care team and, if so, how the team will handle the conflicts and tensions that result from naming the patient as a member.

First, if the patient is a member of the team, what do words like *compliant* and *noncompliant* mean? Are they about the patient, or about the professional members' relationship with the patient, or about the professionals themselves? We believe *compliance* and *noncompliance, adherence* and *nonadherence,* are ethnocentric terms. They imply that the professionals have not taken the patient's realities, perspectives, and values into full consideration. These terms should disappear from our mental models of the professional–patient/family team relationship. They are demeaning toward the patient or the family. In actual use, we believe that the terms are a source of countertransference reactions that clinicians rationalize under stress. Both of these last statements can, and should, be researched.

TABLE 3.2
Summary Concerning the Trial Statement: "The Best Ethical Course is to Place Ms. Mason on Hemodialysis and to Have Her Move to a Nursing Home"

Goals of medicine	Patient perspectives

Promotion of Health and Prevention of Disease
   Favors HD, if HD is more effective than PD, or than
      Ms. Mason's PD.
   Should help prevent other admissions like the current one.
   Favors PD, if switch to HD and more to nursing home would
      disturb Ms. Mason's mental health.
Relief of Symptoms, Pain, and Suffering
   Favors HD, if HD is more effective than PD.
   Favors PD, as switch to HD and move would distress her.
Cure of Disease
   Not applicable; neither diabetes nor ESRD is curable.
Preventing Untimely Death
   Untimely death can come too late or too soon.
   Death-too-soon seems more pertinent in this case.
   This goal favors HD for prevention of death-too-soon, if HD
      is more effective.
Improvement of Functional Status or
Maintenance of Compromised Status
   Favors HD, if HD is more effective than PD. Otherwise, either
      course is permissible.
Education and Counseling of Patients [and Family]
Regarding Condition and Prognosis
   Favors neither option; clinicians have fiduciary responsibility
      to assure that Ms. Mason or her surrogate understands the
      nature and the consequences of the decisions about type of
      dialysis and moving.
Avoiding Harm to the Patient in the Course of Care
   Harm cannot be absolutely avoided.
   Favors HD physiologically; PD may be more associated with
      depression than HD, so HD may also be psychosocially
      preferable.
Summary
   Goals of medicine favor the trial statement for Ms. Mason's
      physical well-being but not for her spiritual or psychosocial
      well-being. By themselves, the goals of medicine would
      justify either choice: accepting the trial statement and
      changing course or rejecting it and keeping the course.
      Overall, on the basis of the goals of medicine alone, the trial
      statement is preferable.
	Ms. Mason tried HD and nursing home placement. She said that she does not want HD and she wants to live with her sons. On hospital admission, she cannot communicate her preferences. In the absence of other information, we presume unchanged preferences. Later, her mental status improves and she can speak for herself.
	Summary: On the basis of patient perspectives alone, both parts of the trial statement would be absolutely prohibited.

Continued on next page

Second, what do the patient and the family contribute to identifying the problem and creating the plan of treatment? In Ms. Mason's case, participation by her and her family was essential to determining the problem and to formulating the care plan.

Third, when the patient and her family are members of the team, who is the patient advocate? All disciplines claim patient advocacy as a task and commitment. Ms. Mason needed an advocate when she was unable to speak for herself.

TABLE 3.2 CONTINUED
Summary Concerning the Trial Statement: "The Best Ethical Course is to Place Ms. Mason on Hemodialysis and to Have Her Move to a Nursing Home"

Quality of life	Contextual features

Fundamental Goal of Medicine
   Improve Ms. Mason's quality of life, maintain it, slow its
   decline, raise its nadir.
Objective Criteria of Quality of Life
   She is presently below her baseline.
   Her baseline is restricted; it is not minimal or below minimal.
   Her quality of life at the moment is between restricted and
   minimal and is expected to improve.
Ms. Mason's Own Assessment of Her Quality of Life
   Not clear.
   Neither the switch to HD nor the move would serve it.
Summary
   Quality of life as a fundamental goal of medicine must include
   Ms. Mason's assessment of her quality of life. Hence, quality
   of life returns us to patient perspectives, which forbid the
   trial statement. JSW's objective criteria do not contribute to
   our assessment.
	Family Perspectives: Family caregivers are willing to help her stay at home, request flexibility from her and for each other so that they can pursue their own life plans.
	Caregiver Perspectives: Clinicians differ about their responsibilities toward Ms. Mason.
	Other Contextual Features: No particular concerns for any of the following:
	   Institutional perspectives and policies
	   Public policy pertaining to the case
	   Legal factors
	   Cost
	   Research
	Summary: Contextual features oppose the trial statement.

Principle of proportionate care	Overall summary

Attending Physician
   Includes Ms. Mason's assessment in determining benefits and
   burdens of renal service's recommendation.
Renal Service
   Recommendation based on what is best for Ms. Mason from
   her prior fall history and their ability to restore access; does
   not include her assessment of benefits and burdens.
Nurse
   Prefers transfer to nursing home, on basis of Ms. Mason's
   history of falls, dislodgments of PD catheter, and disagree-
   ment with attending physician re mental status.
Ethicist-chaplain
   Recommends not moving her until family issues are sorted out
   and not switching her to PD until necessary.
Patient's Children
   Do not address the recommendations at all.
Ms. Mason
   Rejects the recommendations.
   1. Fears infection from HD.
   2. Prefers living with her sons.
The Entire Team
   Does not explicitly arrive at a recommendation.
	1. The renal service's recommendation produces a genuine dilemma. Medically, it is ethically preferable. From the point of view of patient autonomy, it is not ethically permissible, owing to Ms. Mason's perspectives to the contrary.
	2. By itself, the attending physician's rejection of the renal service's recommendation does not meet the ethical needs of the situation, especially avoiding future hospitalizations.
	3. Ethical needs of the situation call for collaboration among health care professionals and Ms. Mason and her family.
	4. Ms. Mason, her family, and her clinicians need to work out a plan that will assure her "good enough" care.

After recovering her mental status, she could be her own advocate. When a decisionally competent patient makes a "bad decision," the professional advocate should continue the educational process and seek her well-being.

If culture is about information that is taught and learned, what do we want and need to teach about the ethics of team care? First, clinicians need to clarify the question(s) that they are working on at any given moment. Second, team members need to remember that ethics examines new situations against established solutions and, if they don't work, creates and tests new proposals for solutions. These proposals are trial statements, not conclusions. In the early stages of discussing the ethics of a case, less censoring of trial statements is best. The early stages of ethical reflection are first drafts, and we continue to "write first drafts" throughout the process, as we revise trial statements and test the new versions. Third, we need to assure that our culture of established solutions is broad enough to seek the greatest possible good for all the stakeholders and does not enforce a traditional ethical solution at the expense of some, especially those who differ with the traditional solution. Fourth, team care offers the opportunity to revisit the great ethical traditions and their contributions to our current ethical solutions—to reconsider duty, the greatest good of the greatest number, virtue, authenticity, and utility. The ethics of team health care requires us to revisit traditional problems in health care ethics. What is the proper use of power? Does ethics, in its faithfulness to its established solutions, misuse power, generate less good than is possible, or produce evil? Fifth, we must remember that when the ethical views of team members collide, that is not a danger. Rather, it is part of the ineluctable tension between cultures of care and a larger culture of care. An ethical challenge of teamwork is for people to articulate their own viewpoints and the viewpoints of their profession, and to reconsider them with one another. Sixth, we need to keep in mind that carrying out fiduciary responsibility alone may seem easier than coordinating it with others, because people have a clear sense of the responsibility of their professions. If people have to negotiate different ideas of responsibility with different professions, the cost in time and recalibration of values may seem unjustifiably high for gains measured in small nuances.

The culture of team care has to overcome some major obstacles: the cultures of care of individual professions; demands of efficiency and cost containment; the tyranny of the urgent; the false need to demonstrate that team care is superior to predecessor cultures; and the need of team care to demonstrate that it is articulating powerful and irreducible realities that have not been sufficiently recognized. There is no care of patients that is not team care, period. The culture of team care needs to be able show that teamwork is essential. Collaborative discussions and deliberations are needed to produce synergistic, novel, and unforeseen solutions; hence, part of the culture of team care, and part of the ethical responsibility of team caregiving, is synergy, the creation together of new solutions unforeseen at the outset.

The culture of team care involves a sophisticated definition or concept of team, a wonderful and appropriate balance of self-respect and respect for others. It is not that sometimes we use teams, and sometimes we do not. Rather, all work on behalf of patients is teamwork, even when only one health care professional is working with a patient and even when the team consists of only one health care professional and the patient—the archetypal therapeutic dyad. Behind every professional is a whole tradition and history of professionals whose teaching has been shaped by their work on teams, most especially by patient-centered teams. The culture of team care is a culture of interprofessional communication, with constant heads-ups and inquiries about what ought to be done with patients. In that sense, the culture of team care approximates the best that ethics seeks when it joins the team to help create the most humane and encompassing solution(s) to the problem(s) at hand.

Discussion Questions

1. Ms. K is an 87-year-old morbidly obese diabetic woman, who has sores on her feet that do not heal and who sits much of the day presiding over her family. She does not take her medication regularly or follow the diet prescribed for her. Her home health nurse tells Ms. K that her cooperation is needed if home care is to continue. Sweetly but definitely, Ms. K replies, "You can't discharge me. You must take care of me. I have my rights."
   a. Which quadrants of JSW pertain to her situation, and what light do they throw on the ethics of team care of Ms. K?
   b. Which specific goals of medicine pertain, and what do they suggest for team care of Ms. K?
   c. How does Ms. K see the team and her role in it?

2. Carolyn is an occupational therapist caring for Mr. J, a 75-year-old who lives alone. He requires therapy after injuring his hand in a fall. He has progressed as far as Carolyn knows how to help him. When Carolyn says, "We've done all that we can, and it's a good job, too," he says that he is afraid of being

left alone. Carolyn reminds him that from the beginning she has said the number of sessions would be limited. She calls for an ethics consultation, saying, "My code of ethics as an occupational therapist requires me to discharge the patient, when the patient has progressed as far as he can."

    a. What are the strengths of this provision of the code? What are its limitations?

    b. What quadrants of JSW pertain to this decision and why?

    3. Alex Casey, R.N., and Michelle Goode, M.D., are at an impasse about whether to tell their patient, Dorothy Wu, an 80-year-old immigrant from Taiwan who speaks passable English, that she has cancer. Dr. Goode says that Ms. Wu's son says that in their culture, they do not tell their loved ones that they have an illness that is likely to result in death, and she wishes to honor Mr. Wu's request not to tell his mother about her cancer. But Mr. Casey experiences great pressure from Ms. Wu for an explicit answer, and he has great difficulty not telling her. He has called for an ethics consultation. This bring Dr. Goode's wrath down on him. Dr. Goode has always pegged Mr. Casey as a stickler for dotting the I's, and Mr. Casey considers Dr. Goode maternalistic on her best days.

When they are able to discuss the issue somewhat rationally, Dr. Goode notes to Mr. Casey that Immanuel Kant said that people should test their maxims (or trial statements) against the categorical imperative. One version of the categorical imperative says that we should treat our trial statements (maxims) as if they would be universalized. Dr. Goode says that Mr. Casey is mistakenly universalizing U.S. standards of informed consent, when he should be universalizing respect for other cultures' solutions to the problems of giving patients bad news.

Dr. Goode also cites John Stuart Mill, who wrote, "The non-existence of an acknowledged first principle has made ethics not so much a guide as a consecration of men's actual sentiments." Mr. Casey then says he has not studied ethics, but he can recognize a viewpoint that is stuck at the starting point: "Don't tell the patient." He also points out that he has not delegated his moral responsibility to Dr. Goode.

    a. Sort out the parts of this conflict that are personal, the parts that reflect cultures of care, and the parts that reflect cultures of ethics. What would the JSW model contribute to the discussion? What would be the limitations of that model?

    b. What would be the responsibilities of an ethics consultant or ethics committee toward each of the actors in this case?

REFERENCES

Burck, R. 1996. Feeding, withholding, and withdrawing: Ethical perspectives, invited review. *Nutrition in Clinical Practice* 11:243–53.

Hill, R. F., J. D. Fortenberry, and H. F. Stein. 1990. Culture in clinical medicine. *Southern Medical Journal* 83:1071–80.

Jonsen, A., M. Siegler, and W. J. Winslade. 1998. *Clinical ethics,* 4th ed. New York: McGraw-Hill.

Kant, I. 1983. *Grounding for the Metaphysics of Morals.* In J. W. Ellington, ed. and trans., *Kant: Ethical philosophy.* Indianapolis: Hackett. (Original work published 1785.)

Kleinman, A., L. Eisenberg, and B. Good. 1978. Culture, illness, and care: Clinical lessons from anthropological and cross-cultural research, *Annals of Internal Medicine* 88:251–58.

Levine, C., and C. Zuckerman. 1999. The trouble with families: Toward an ethic of accommodation. *Annals of Internal Medicine* 130(2):148–52.

Mill, J. S. 1998. *Utilitarianism.* In L. P. Pojman, *Ethical theory: Classical and contemporary readings,* 4th ed. Belmont, Calif.: Wadsworth. (Original work published 1863.)

Poortinga, Y. H. 1990. Towards a conceptualization of culture for psychology. *Cross-Cultural Psychology Bulletin* 24(3):2–10, cited in Paul B. Pederson, *Culture-centered counseling interventions: Striving for accuracy.* Thousand Oaks, Calif.: Sage Publications, 1997.

Rasmussen, D. B. 1999. Human flourishing and the appeal to human nature. In E. F. Paul, F. D. Miller, and J. W. Paul, eds., *Human flourishing.* Cambridge: Cambridge University Press.

Rawls, J. 1971. *A theory of justice.* Cambridge, Mass.: Belknap Press of Harvard University Press.

Rodwin, M. A. 1992. The organized American medical profession's response to financial conflicts of interest, 1890–1992. *Milbank Quarterly* 70 (4):703–41.

Segall, M. H., P. R. Dasen, J. W. Berry, and Y. H. Poortinga. 1990. *Human behavior in global perspective: An introduction to cross-cultural psychology.* New York: Pergamon.

Senge, P. M. 1994. *The fifth discipline: The art and practice of the learning organization.* New York: Doubleday/Currency.

Smith, R., H. Hiatt, and D. Berwick. 1999. A shared statement of ethical principles for those who shape and give health care: A working draft from the Tavistock Group. *Annals of Internal Medicine* 130:143–47.

Webster's second new international dictionary of the English language unabridged. 1961. Springfield, Mass.: G & C Merriam.

CHAPTER 4

Professional Attitudes Toward End-of-Life Decision Making

Eileen R. Chichin, R.N., Ph.D., and
Mathy D. Mezey, R.N., Ed.D.

Making decisions about health care, particularly those associated with end-of-life care, is a highly complex endeavor. Even when made before disability by an individual via an advance directive, health care decision making is fraught with emotion. And when it comes to end-of-life treatment issues, the implications of health care decisions are always profound.

In the nursing home setting, making health care decisions assumes an even higher level of complexity. In addition to the fact that decisions made in nursing homes most often involve a life-or-death situation, the patient generally is not able to participate in the decision and make his or (more likely) her treatment preferences known. Interdisciplinary teams play significant roles in health care decision making in nursing homes. As well, the disparate views of professionals from different disciplines toward respect for patient autonomy influence how the team arrives at end-of-life treatment decisions. Further compounding the complexity of decision making in this setting are the close relationships that develop over time between nursing home residents and their institutional caregivers. Making treatment decisions whose outcome is associated with the death of a resident can be particularly distressing to caregiving staff.

The following case illustrates some of the issues associated with health care decision making in the institutional long-term care setting. The case is followed by an analysis that focuses on professional attitudes and perspectives and how they impact on team decision making.

Case Description

The case described here illustrates differing attitudes toward respect for autonomy versus paternalism, as well as individual personality and some discipline-specific perceptions that can have a negative impact on team functioning.

Mrs. Levy is an 80-year-old widow who was admitted to a nursing home in New York City from a nearby acute care hospital approximately one year ago. She was hospitalized for treatment of a fractured hip she sustained when she fell at home. In addition, she suffers from Gaucher disease and chronic lymphocytic leukemia, as well as hypertension, ASHD, and dementia. Before her fall, Mrs. Levy lived alone at home. She has a close relationship with her sister, who also lives in New York City.

Mrs. Levy seemed to adapt relatively well to the nursing home, although the manifestations of her dementia increased. She tended to pace incessantly, usually babbling softly to herself. On several occasions, the team responsible for her care questioned the advisability of having her transferred to a dementia unit. But Mrs. Levy's medical status was rather unstable, and periodically she needed blood transfusions to control her leukemia. In fact, about every month or so, Dr. Reynolds, the physician caring for her, would call her sister to inform her that Mrs. Levy would be given a transfusion.

The decision to transfuse Mrs. Levy was made by Dr. Reynolds, and Ms. Brown, the head nurse on the unit, assisted him in starting the transfusion. Although the staff attempted to constantly reassure Mrs. Levy before and during the transfusions, sitting with her and holding her hand, she was quite resistant to the procedure. This resistance was becoming an issue of concern to some of Mrs. Levy's direct caregivers, particularly Ms. Brown, as well as Mrs. Levy's primary nursing assistant, Ms. Douglas. Before administering the blood to Mrs. Levy, it became necessary to give her a dose of lorazepam. Then nursing staff had to physically hold Mrs. Levy in her bed while the transfusion was started. If they left her alone, she would remove it. Ms. Brown was particularly distressed by this but was reluctant to question the physician about it. Ms. Brown mentioned to Ms. Douglas that she was very upset about Mrs. Levy, the periodic transfusions, and what was required in order to administer them. But Ms. Brown was very reluctant to bring this up to Dr. Reynolds because in the past he had made it clear that he did not like to have his decisions questioned. Ms. Brown was very concerned about having a "good" working relationship with Dr. Reynolds and was cautious about doing anything that might rock the boat. She didn't mention her concerns to other members of the team because she felt this was a medical-nursing issue only. She had considered bringing the case to the ethics committee but again felt that Dr. Reynolds would be annoyed if she did so. Thus, while she was distressed about Mrs. Levy, Ms. Brown's concerns about maintaining an amicable relationship with the physician assumed greater prominence.

Ms. Brown was doubtful that Mrs. Levy would have accepted the transfusions if she were cognitively intact. Five years before the fall that precipitated her admission to the nursing home, Mrs. Levy had executed advance directives. In addition to a health care proxy naming her sister as her agent, Mrs. Levy also delineated her treatment preferences in a living will. Of note were the following statements in Mrs. Levy's living will:

In the event I am unable to make health care decisions for myself, my wishes are as follows:

Medication and treatment should not be or continue to be administered to me for therapeutic reasons or to prolong my life, if . . . I have an incurable or irreversible condition which is not terminal, but which causes me to experience severe or progressive physical or mental deterioration and loss of capacities I value, so that the burdens of continued life (with treatment) are greater than the benefits I experience.

If I am in (such a condition), I do not want mechanical respiration, cardiopulmonary resuscitation, electrical or mechanical resuscitation of my heart when it has stopped beating, pulmonary resuscitation, antibiotics, dialysis, artificial nutrition and hydration or any other treatment or procedure that might prolong my life to be or to continue to be administered to me under any circumstances. (However,) . . . I want to be as free from pain or discomfort as is possible, even if the administration of medication or treatment for this purpose (other than mechanical respiration, cardiopulmonary resuscitation and artificial nutrition or hydration) may render me unconscious or may shorten my life, or alternatively have an incidental therapeutic effect or may tend to prolong my life.

Ms. Brown was aware of the existence of Mrs. Levy's living will, as was Dr. Reynolds. That Mrs. Levy had taken the trouble, several years earlier, to clearly document her treatment preferences contributed to Ms. Brown's discomfort about what was being done. Dr. Reynolds, on the other hand, a devout Catholic, said he believed that the transfusions constituted good medical treatment, and he would not even consider not ordering them. In fact, when he called Mrs. Levy's sister each month to announce that he was giving Mrs. Levy a transfusion, it was never to seek her approval but simply to inform her.

Unfortunately, the other members of the health care team were unaware of what was being done. Since, as noted earlier, Ms. Brown considered this a medical-nursing issue, she never brought it up at a team meeting or discussed it informally with any other team members except Mrs. Levy's nursing assistant. Accordingly, only she, the physician, and Mrs. Levy's nursing assistant were aware that Mrs. Levy was receiving a treatment that she most likely would have refused if she were cognitively intact and that she was clearly refusing in her current state.

One day members of the ethics committee were visiting another resident on Mrs. Levy's unit, at the same time that Dr. Reynolds and Ms. Brown were starting Mrs. Levy's transfusion. The ethics committee members asked one of the nursing assistants about the screaming that could be heard from Mrs. Levy's room, and she told them about Mrs. Levy and the transfusions. Later, a member of the ethics committee returned to the nursing unit and mentioned to Ms. Brown that she had heard the screaming earlier. Apologetically, Ms. Brown began to tell the ethics committee member the story of Mrs. Levy, and why she had been unable to bring it to anyone's attention. When asked why she didn't at least bring it up at a team meeting, Ms. Brown reiterated yet again her concerns about her relationship with Dr. Reynolds. She very sheepishly agreed that she felt very bad about the entire situation, not only because she felt Mrs. Levy's wishes were not being respected but also because she felt Mrs. Levy was suffering. The ethics committee member urged Ms. Brown to discuss the issue with other members of Mrs. Levy's team, and Ms. Brown brought up the situation at their next regularly scheduled team meeting.

Resolution of the Ethical Dilemma

At the team meeting, after each member discussed what they felt was appropriate for Mrs. Levy, the team decided to access the ethics committee. While no member of the team felt there was an ethical dilemma per se, they wondered why some of them felt troubled, if what they were doing and planning to do was in fact "ethical."

Two members of the ethics committee joined the interdisciplinary team, which included Dr. Reynolds, Ms. Brown, Ms. Magee (the social worker), and Mrs. Rubin (Mrs. Levy's sister), to discuss Mrs. Levy's case. As recommended by Jonsen, Siegler, and Winslade (1998), those present reviewed Mrs. Levy's condition, including her medical problems, history, diagnosis, and prognosis, noting her steady downward spiral. Everyone present agreed that, unfortunately, Mrs. Levy's condition was irreversible, and that there would be no benefit to continued attempts at curative medical treatment.

Jonsen, Siegler, and Winslade (1998) suggest focusing on patient and family preferences, as evidenced either by conversation at the time a decision is being made, or by advance directives in a case of decisional incapacity. Clearly, at this time, Mrs. Levy could not tell the team what she would like as far as treatment preferences were concerned. Thus, her advance directive was reviewed. Both Mrs. Levy's caregiving team and the members of the ethics committee unanimously felt that Mrs. Levy's condition met the description, in her living will, of conditions where she would not want life-prolonging treatment. While everyone at the meeting was in agreement, however, not all present were entirely comfortable. Finally, after a few minutes of silence, Dr. Reynolds spoke up, noting that "not doing anything" was very hard for him. Further, he stated, he was somewhat resentful at having his opinions and his treatment plan challenged. He felt as if he were losing control of the situation, and this was not how he liked to practice medicine. Yes, he said, he understood the law and the resident's right to make her own treatment decisions (in Mrs. Levy's case, through her advance directives), but he still did not have to like it! Also he believed that, as a Catholic, he was mandated by his Church's teaching to provide life-sustaining treatment in every case. Dr. Reynolds's reaction is a textbook example of a health care provider's issues influencing a treatment decision (Jonsen, Siegler, and Winslade 1998).

Ms. Brown's feelings are another example of a provider issue that might influence a decision. She noted that she, too, was having some trouble respecting Mrs. Levy's previously stated wishes. But Mrs. Levy's reactions to the periodic blood transfusions truly did make her question the advisability of continuing the treatment, particularly given her progressive decline. It was this reaction, Ms. Brown said, that most influenced her feelings about continuing the treatment for Mrs. Levy. The preferences Mrs. Levy had outlined in her living will were secondary, in Ms. Brown's opinion. In fact, she would have liked to try everything possible to keep Mrs. Levy alive—she had become very attached to Mrs. Levy during her one-year stay at the nursing home, and she was dismayed at the thought that stopping the blood transfusions would eventually result in her death.

Further muddling her thinking about the entire situation, though, Ms. Brown had also been considering the appropriateness (or lack thereof) of giving regular blood transfusions to someone with an irreversible dementing illness. Should the team be concerned about the allocation of scarce health care resources, and should they be using such treatments in this situation? She decided to share her concern with the others at the meeting.

Dr. Reynolds stated that he felt very comfortable with using blood for an end-stage dementia patient, but mostly because of his feeling that he should provide treatment in all cases—he rarely found death an acceptable outcome. Additionally, he said, there was the possibility that the transfusions gave Mrs. Levy more energy and made her feel better and therefore, were a comfort measure—arguably, a quality-of-life (and perhaps palliative) issue that must be considered (Jonsen, Siegler, and Winslade 1998).

Jonsen, Siegler, and Winslade suggest taking note of resource allocation issues. Ms. Magee, the social worker, noted that she had considered the principle of justice when she learned of Mrs. Levy's periodic transfusions. While blood is more available than human organs, isn't it a relatively scarce resource? she wondered. Shouldn't what we have be used for those who will benefit more?

Ms. Magee also offered her opinion about stopping the transfusions from the perspective of Mrs. Levy's wishes. She understood the feelings of the other team members, she said, but they were clearly counter to her own. While she, too, was quite attached to Mrs. Levy, she believed very strongly that Mrs. Levy's right to make her own treatment decisions took precedence over whatever the team wanted for her. In discussing this with the other members of the team, she tried to emphasize her awareness of the difficulties Ms. Brown and Dr. Reynolds were having, as well as noting that she knew they both had Mrs. Levy's best interests at heart.

Again in following Jonsen, Siegler, and Winslade's (1998) recommendations, the team focused on resolving the ethical issues by creating a treatment plan, using the team process. After talking with members of the ethics committee, Mrs. Levy's team began to develop a plan for Mrs. Levy that eliminated the use of blood transfusions and maximized palliative care. Included among the decisions they made—in collaboration with Mrs. Rubin, Mrs. Levy's sister and health care agent—were no more acute care hospital transfer, no blood work, and no other treatments or diagnostic procedures unless they were required to provide comfort.

Ethical Issues to Consider
Respect for Autonomy

Theoretically, respect for patient autonomy is the dominant ethical principle in health care today. But as this case illustrates, recognition of this principle often falls by the wayside, giving further credibility to reports in the lay press as well as in scholarly journals that suggest that health care providers do not respect advance directives (e.g., Danis et al. 1991). What we are seeing in this case is an extreme example of the medical authoritarianism that was prevalent in health care for so many years before the pendulum swung toward autonomy. The physician typifies, at least in some respects, physicians of old, who believed they knew what was best for the patient and acted accordingly. In fact, Dr. Reynolds's allegiance to his own values and beliefs prevented him from approaching each case in terms of what was best for *this* patient. This, then, was more than medical authoritarianism—it was an impediment to patient care.

Similarly, the nurse in this case functioned in a fashion illustrative of some of her early counterparts as described by nurse-ethicist Catherine Murphy. When Murphy (1984) studied the moral reasoning of nurses in the 1970s, she found that a substantial number of nurses saw their loyalty to the hospital or to the physician. While Ms. Brown's motivation does not appear to have been loyalty to the physician, it certainly appears that she valued her concerns about her relationship with him more highly than her concern about respecting her patient's autonomy or her feelings about the patient's suffering. As well, Ms. Brown's concern with her own interests prevented her from focusing on what was in the patient's best interest.

What is very obvious in this case is that, while Mrs. Levy was unable to articulate her treatment preferences, she had left very clear evidence of her wishes in her living will. This was not a case in which the team would have to conduct an extensive search to determine Mrs. Levy's wishes, speaking to any family members or friends to whom Mrs. Levy may have communicated her views on quality of life in general and specific treatments in particular. Therefore, all members of the primary care team responsible for Mrs. Levy's care were obligated to respect her wishes. This clearly was not done, for a variety of reasons.

Professional-Patient and Professional-Proxy Relationships

A key feature of the relationship between health care professionals and patients should be veracity. In Mrs. Levy's case, where her agent was acting in her stead, that same requirement for truthfulness was necessary. Mrs. Rubin, functioning as Mrs. Levy's proxy, should have been treated by clinicians in the same way that Mrs. Levy would have been treated with respect to issues around truth-telling in diagnoses and prognoses as well as informed consent regarding any proposed treatments or procedures. This would have best protected Mrs. Levy's interests and ensured that she would receive appropriate care.

Thus, inherent in the principle of truth telling was Dr. Reynolds's responsibility to be completely open with Mrs. Rubin. But as described earlier, his dealings with Mrs. Levy's sister were not appropriate. Mrs. Rubin had the right to know everything about Mrs. Levy's condition and any proposed treatment, including all treatment options. Optimally, Dr. Reynolds, in collaboration with other members of the team, should have discussed with Mrs. Rubin all the pros and cons of periodic blood transfusions for a person with a progressively deteriorating condition and her option of refusing a particular treatment, particularly one rejected by Mrs. Levy in her living will.

Justice

One additional issue that could also be considered when thinking about the appropriateness of monthly blood transfusions for someone with advanced dementia is the principle of justice, particularly as it relates to the allocation of scarce resources. While the American health care system is not yet formally rationing health care resources, it seems logical that some of our more scarce health care assets should be conserved. Given Mrs. Levy's advanced, progressive, and incurable dementia, blood transfusions almost seem futile. In Mrs.

Levy's case, they might be logically characterized as a misuse of health care resources that could better be used by individuals to whom they would be of benefit.

Individual Values

Rempusheski (1989, 722), in addressing the subject of ethnicity in elder care, reminds us that "there are Western scientific beliefs, and individuals' ethnic and religious beliefs, and ethical beliefs underlying [one's] profession." Thus, all the players in this case were influenced by the personal and professional values to which each participant subscribed. Patients and health care professionals from different cultures often have disparate beliefs about health and health-related issues (Caralis et al. 1993; Tripp-Reimer and Affifi 1989), and every individual brings to the situation his or her own set of values.

Cultural background and, as in the case of Dr. Reynolds, religious beliefs transcend the boundaries of disciplines. The feelings of a social worker whose religion or culture mandates that life must be preserved at all costs will likely mirror the feelings of a physician or nurse from the same religion or culture. What is seen as beneficence in one country may be maleficence in another (Pellegrino 1992). Awareness of and sensitivity to these issues are key to smooth-running teams. Team members must exercise care to acknowledge these beliefs, while at the same time stressing patient autonomy and their mandate to respect it.

The values of a discipline may influence its members as much as or even more than cultural and religious factors. Despite the trend toward respect for patient autonomy, the values historically associated with each profession clearly influence the views of some professionals with respect to treatment issues. For example, physicians have historically been paternalistic. As well, their training imbues them with a focus on cure and the preservation of life. Thus, they may be troubled when a patient opts to forgo treatment that may extend life. Many nurses continue to find it difficult to "allow" someone to die rather than attempting some life-prolonging treatment. Bartholeme (1992) describes nurses' need to "protect" and care for their patients as "maternalism," a quality that may make it difficult for some nurses to accept a treatment plan that may be associated with the death of the patient.

Together, Bartholeme (1992) suggests, physicians' paternalism and nurses' maternalism become parentalism, an attitude that, like paternalism and maternalism, is rooted in the positive principle of beneficence. Parentalism may cause discomfort in these members of the health care team when they are required to participate in any act they consider to be harmful (i.e., an act that will result in the death of the patient).

On the caregiving team in the nursing home, physicians and nurses must work in concert with social workers. The social work profession is based on the principle of self-determination, and social workers are thus clearly invested in respect for patient autonomy. As well, although they are integral to the care of the nursing home resident, their involvement is less intense than that of physicians and nurses and in most cases less intimate. This combination of factors may facilitate their acceptance of residents' choices to limit life-sustaining treatment. It may also, however, make them less sensitive to the intense feelings of nurses and physicians when it comes to certain aspects of resident care.

The issue of withholding or withdrawing life-sustaining treatment is fraught with emotion. In numerous instances where therapies such as tube feedings or antibiotics are withheld or withdrawn, the patient continues to live for months or years, but very often the decision to withhold or withdraw these treatments results in death. When a patient indicates (either at the time the decision needs to be made or in advance through an oral or written directive) that he or she would want treatment withheld or withdrawn in certain instances, the team needs to be apprised of the patient's preferences and supported through the implementation of a treatment plan that incorporates those wishes. The team as a unit or its individual members may perceive this information as either depriving the patient of a needed treatment or protecting him from ineffective and burdensome interventions. Nonetheless, the bottom line is that the patient's preferences take precedence, and team members who find this difficult to accept need to be supported and educated to do so. As well, they need to implement a care plan that maximizes patient comfort and dignity, and recognize that care that emphasizes low-tech comfort measures is as important if not more important than the use of higher technologies that often prolong a dying process rather than improve quality of life.

Team Issues to Consider

A few decades ago, Ducanis and Golin defined an interdisciplinary health care team as "a functioning unit, composed of individuals with varied and specialized training, who coordinate their activities to provide services to a client or group of clients" (1979, 5). The operative words here are unit and coordinate. These terms differentiate an interdisciplinary team from a multidisciplinary team, where "member of diverse disciplines . . . more or less informally interact with—or tolerate—each other" (Bloom and Parad 1976, 676).

Reviewing the case of Mrs. Levy, it seems apparent that her care was essentially being delivered by a multidisciplinary team. Nowhere is there evidence of teamwork per se. Rather, we see two health care professionals who, while they may perceive themselves to be part of a team, were in reality simply two individuals providing care to the same patients.

Nowhere, either, in the case description, is there evidence of any other team members, with the exception of the family, which is relegated to the passive role of information receiver. Dr. Reynolds makes an autonomous decision, then tells Mrs. Rubin what that decision is. While a team may theoretically consist of only two members, in Mrs. Levy's case her team had a number of other members. Prominent among them should have been the social worker, Ms. Magee. In this case description, however, there is no evidence that a social worker existed, let alone played any part in resident care and decision making.

Over time, interdisciplinary teams must go through a process of growth and development, and through that process find mechanisms to overcome barriers to communication and to develop methods for group decision making (Bennis and Shepard 1974). Although Mrs. Levy's physician, nurse, and social worker had been assigned to her care since she entered the nursing home a year before, there is minimal evidence that these three individuals functioned as an interdisciplinary team.

It has been suggested that personality and power struggles may be barriers to smooth team functioning (e.g., Fry and Miller 1974; Tsukuda 1990). Ms. Brown's passive, rather subservient manner, as well as her desire to maintain peace at any cost, in concert with Dr. Reynolds's view of himself as sole decision maker, prevented this group of individuals from functioning as a team.

Tsukuda (1990) reminds us that some key features of an interdisciplinary team are leadership and the ability to make decisions. Clearly, there is little, if any, evidence of leadership among Mrs. Levy's providers. As well, while decisions were made, they appear to have been made in a vacuum and obviously were not team decisions.

Overlapping knowledge bases can sometimes lead to conflict or power struggles. Who knew what was best for Mrs. Levy: the doctor, who had the most medical knowledge; the nurse who had strong grounding in medical knowledge; the social worker, who would have liked to support whatever Mrs. Levy wanted for herself; or Mrs. Rubin, Mrs. Levy's sister and health care agent? Optimally, if these individuals had functioned as an interdisciplinary team, a plan of care that was in Mrs. Levy's best interest would have evolved. Clearly, it would have involved some give and take, but for an interdisciplinary team to function at an optimum level its members must have common value base and mutual understanding (Abramson 1984; Billups 1987; Sands, Stafford, and McClelland 1990).

Frequently, in teams that have physicians as members, the physician may either be the leader or be perceived as the leader. Thus, in this case Dr. Reynolds may have seen himself as the leader. Even if others did not see him in this role, his influence was still felt.

Another factor that may have impeded this "team's" functioning is the organization in which it was located. In contrast to most nursing homes, where a nursing department wields the most power, Mrs. Levy lived in a large academic nursing home with a large medical staff. In the hierarchy here, the medical department was viewed as being "at the top." This further affirmed Dr. Reynolds's position as the leader of the team. And while team leadership can be a "movable" role, with one person assuming leadership for a particular task and another assuming leadership for "maintenance and self-renewing" functions (Tsukuda 1990), here we see little evidence of any team functioning at all.

Another major issue evident in this case is the absence of the social worker from any discussion. The dilemma raised in this case—failure to respect the resident's previously stated wishes—would most likely not have been a dilemma had it occurred several decades ago. Not only were teams not in existence then, but for the most part geriatric settings were not in existence either. Moreover, the wishes of the patient were considered of no relevance; medical treatment was dictated by the physician, sometimes with family input. Now, however, when we ostensibly perceive respect for patient autonomy as the cornerstone of medical ethics, the patient's treatment preferences are paramount. A nurse on a team with an overly paternalistic physician would clearly have been supported by a social worker whose discipline was founded on self-determination. But the physician in this case, who opted to make his own decisions absent team input, and the nurse, who saw the use of blood transfusions as a medical-nursing issue only, consciously or unconsciously chose not to include the social worker. Ms. Magee became aware that there was an issue only when a member of the ethics committee approached her, seeking her opinion on the case.

Conclusion

The case of Mrs. Levy describes just one issue associated with end-of-life decision making and interdisciplinary teams. Obviously, there are many others,
including such things as decisions about hospital transfer, decision making for
patients without families or advance directives, and demands by patients or
families for continued treatment that the team feels would not be in the best
interest of the patient. Each of these issues requires careful analysis.

This case of Mrs. Levy presented two dilemmas: one involving treatment
decisions for a nursing home resident at the end of life, and the other involving
a dysfunctional team. In many ways, resolving the ethical dilemma seems to
have been easier and more clear cut. Restructuring the functioning of the team
appears to have been the greater challenge. This team clearly needed to work
on its "teaming" skills, particularly those involving communication. Assistance
from facility leadership may have been necessary to enhance individual team
members' awareness of and reaction to one another's personal and discipline-
specific values. Clearly, this team had a long way to go to reach optimum functioning, but aiming for that goal would enhance not only the quality of their
work environment but also, more important, their ability to provide quality
care to their nursing home residents.

Discussion Questions

1. Are there any other facts or issues that the team should have considered
when developing a plan of care for Mrs. Levy?

2. Given the feelings of some of the team members with respect to Mrs.
Levy's care and her stated treatment preferences, is there anything that the other
team members could do to help them when they are presented with such issues
in the future? Is there anything the institution could or should do?

REFERENCES

Abramson, M. 1984. Collective responsibility in interdisciplinary collaboration: An ethical
perspective for social workers. *Social Work in Health Care* 10(1):35–43.
Bartholeme, W. G. 1992. A revolution in understanding: How ethics has transformed health
care decision-making. *Quality Review Bulletin* 18(1):6–11.

Bennis, W. G., and H. S. Shepard. 1974. A theory of group development. In G. S. Gibbard, J. J. Hartman, and R. D. Mann, eds., *Analysis of groups.* San Francisco: Jossey-Bass.

Billups, J. O. 1987. Interprofessional team process. *Theory into Practice* 26(2):146–52.

Bloom, B. L., and H. J. Parad. 1976. Interdisciplinary training and interdisciplinary functioning: A survey of attitudes and practice in community mental health. *American Journal of Orthopsychiatry* 46:669–77.

Caralis, P. V., B. Davis, K. Wright, and E. Marcial. 1993. The influence of race and ethnicity on attitudes toward advance directives, life-prolonging treatment, and euthanasia. *Journal of Clinical Ethics* 4(2):155–65.

Danis, M., L. I. Southerland, J. M. Garrett, J. L. Smith, F. Hielema, C. G. Pickard, D. M. Egner, and D. L. Patrick. 1991. A prospective study of advance directives for life-sustaining care. *New England Journal of Medicine* 324(13):882–88.

Ducanis, A. J., and A. K. Golin. 1979. *The interdisciplinary health care team.* Germantown, Md.: Aspen Systems Communication.

Fry, L., and J. P. Miller. 1974. The impact of interdisciplinary teams on organizational relationships. *Sociological Quarterly* 15:417–31.

Jonsen, A. R., M. Siegler, and W. J. Winslade. 1998. *Clinical ethics,* 4th ed. New York: McGraw-Hill.

Murphy, C. 1984. The changing role of nurses in making ethical decisions. *Law, Medicine and Health Care* 12:173–74, 184.

Pellegrino, E. D. 1992. Intersection of western biomedical ethics and world culture: Problematic and possibility. *Cambridge Quarterly of Healthcare Ethics* (3):191–96.

Rempusheski, V. F. 1989. The role of ethnicity in elder care. *Nursing Clinics of North America* 24(3):717–24.

Sands, R. G., J. Stafford, and M. McClelland. 1990. "I beg to differ": Conflict in the interdisciplinary team. *Social Work in Health Care* 14(3):55–72.

Tripp-Reimer, T., and L. A. Affifi. 1989. Cross-cultural perspectives in patient teaching. *Nursing Clinics of North America* 24(3):613–19.

Tsukuda, R. 1990. Interdisciplinary collaboration: Teamwork in geriatrics. In C. K. Cassel, D. E. Reisenberg, L. B. Sorenson, and J. R. Walsh, eds., *Geriatric medicine,* 2d ed. New York: Springer-Verlag.

PART III

Care Recipients

CHAPTER 5

Protecting the Patient's Voice on the Team

Nancy L. Smith, Ph.D., A.P.R.N., C.S.,
Ernestine Kotthoff-Burrell, M.S., R.N., C.S. and
Linda Farber Post, J.D., B.S.N., M.A.

Major advances in medical technology and public health have increased life expectancy from an average of 50 years in 1900 to more than 75 years today. While the quantity of years can be prolonged, however, the quality of those later years is threatened by numerous factors. For example, chronic debilitating conditions, cardiovascular and cerebrovascular diseases, cancer, Alzheimer disease, and the use of multiple medications that combat their symptoms can impair cognitive, expressive, and motor abilities.

The result for many older adults is not simply the loss of independent functioning but the decreasing ability to form and communicate thoughts and feelings. In general, people's expressions, whether oral, written, or behavioral, are more than vehicles for the exchange of information. Over time, they commonly develop a characteristic quality that allows people who know them to say, "Oh, that sounds just like him," or, "She would never do that." An individual's expressive capacity, or *voice*, is thus both an interactive link to others and a type of identity authentication. Without it, individuals lose their ability to participate in their environment and assert their autonomy. Arguably, nothing else so profoundly diminishes and isolates the elderly or increases their vulnerability as its loss.

The importance of voice is heightened in the health care setting, where it is critical to elicit patient values, health beliefs, and preferences. Health care professionals often lack the appropriate knowledge and skills to adequately address the sensitive and unique care needs of aging adults. Regrettably, paternalism, ageism, and negative stereotypes are commonly seen among health professionals and staff members as well as among the general public. On an interdisciplinary team and in a variety of settings, these problems pose daunting obstacles to protecting the voice of the older individual.

Measures to combat these barriers include incorporating geriatric, gerontological, cultural, and bioethical content into health professional educational programs; using values histories and advance directives in the event of decisional incapacity; and forming interdisciplinary teams to provide comprehensive high-quality health care for older adults. Frequently, when a patient's wishes are not known, they can be elicited from the family or other surrogates who know the patient well. Each of these measures can help preserve the patient's voice and incorporate it into the health care deliberation process, enhancing the likelihood that decisions will authentically reflect the individual's values and preferences.

While these measures can assist in safeguarding patient autonomy and promoting self-determination, certain constraints also influence the process. For example, the pluralism and increasingly global nature of our society mean that patients often do not have English as their primary language. They may also have vastly different health beliefs and practices from those of their providers. Although the education of health professionals has begun to address multiculturalism, there is still insufficient sensitivity to these issues. In addition, the imperatives of managed care have exacerbated conflict about therapeutic goals and cost effectiveness, dilemmas that have particular resonance in the geriatric setting.

Given the special needs of older patients in the current health care setting, it is critical that professionals on interdisciplinary teams (1) acquire adequate knowledge of geriatrics, gerontology, and ethics; (2) elicit, respect, protect, and attend to the voice of the patient and, when appropriate, the family; (3) learn about and act in accordance with the patient's cultural traditions and health beliefs; (4) identify actual or potential ethical dilemmas; and (5) learn and use models for ethical decision making and conflict resolution to promote patient-specific, therapeutically appropriate, and culturally sensitive plans of care.

This chapter discusses the patient and family or other surrogate decision maker as *active voices* and *participatory members* of the interdisciplinary team. A case study of an elderly Native Hawaiian man will demonstrate several key elements, including (1) the role of the family or other surrogate in enhancing and preserving the voice and protecting the autonomy of the patient; (2) the importance of cultural beliefs and practices in health care, especially at the end of life; (3) the interdisciplinary team process that allows the expression and exploration of different philosophies and perspectives; and (4) the use of an ethical decision-making model and its integration into the plan of care. The desired outcome is a comprehensive treatment plan that meets the patient's health care needs and incorporates the cultural values, beliefs, and wishes he shares with his providers, surrogates, and family. A plan should respect and accommodate the patient's, the family's, and each professional's viewpoints.

Case Description

Mr. Umilani, an 85-year-old Native Hawaiian gentleman, was a resident of the Mid-Pacific Nursing Center. He was transferred four months previously from an acute care hospital to which he had been admitted after he had suffered a stroke. During his initial hospital treatment, he was aphasic and could not swallow. In the hospital, he was fed through a nasogastric tube, but just before his transfer to Mid-Pacific, a percutaneous endoscopic gastrostomy (PEG) tube was inserted. The PEG was his only source of nutrition and hydration. He was transferred to the long-term care facility so that he could receive supportive nursing care.

Mr. Umilani was the head of a large extended family comprised of five grown children and several grandchildren. His wife of sixty-five years was active and healthy. Although she was not Native Hawaiian, Mrs. Umilani had participated in all of the Native traditions throughout their marriage, and their children had been taught the Native beliefs and customs that were a central part of Mr. Umilani's life. It is worth noting that today Native Hawaiians represent only 18 to 22 percent of the population of the islands. Although the Hawaii Medical Society has more than 2,400 actively practicing physicians, only 103, or 4 percent, are Native Hawaiian (Else, Palafox, and Little 1998). This disproportion exacerbates the problem of providing culturally sensitive health care.

At the time of Mr. Umilani's initial hospitalization, the family had met. The meeting began with a *pule* (prayer). Hawaiians traditionally believe the *pule* creates an environment for *mana* (power, life force) to be used for self-healing, spiritual empowerment, and maintaining *pono* (goodness). The *'ohana* (family) is central to the culture. The *kupuna* (elders) are the source of wisdom. The *keiki* (children), who are the hope for the future, learn from individuals senior to them.

Mr. Umilani had no written advance directives. But he and his wife had previously agreed that, if the need arose, their eldest son, Josh, would assume the responsibility of surrogate decision maker and speak on behalf of either or both of them. Accordingly, while it is most common for the spouse to assume this role, Mrs. Umilani requested that their firstborn child speak for his father and the family. During the time of the initial family meeting, other family members concurred with Josh's role as Mr. Umilani's surrogate decision maker.

Since his initial admission to the hospital, Mr. Umilani had shown no improvement. His family frequently visited and engaged his care providers in *talk story*, an integral part of the Hawaiian social culture. Through *talk story*, Hawaiians share information about current issues, life events, and problems. They also use the process to make decisions. In fact, during his four-month stay at the nursing facility, this had been the only mechanism through which the providers had gleaned an understanding of Mr. Umilani's beliefs and values.

As Mr. Umilani's birthday approached, members of his family expressed the desire to take him to a local restaurant to celebrate the occasion. The staff had concerns about the plan. His swallowing reflex had not returned, and he remained aphasic, with a right-sided hemiparesis. He was unable to communicate in any way. When awake, he showed a blank stare with an occasional smile. He had not given any indication that he was aware of his circumstances. The staff knew he would be unable to participate in the festivities or eat any of the food. Yet the family remained steadfast in its request.

During the birthday party, Mr. Umilani sat in his wheelchair and did not participate. At previous family celebrations, as the patriarch of the large family, he would extend *aloha* to all the guests, lead the events, and ensure that everyone was having fun. He would play the ukulele and guitar and lead the singing. This time was very different. When Josh returned Mr. Umilani to the facility, he said to the nurse, "This is not right. Our father would not want to live any longer." After some discussion among Josh, the nurse practitioners and the social worker, it was decided to convene a meeting of the interdisciplinary team and the extended family to explore the issues in more detail.

Case Discussion and Analysis

Ethical principles and concepts provide a framework for identifying and analyzing dilemmas, and they serve as guides for individual, professional, and institutional behavior. Considering the interests of all the parties, weighing the benefits, burdens, and risks of the various options, and arriving at a principled resolution are facilitated by using a decision-making model such as the one proposed by Jonsen, Siegler, and Winslade (1998). This model will be used to frame the discussion of Mr. Umilani's case.

Gather the Clinical Information

Developing a care plan that is responsive to the needs of the patient begins by exchanging information among the key parties. The interdisciplinary team approach is ideal for this endeavor because of its potential to reach a wide variety of people who differ in terms of age, gender, culture, religion, education, and relation to the patient. Through the process, information can be elicited from the patient, the family, or other surrogate decision maker; friends; and other close associates, such as a spiritual leader or, in this case, the Native Hawaiian healer. In turn, the patient and, as appropriate, the family or surrogate can be given information about the patient's current health status and prognosis, the therapeutic options and their relative benefits, burdens, and risks, and the potential for rehabilitation and the likely course of the illness.

The core professional team providing care to Mr. Umilani consisted of a physician, two geriatric nurse practitioners, a social worker, a physical therapist, several licensed practical nurses, and a number of nursing assistants. The entire team evaluated Mr. Umilani at the time of his admission to Mid-Pacific Nursing Center and periodically throughout the subsequent four months of his residence. The nursing assistants were responsible for providing his daily care (bathing, dressing, grooming, toileting, and transferring him from bed to chair). His medications, nutrition, and hydration were administered through his PEG tube.

At the first team meeting held after Mr. Umilani's birthday celebration, Josh, his surrogate decision maker, expressed the family's wishes. He said that, on behalf of their father, the family had agreed that his extraordinary care measures should be terminated. The team members then reviewed with the family the results of their initial and periodic assessments of Mr. Umilani's condition and likely future course. The physician noted that Mr. Umilani had suffered a massive stroke that left him paralyzed on his right side. His inability to chew or swallow had necessitated the nasogastric tube and the subsequent PEG tube. Mr. Umilani was unable to communicate either verbally or nonverbally through the use of gestures, a storyboard, or any other means. His affect had not changed, despite treatment with antidepressants. He had not indicated any awareness of his surroundings or any understanding of what had happened to him. Perhaps most significant, there was no reason to expect that his condition would improve.

Both nurse practitioners concurred that Mr. Umilani had not shown any physical, cognitive, or affective improvement since his admission. The primary goals of his care had been to provide comfort, nutrition, and hydration and to prevent any iatrogenic complications. He showed no signs of pain or discomfort. His blood pressure was being adequately controlled. His nutritional needs were being met. Although he needed total care for all of his personal needs, the nursing assistants had been successful in preventing any skin breakdown or infections.

The physical therapist related that attempts to improve Mr. Umilani's independent mobility with the aid of a walker or wheelchair had been ineffective. Because he was unable to comprehend directions or participate in rehabilitation, her plan was to provide passive range-of-motion exercises to prevent contractures and other complications.

In summary, Mr. Umilani's current health status was stable. He had little rehabilitation potential and would not return to his prestroke level of physical or cognitive functioning. He was not in any pain or discomfort. If the PEG tube were removed, Mr. Umilani would not survive. But with continued care at the current level, he could live for an indeterminate amount of time in his present state. Although Mr. Umilani would ultimately succumb to his illness, the trajectory could be protracted and the dying process lingering.

Identify Patient and Family Preferences

I paʻa i kona kupuna ʻaʻ ole kakou
Had our ancestors died bearing our grandparent, we would not have come forth.

HAWAIʻIAN PROVERB

The next step in the ethical decision-making process involves determining and incorporating the patient's care preferences. Because Mr. Umilani lacked the capacity to participate in discussion and decision making and did not have advance directives to provide insight into his wishes, it was necessary for the team to listen to other sources for his voice. It was important for them to elicit information about prior statements, decisions, behavior patterns, or other characteristics that might indicate his thoughts about illness, dependence, acceptable quality of life and death, as well as his preferences about life-sustaining treatment and care at the end of life. How had he lived his life when he was healthy? What did he consider most important? What were his cultural, religious, or foundational values and beliefs? If he were able to communicate, what would he articulate as his personal preferences?

In Mr. Umilani's case, his cultural traditions greatly facilitated the information-gathering process. Through recollections and anecdotes, *talk story* allowed the family to share his wishes, often in his own voice. Fortunately the team recognized this medium as a subtle but gentle means of finding out about the patient-as-he-had-been and a comforting way to communicate with the family about difficult and sensitive issues. If the health providers had not appreciated this shared communication approach and insisted on a more linear monologue style or the traditional provider-directed interviewing process, the result might have been a breakdown in communication and possibly the family's withdrawal from the therapeutic relationship.

The team met with the family. After the opening *pule,* Josh and the other family members began to describe their perceptions of Mr. Umilani and his values. They shared the above proverb to illustrate the importance of the family, especially elders, in the Native Hawaiian culture. Culture has been defined as the civilization of a given people or nation at a given time in its customs and arts; or behavior that is socially taught rather than instinctive or individual (Thorndike and Barnhart 1991, 270). The very existence of the family or *ʻohana* originates with the elders and is reflected through respect and caring of all extended members. In a study of *kanaka maoli* (Native Hawaiian) women, one woman stated, "We want [members in our families] to respect everyone. It doesn't matter [to whom] show respect. And that is where the love comes from. . . . Love and respect" (Browne and Braun 1994).

Central to the Hawaiian culture is 'ohana, through which the values, history, and traditions are communicated to the individuals. The traditional 'ohana is multigenerational, and grandparents traditionally live with their adult children and their children. Family members are expected to share in household activities, pool resources, and support and assist one another in times of need.

For knowledge to be passed from parents to the keiki (children), the parents must have enough mana (spirit or life force) to teach keiki cultural truth, practices, and the true meaning of aloha. Aloha originates in the family, and it is through the family teachings of rituals and the developed pohai ke aloha (circle of aloha) that the roots of one's existence are acknowledged and pono (right behavior) is maintained. The ability to self-determine, to be sovereign, begins with self, which includes the collective history of one's 'ohana.

Mr. Umilani's family shared the proverb to express the love and respect they felt for him. They related that, throughout his life, he had taken pride in his Native heritage and had been an actively participating member of his cultural community. When he and his wife were young, they had cared for his parents and extended 'ohana, which remained the central core of his life. He had taught his children and grandchildren about their ancestors, often relating stories of his parents and grandparents. He spoke of the beautiful and uncluttered landscape before the commercialization of the islands. He hoped that his children and grandchildren would remain on the islands and continue to pass the stories and the customs on to their descendants.

The family described Mr. Umilani's warm and gregarious nature. Despite his hypertension and other chronic diseases, he had never complained. He was the life of the party. He wanted everyone to feel welcome in his home and to participate in family celebrations. Each person spoke of their love and regard for Mr. Umilani and described the family meeting after his birthday celebration when they had discussed with sadness his inability to communicate or to take part in the festivities. Seeing him in this condition and knowing that he would not return to his former gusto for life, they agreed that he would not have wanted to live under these circumstances.

An additional consideration was the importance of 'ohana. None of the family had thought that a loved one would have to be in a nursing home. Yet despite the central value of family and the deeply held traditions, they realized that they could not provide his care. After careful consideration, they decided that Josh, on behalf of Mr. Umilani and the other family members, should authorize the termination of Mr. Umilani's life-sustaining measures. They reasoned that the father and husband they had known and loved was no longer alive. Although he might not be in discomfort, his current and likely future condition was a source of great pain and suffering to those who knew and cared about him.

They had listened respectfully to the team's assessment of Mr. Umilani's condition and the predictions for his remaining life. According to Hawaiian philosophy, time functions in a spiritual context; the past, present, and future of every individual in the 'ohana are all contained in the present. Although ancient Hawaiians marked time according to the cycles of nature, their descendants also acknowledge and respect the sense of physiological timing through the individual's relationship to his internal clock. The family was adamant that the feeding tube be removed. It was agreed that, on his death, he would be buried as he had lived—in the traditional style of his culture.

Evaluate Quality-of-Life Issues

Injury or illness can threaten not only an individual's life but also its quality. The goal of medical intervention is to restore, maintain, or improve the quality of life (Jonsen, Siegler, and Winslade 1998). In discussing quality of life, however, it is important for health care professionals to remember that such evaluations are intensely personal. What may be unacceptable to one individual in terms of comfort or function may be precious and even sacred to another. To characterize a person's existence as having a particular quality is to risk imposing one's own values, a reminder with special significance for health care professionals, whose assessments may carry weight in patient and family decision making.

While the concept of quality of life (QOL) may be subjective and therefore somewhat elusive, some objective parameters may be usefully considered. These include the patient's level of comfort or discomfort, cognitive abilities, mental and emotional capacity, mobility, independent functioning, ability to recognize and relate to others, and pleasure derived from life as it is in the present.

Using these objective parameters and guided by the family's description of Mr. Umilani as he had been before his stroke, it is possible to infer that the current quality of his life would likely have been unacceptable to him. Although he appeared to be free from pain and physical discomfort, his stroke had taken all of the remaining capacities that had given his life meaning and pleasure—mental capacities, independence, mobility, and perhaps most important, the ability to communicate with and relate to others. Based on their conviction that Mr. Umilani would not want to live in his current condition, Josh (his surrogate), his wife, his other children, and his grandchildren continued to request the removal of his PEG tube. They planned to say their good-byes before the tube was disconnected and remain at his side during his final days.

While his physician agreed that the patient had significant impairments in his ability to function and communicate, in her opinion the most important fact was that he was alive. She pointed out that he was not in pain, he had a loving family that came to visit and participate in his care, he had not suffered any further complications from his stroke or other problems, and his current medical needs were being adequately addressed. What more could the family ask?

The physician had some significant disadvantages as a member of the team and as a conscientious provider of care to this specific patient. She was still somewhat new to her role, having completed her residency just two years earlier. She was a product of her medical education and culture, in which she learned that the physician's goal is to cure the patient. In addition, she had not had much exposure to long-term care because most of her training had been spent in the acute care setting. She was unfamiliar with palliative care and end-of-life care. She had difficulty breaking any bad news to families, much less discussing the termination of life-sustaining interventions. She had not grown up on the island, nor had she had any previous exposure to Native Hawaiian culture and practices. She felt that, if this were her father, she would want to share more time with him. She was satisfied that both the hospital and the nursing center care teams had met their obligations to the patient by preserving his life.

In contrast, the two geriatric nurse practitioners were seasoned and highly skilled clinicians, both of whom had lived and worked on the islands for many years. One had worked at a local clinic that was funded by the U.S. Public Health Service. This facility was unique in having a Native Hawaiian nursing administrator who had been able to engage a Native healer to work in the clinic and provide traditional services. This had greatly increased the local community's trust in the clinic and its providers. The nurse practitioner had witnessed the difference that the inclusion and acceptance of a Native healer had made at the clinic. The second nurse practitioner had worked in hospice during her graduate program and was very comfortable talking to patients and their families about death, dying, and spirituality.

During Mr. Umilani's stay at Mid-Pacific, both nurse practitioners had engaged in numerous conversations with individual family members, who had articulated their distress at his inability to communicate or return to a higher level of functioning. One daughter had even expressed her belief that her father had died on the day of his stroke. The nurse practitioners agreed that the patient's physical health needs were being addressed and that the focus now was to provide supportive care for the family as well as the patient.

Likewise, the social worker spoke of her visits with the many caring and loving family members who often came by her office for informal chats about Mr. Umilani's lack of progress. One of his younger children and her husband had recently given birth to their first child, and she would grow tearful when she talked about her father never being able to see his newest grandchild.

The members of the care team all viewed Mr. Umilani's quality of life through the lens of their respective personal values and professional experiences. Because the physician's assessment was based on objective parameters and informed by her recent medical education, she wanted to maintain his life by keeping the PEG tube in place to provide nutrition, hydration, and medications. The nurse practitioners appreciated the physician's perspective, but they also understood the family's view. Recognizing the irreversibility of Mr. Umilani's condition, which was especially sad in light of how he had been described, and having witnessed the family's continuing distress, they both supported removing the PEG tube. The social worker considered the family's requests to be appropriate, especially their wish to have a Native healer present when the tube was removed and to hold a service that would be a celebration of Mr. Umilani's life. She had been asked to assist in making the necessary arrangements with the nursing center administrator. By listening closely to the family's request, most of the interdisciplinary team members had heard, understood, and protected the patient's voice.

Consider Contextual Factors

Contextual features are medical, ethical, and legal issues that implicate the interests and perspectives of the patient, the care providers, the family, and the institution. When there is dissonance in how the interested parties view and value these issues, conflicts may arise.

Central to principled health care decision making is an evaluation of the care goals in terms of their potential advantages and disadvantages to the patient. This assessment considers the patient's wishes in light of the diagnosis, the current condition and likely prognosis, the treatment choices, and their probable outcomes. The aim is to provide care that will effectively promote the patient's well-being while minimizing its untoward effects. The subjective (personal values) and objective (clinical) evidence and information determine the therapeutic options in terms of the benefits and burdens they represent *to the patient.* It is how the relative benefits and burdens are perceived and analyzed by the concerned parties that often creates conflict.

In this case, the physician disagreed with the perspectives of her colleagues and the patient's family. Although she had listened respectfully to their reasoning, her moral, theological, and professional values precluded her removing the PEG tube. Because her personal ethic held the sanctity of life as the core tenet, she believed that the benefit of continued life far outweighed the burdens of its diminished quality. She took seriously the obligations of her profession, especially the maxim, "Above all [or first] do no harm." In this context, she saw the removal of the PEG tube as gravely and irreparably harming the patient, rather than benefiting him by honoring his wishes and easing his family's suffering. For these reasons, she concluded that she personally could not comply with the family's request.

She referred the case for consideration by the long-term care facility's ethics committee. The committee members heard the opinions and concerns of the physician, the nurse practitioners, the social worker, and the family members. Review of the medical records provided information about Mr. Umilani's current and probable future condition. The various perspectives informed the discussion of quality versus quantity of life and the importance of Native customs and beliefs.

In addition to the ethical issues, this case also had two competing legal constraints concerning provider obligations and decision-making authority. The attending physician had decided that she could not be personally responsible for removing the PEG tube. It would be important, however, to ensure that her decision was informed by a clear understanding of the relevant law. Often physicians mistakenly believe that any action that does not prolong or—worse— that shortens life is illegal and makes them vulnerable to malpractice suits. In fact, the well-settled doctrine of informed consent is grounded in the law of assault and battery, which makes any unconsented-to touching legally actionable. In the health care setting, this means that treating a patient over his objection is both ethically and legally unsupportable. Physicians and health care institutions should be reassured that honoring the prior or contemporaneous wishes of a capacitated patient or surrogate to forgo treatment, even life-sustaining treatment, should not result in legal liability.

When, as in this instance, the physician's convictions prevent her from honoring the wishes of the patient or surrogate decision maker, she can and should remove herself from the case. Determining the goals of care should be a collaborative enterprise, drawing on the professional judgments of the providers and the personal insights of the patient and family. When these perspectives cannot be reconciled, promoting the patient's well-being may be hindered. While the physician is under no obligation to provide care that she finds unacceptable, she is obliged to ensure that her patient's care is undertaken by another provider. Explaining to the patient or family her inability to continue the therapeutic relationship and making arrangements to transfer the case to a different physician or even a different institution fulfills the doctor's professional obligation to her patient and protects her and the hospital from a charge of abandonment.

From a legal as well as an ethical perspective, the most important determination is that of decision-making authority. The informed wishes of the capacitated patient, especially about refusing treatment, are controlling and should always be honored. To ensure that health care preferences are communicated and implemented, it is recommended that they be articulated in legally binding advance directives, either a living will or a health care proxy appointment. This is the most effective way for patients to have their voices heard, even after they have lost the ability to speak for themselves. But even within the United States, groups from different cultural backgrounds do not yet use or value written advance directives. As such, providers must be aware of and ready to encompass alternative methods for obtaining information about the wishes of the patient or family.

When health care wishes are not expressed through an appointed proxy or living will, the authority to make decisions on behalf of an incapacitated patient varies widely, depending on the state in which the patient is being treated. Some states accord considerable decision-making latitude to surrogates, especially next of kin and even close friends, while others are very restrictive and require written or documented evidence of the patient's wishes, particularly when it comes to withholding or withdrawing life support. Because the relevant laws in Hawaii permit surrogate decision making in the absence of advance directives, Mr. Umlani's family had the authority to make treatment decisions on his behalf.

In this case, Mr. Umilani had not expressed his health care wishes through an advance directive. But the family revealed that he and his wife had had some previous informal discussions about their eldest son, Josh, assuming the role of surrogate decision maker if and when the need arose. During subsequent discussions with members of the interdisciplinary team, none of the family members had expressed any objections or offered differing opinions. The family remained unified and adamant in requesting that the life-sustaining measures be removed as a way of honoring Mr. Umilani's wishes.

It should be noted that Mr. and Mrs. Umilani's agreement that Josh would be their spokesperson and decision maker would have been most effectively secured by appointing him to be their health care proxy. In this role, his decisions would have been legally and ethically binding, even if there had been disagreement within the family or if his father had needed treatment in another state with more restrictive laws about surrogate decision making. This appointment ideally should have been made before the onset of illness and mental decline, when health care plans and wishes could have been fully discussed. Appointing a proxy requires a lower level of capacity than is required to make the health care decisions the proxy will make. Thus, even after Mr. Umilani's stroke, it might have been possible for him to appoint Josh to be his proxy if he had retained the ability to understand the possible future need for someone to make decisions for him and could identify the person he wanted to assume that role. The care provider can and should take the responsibility for engaging every patient in discussions about advance directives and end-of-life care planning.

Although it is common for the patient's spouse to be the surrogate decision maker or appointed proxy, it is not unusual for an adult child, sibling, or even close friend to assume that role. It is important, especially in a family-oriented culture, to note that the selection or even the legal appointment of one person to speak for the patient does not preclude family discussion. It does, however, tend to give decisions greater consistency and makes interaction with care staff more efficient. When there is disagreement between or among members of the family or care team, a bioethics consultation can be useful in clarifying issues, identifying interests, articulating preferences, and facilitating consensus.

Resolve the Ethical Issues

The ethical issues to be considered in this case include respecting the autonomy of both Mr. Umilani and his physician, determining the patient's goals for care, identifying and supporting the decision-making authority, and promoting a care plan consistent with the patient's best interest.

An ethical analysis considers the goals of care in light of the patient's wishes, condition, and likely prognosis, and the therapeutic options and their benefits, burdens, and risks. The objective is to provide care that will enhance the patient's well-being and avoid interventions that would increase suffering without providing benefit. These considerations demand heightened scrutiny when, as in this case, the patient's condition is irreversibly deteriorating and he is unable to participate in treatment discussions or decisions. The analysis must be kept patient centered, with the focus on the overall goals of care rather than on the goals of individual interventions. The understandable desire of care providers to provide care often leads to the initiation or continuation of treatments simply because they are available and can delay death. When the objective becomes maintaining life at any quality, it is appropriate to ask whether it is the patient's or the provider's goal that is at stake. In this case, continuing to provide artificial nutrition would have effectively prolonged a life that the family was convinced would have been unacceptable to Mr. Umilani.

If Mr. Umilani had been decisionally capable and had asked to have the PEG tube removed, his request should have triggered an extended discussion to evaluate whether he fully appreciated the consequences, including his likely death. If he had demonstrated his understanding, then his informed refusal of treatment, even if it conflicted with the advice of his care team or the preferences of his family, would have been honored. Because he was not able to advocate for himself, however, his wishes as interpreted by his family and articulated by his surrogate commanded the same respect. The decision-making authority was assumed by his son, in accordance with his previously expressed intentions.

Respect for autonomy, a singularly important ethical principle, assumes a central role in any discussion of decision making because of the high value often placed on liberty, privacy, individuality, and self-determination in Western culture. It is worth noting, especially in the context of cultural diversity, that these concepts are not universally revered. In many cultures, the value of individual autonomy may be secondary to the importance of the needs of the collective, and group decision making may take precedence over self-governance.

Still, even in Western cultures, it would be an impoverished notion of autonomy that focused only on rights, even the right to make choices. A richer conception is that autonomy represents the freedom to express one's true self through defining behaviors, the idea that an individual's values, beliefs, and/or preferences are authentically reflected in considered and voluntary actions. In this view of autonomy, what one chooses to *do* affirms what one *is*.

Mr. Umilani's story illustrates this perspective. Native Hawaiian culture places great significance on the group, especially the family. It is from the family and or the group that the individual draws strength, wisdom, and the connection that comes with shared heritage. This family knew its patriarch—his beliefs, values, concerns, and preferences. Precisely because he had been such an integral part of the group, there was no doubt or differing opinion about what he would want. Even without the benefit of explicit instructions, the way he had lived his life made clear how he would want it to end.

On reflection, it may not be surprising that he had not executed an advance directive. In the tradition of oral communication, he and his wife had talked about how matters should be handled in the event of their illness or death, a process that, in their view, made these arrangements as secure as they would have been on paper. His voice had been heard for years by those around him, and they now considered it their obligation to him to communicate his wishes and make sure they were honored.

Likewise, respecting the physician's professional autonomy demands respecting the concerns of conscience that dictated her clinical choices. Although her personal ethic prevented her from terminating the PEG feedings, it also prevented her from abandoning her patient. Recognizing that patients and physicians bring to their interaction different perspectives that may collide, both ethics and law insist on the transfer of care to providers who can more comfortably accommodate patient and family wishes. In this way, both the integrity of the therapeutic relationship and the quality of health care are maintained.

In this case, the interdisciplinary team and the ethics committee worked with the family to enhance, protect, and attend to the voice of the patient. A plan was developed that responded to his best interest within the framework of good medical practice and respect for patient autonomy.

Implement the Plan

At the conclusion of the ethics committee meeting, Mr. Umilani's physician transferred his care to a colleague who was able to comply with the request to terminate the PEG feedings. The family said its farewell and remained with Mr. Umilani until his death. A Native Hawaiian healer was present as chants and *pule* were offered in celebration and recognition of the connections to *'ohana* both living and dead, as well as the yet unborn.

Conclusion

An important step in the resolution of ethical dilemmas is taking the time to reflect. Unfortunately, this critical process is often overlooked, especially in the pressured clinical setting of an acute or long-term health care facility. Reflecting on this case highlights a number of critical issues.

1. Health care professionals have an obligation to develop and demonstrate a working knowledge of ethical theories and principles, as well as their practical application in the clinical setting.

2. Health care professionals need to conceptualize and utilize models for ethical decision making.

3. The patient and family or other decision-making surrogates play a key role in collaborative evaluation and management of complex health care problems.

4. Enhancing, protecting, and attending to the patient's voice is an imperative for the interdisciplinary team.

5. Patients and families need to teach and professionals need to learn about different cultural values, beliefs, customs, and practices.

6. Clinical ethics intervention, either by a clinical ethics consultation service or an institutional ethics committee, can be a useful resource in resolving conflicts between and among the perspectives of the patient, family, and care providers.

This case illustrates both the real and the ideal of the interdisciplinary team process. The process reflected the shared team leadership and collaboration among the professionals and the family. Mr. Umilani's family drew on its intimate knowledge of who and what he was and advocated forcefully for what he would have chosen. The physician, in light of her personal and professional values, demonstrated respect for her patient by transferring his care to a colleague who was more comfortable honoring his wishes. The care team was receptive to and flexible in accommodating the different perspectives. The knowledge and application of ethical principles through an effective and respectful team process achieved the outcome that most authentically echoed the patient's voice.

Discussion Questions

1. What is the responsibility of health care professionals in identifying, enhancing, and protecting the patient's voice in health care discussions and decisions? How does this responsibility differ when the patient is capacitated or incapacitated? the patient is alone or has involved family?

2. How is the voice of the patient identified, enhanced, and protected when it reflects values that differ from those of the attending physician? other providers on the care team? the prevailing culture? the family?

3. How does the health care professional identify the patient's values and incorporate them into the decision-making process?

4. How does the health care professional distinguish the voice of the patient from the needs of the patient? How does this implicate the professional's ethical obligations to respect the patient's wishes and values (autonomy) and promote the patient's well-being (beneficence)?

5. Under what circumstances might a health care professional consider transferring the patient's care to another clinician whose values are more consistent with those of the patient? How can this be accomplished in a way that does not appear to reflect negatively on the patient's values? suggest that the clinician's values prevent attending to the patient's health care needs? irreparably damage the therapeutic relationship?

TEACHING RESOURCES

Alu Like, Inc. 1990. *The Native Hawaiian elderly needs assessment report.* Honolulu: Alu Like, Inc.

American Medical Association, Council on Ethical and Judicial Affairs. 1995. Ethical issues in managed care. *Journal of the American Medical Association* (273):331–35.

Blustein, J. 1999. Choosing for others as continuing a life story: The problem of personal identity revisited. *Journal of Law, Medicine and Ethics* 27(1):20–31.

Hawaii Medical Treatment Decisions Act, Haw. Rev. Stat. §327D-211 (1993 and Supp. 1997), as interpreted by *In re Guardianship of Crabtree,* No. 86-0031 (Hawaii Fam. Ct. 1st Cir. April 26, 1990) (Heeley, J.) (Chapter 327D repealed effective 5/7/99 by H.B. 171, signed by Governor 5/7/99).

Judd, N.L.K.M. 1998. Laau Lapaau: Herbal healing among contemporary Hawaiian healers. *Pacific Health Dialog: Journal of Community Health and Clinical Medicine for the Pacific* 5 (2):239–45.

Post, L. F., J. Blustein, E. Gordon, and N. N. Dubler. 1996. Pain: Ethics, culture and informed consent to relief. *Journal of Law, Medicine and Ethics* 24(4):348–59.

Right-to-Die Law Digest. 2000. New York: Partnership for Caring.

Sabatino, C. P. 1999. The legal and functional status of the medical proxy: Suggestions for Statutory Reform. *Journal of Law, Medicine and Ethics* 27:52–68.

The Uniform Health-Care Decisions Act (Effective 5/7/99. H.B. 171, signed by Governor 5/7/99).

REFERENCES

Browne, C., and K. Braun. 1994. Unpublished transcripts from a study, *Cultural variations in values on aging.* Honolulu: University of Hawaii at Manoa, Schools of Public Health and Social Work.

Else, I., N. Palafox, and D. Little. 1998. Where are the Native Hawaiian physicians? *Pacific Health Dialogue: Journal of Community Health and Clinical Medicine for the Pacific* 5(2):246–52.

Jonsen, A. R., M. Siegler, and W. J. Winslade. 1998. *Clinical ethics,* 4th ed. New York: McGraw-Hill.

Thorndike, E. L., and C. L. Barnhart. 1991. *Thorndike-Barnhart student dictionary.* New York: HarperCollins.

6

CHAPTER

Guarding Patients' Secrets: Clinicians' Responsibility to Protect Patient Confidentiality

Ellen Olson, M.D.

Patient confidentiality has been a cornerstone of medical care dating back to Hippocrates. The Hippocratic oath states, "And whatsoever I shall see or hear in the course of my profession, as well as outside my profession . . . if it be what should not be published abroad, I will never divulge, holding such things to be holy secrets" (Hippocrates 1923, 301). In modern-day practice, continued adherence to the principle of confidentiality is based on respect for patient autonomy, fidelity on the part of the physician, and the concern that disregard for confidentiality will discourage patients from revealing all information relevant to their care (Jonsen, Siegler, and Winslade 1998). Historically, the concept of confidentiality has been nearly absolute. The only exceptions were when there was concern over the safety of the patient or other individuals, or the public welfare. While near-absolute adherence to confidentiality remains the goal, modern-day medicine, with computerized data and multiple consultants and care providers, makes confidentiality a difficult ideal to achieve (Siegler 1982). Information is shared daily not only among consultants and members of health care teams but also with persons with no caregiving status, such as medical records and billing personnel. The advent of ethics committees and ethics consultation teams within nursing homes and hospitals provides another opportunity where sensitive patient information may be shared with persons who have no direct caregiving role for an individual patient. Ethics committees must grapple with the issues of what information is necessary to their deliberations and what information they should share with others on a regular basis (Hoffman, Boyle, and Levenson 1995).

When the patient in question has decision-making capacity, the patient can and should help decide what information can be shared. When the patient lacks capacity or an appropriate surrogate decision maker, individual caregivers are often uncertain as to how much information to share among themselves or provide to others. Although most professional health care organizations have ethical codes that support patient confidentiality, it is usually left up to the individual care providers to determine what information could impact patient care and needs to be shared with others. How can interdisciplinary team review, either by a primary care team or by an ethics review committee, facilitate the appropriate sharing of information, especially for patients who lack capacity? Does the interdisciplinary nature of such groups help or hinder this process? The following case studies will explore these questions.

Case Description

Lillie Johnson is an 84-year-old woman who has been living in a nursing home for five years. She was admitted by family members who stated that she could not take care of herself any longer due to a progressive forgetfulness. She is alert and ambulatory but no longer speaks. She seems to respond appropriately to simple questions with a smile or a nod, but she cannot complete even the nonverbal aspects of a mental status exam. Recently, Lillie seems to have developed a relationship with a male patient, Eli Carson, who is alert and without cognitive deficits but is wheelchair dependent for ambulation due to a stroke that has left him paralyzed on his left side. The two residents are often seen sitting together in the dining room after meals, and on several occasions Lillie has appeared to be fondling Eli.

The staff responds initially by finding an excuse to move Eli from the dining room to the hallway or off the unit. They do not confront him with what they have seen. Several weeks later, however, they find Lillie in his bed, where they are attempting sexual relations. The staff feels that in theory it is the residents' right to have a sexual relationship, but they are bothered by the facts that (1) Eli is married (although his wife seldom visits) and (2) Lillie has a significant dementia.

Lillie is taken from the room, and the social worker is called to speak with Eli. He states that he does not know how the relationship started but that he does not seek out Lillie. On the contrary, she seems to seek him out, and he has no desire to rebuke her advances. He does not seem bothered by her inability to communicate verbally with him, and he shows limited understanding of dementia. He is also not concerned that his wife might visit and find them in a compromising situation. The floor social worker has strong feelings that Lillie should not be allowed to continue a sexual relationship with Eli, but if the floor staff feels differently, she at least wants to tell his wife what is happening. Eli states that he has no problem with that.

When the attending physician, Dr. Short, is notified of the issue involving Lillie and Eli, he becomes troubled. He recalls a conversation with a social worker on the floor several years earlier in which she told him that Lillie had run a brothel in her younger years. He did not recall the source of that information but wonders if it provides at least some explanation for Lillie's behavior. He wonders whether he should share this information with the rest of the team. He did not include it in the medical record, as he felt it was not relevant to the patient's care and that it might stigmatize her in some way if generally known. To his knowledge, the information is not known to anyone but himself. The social worker who confided in him left the nursing home shortly after their conversation, and he is not sure if she shared this information with any other staff members. Dr. Short decides that the information is relevant to the discussion, as the patient may only be engaging in behaviors that were once commonplace for her and are not the source of any distress. He knows that freedom of sexual expression is a right that should be respected in the nursing home setting, with certain constraints. He is not sure, however, what role her dementia should play in deciding whether this activity should be supported. He decides to share this information regarding Lillie's former profession with the health care team at their next weekly meeting and ask for their input.

Assess the Team Structure

The team consists of two floor nurses, a primary care physician, a social worker, a psychiatrist who covers several floors in the nursing home and does not know Lillie well, nursing assistants who have cared for Eli and Lillie, a dietitian, a recreational therapist, and a physical therapist. The certified nursing assistant assigned to Lillie also attends that part of each team meeting. Lillie and Eli are on the list of patients to be reviewed because of continuing staff concerns about their relationship. The psychiatrist functions as the team leader. At the team meeting, the social worker on the unit continues to express concern about Eli's wife. She reiterates her desire to speak with the wife, if the team decision is to allow Eli and Lillie to continue their relationship. One of the nurses and Lillie's nursing assistant express concern that the institution should not be condoning a sexual relationship between a married man and a woman who is not his wife. They feel that Lillie and Eli should not be allowed to continue their relationship on moral grounds. When Dr. Short shares his information about Lillie's former profession, they are uncertain as to whether it should have any bearing on the decision. They are concerned more that her current behavior is a reflection of her dementia than about the possible life experiences that might be behind that behavior. They feel that Eli is taking advantage of how Lillie's dementia is manifesting itself. No one feels qualified to judge if Lillie is deriving any pleasure from her behavior.

Identify Patient and Family Preferences

Lillie's preferences can only be inferred from her behavior. The staff agrees that Lillie probably sought out Eli. The psychiatrist briefly interviews Lillie and concurs that she can express no meaningful preferences. Lillie's sisters rarely visit, and the primary care team does not feel they should be involved in this situation, given their apparent disinterest. They also note that neither of them is formally appointed as health care agent, so they are unclear what their status as decision makers should be in situations such as this. Because Dr. Short cannot tell the team if the sisters were the original source of what they feel is very sensitive information regarding her past, no one feels comfortable confronting the sisters until the team determines if the information should in any way guide the discussion. Because Lillie's dementia is the main reason for staff concern, Eli's preferences in this matter are deemed irrelevant.

Evaluate Quality-of-Life Issues

Lillie's quality of life, although devoid of verbal communication, appears to be free of any physical discomfort. She never appears in any emotional distress and is never physically withdrawn. She eats and sleeps well. She still toilets herself most of the time. When the nursing home staff separated her from Eli after their encounters, she showed no signs of distress or anger, as opposed to Eli, who seemed quite perturbed. While she showed no signs of discomfort or distress during what was observed of their encounters, she also did not show signs of pleasure. Again, the team feels that although Eli's quality of life is clearly enhanced by his relationship with Lillie, there are too many issues surrounding the propriety of the relationship to make Eli's quality of life a significant factor.

Consider Contextual Factors

This case has several contextual issues. The first involves the physician, and the question of whether he should reveal his knowledge of Lillie's former profession to the whole team, especially the dietitian and the recreational therapist, who are less intimately involved with Lillie's care. Lillie can no longer express her current food preferences, and therefore the dietitian has to use nonverbal cues to assess them. Likewise, as Lillie is only a passive participant in activities, the recreation therapist can only guess as to which activities Lillie would enjoy. But can certain care providers be excluded from the full discussion? Whose role is it to decide who can receive privileged information and who cannot? Who is to know if even peripherally involved staff have information relevant to patient care, if they are not included in all deliberations involving the patient? A nursing home resident may develop a relationship with a staff member over time that does not necessarily reflect the latter's caregiving role. Such relationships may be characterized more as friendships, which create a different level of trust and intimacy and therefore the opportunity for the sharing of sensitive information. Whether this has occurred can be ascertained only if all staff who have contact with the patient are included in the discussion. The physician has traditionally been the recipient and gatekeeper of most patient information. When a team of professionals cares for a patient, as is now more commonly the case, how is the sharing of information monitored and controlled? The social worker's allegiances in this case are also felt to be problematic, as she more clearly identifies with Eli's wife than with the two nursing home residents entrusted to her care. When persons are cared for in institutions, their families develop relationships with staff members as well. Who is the client—the nursing home resident, the family members, or both? What are employees of health care facilities to do when the interests of the patient and the family conflict? What are other staff to do when they feel patient needs are not being appropriately addressed by persons outside their own profession?

Address Other Ethical Issues

This case presents several issues involving patient autonomy. Should a demented person be allowed to continue apparently consensual sexual behavior? In other words, is a severely demented individual still capable of some autonomous behaviors, or does Lillie require special protection because of her mentally impaired state? Does Eli lose his right to engage in relationships, illicit or not, merely because he now resides in a nursing home?

The case also presents concerns about assessments of burdens and benefits, as well as the aforementioned concerns about confidentiality. Should Eli's wife be informed of his extramarital behaviors to protect her from the potential harm that she might experience if she found him with Lillie during one of her infrequent visits? Despite Eli's apparent consent to the social worker to reveal his relationship to his wife, does the potential for harm to Eli's wife justify this action, or is this a matter better left to Eli to deal with? Does any one team member have the training or insight to determine the harm for Lillie? Or is the beauty of the team approach that it can create a consensus that reflects community standards, and no one person or profession has to determine what is harmful and what is beneficial? Is this feature of particular value when patient values cannot be determined, as happens so frequently with older, cognitively impaired individuals? Or should Lillie's family play a greater role in these deliberations, despite their lack of involvement to date in her care? Can they, as family, better represent her values, or at least her best interests, than the staff who have been caring for her daily for the last five years? Who are the best surrogate decision makers? Should Dr. Short have sought the family's consent before sharing any privileged information regarding Lillie with the team?

Resolve the Ethical Issues and Create the Plan

At the end of the first team meeting in which Eli and Lillie are discussed, the team decides on a plan that allows their relationship to continue, until they can better determine if Lillie's active role in the relationship is based on more than just reflexive behavior secondary to her dementia. Nursing expresses the concern that the family has not been involved in the discussions to date. They disagree with the physician that this situation is different from other situations involving patients with dementia, and that the family should be there to represent the interests and wishes of the patient. They also feel that although Lillie's former profession is of some relevance to the case, the doctor should have verified the accuracy of that information and consulted the family before sharing it with the team. In the case of Eli, the psychiatrist feels that if he is capable of making his own decisions, it would be a violation of his rights to confidentiality if his wife were notified of his behavior, and that the responsibility rests with him to do so. But staff can continue to encourage him to speak with his wife or cease the relationship.

The team agrees to meet the next week and invite Lillie's family. Before the meeting, the physician verifies Lillie's former profession with the sisters. Lillie's sisters also state that she has distanced herself from them as a result. This information is also shared with the team. The sisters are, however, still concerned for her welfare. They describe her as a very private person and do not feel she would want to be the focus of so much ongoing attention. Given the team's existing concerns over Lillie's ability to comprehend her actions, and her family's concern for her privacy, the team decides to move Eli to another part of the nursing home.

Implement the Plan

The social worker discusses the team decision with Eli, who reacts with little emotion and agrees to be transferred to another unit. The social worker also asks for Eli's permission to be honest with his wife, if she asks why he is being moved. After Eli leaves, Lillie makes several visits to his old room, then quits going there. She expresses no outward signs of sadness. Eli reportedly shows little response to his move, either.

Case Description

Ed Samuels is the only child of Sam and Sarah Samuels. Sarah has Alzheimer disease and has resided in a nursing home for four years. She came there from home, where she had been cared for by her husband, Sam, until he could no longer manage her alone. Her interest in food has diminished to the point where she is not eating enough to sustain herself. She has been evaluated for reversible causes of poor appetite, but nothing has been found. She does suffer from a chronic back problem that requires opioid pain medication, but this medication is necessary for her comfort and is not felt to be responsible for her declining appetite. She also has failed to respond to antidepressants and appetite stimulants. Sarah is incapable of making health care decisions. She is nonverbal. She makes eye contact on questioning but shows no signs of comprehension when asked questions. She expresses discomfort by grimacing. She usually refuses to open her mouth during feeding attempts, and she rarely swallows even when she accepts a spoonful of food. Sam came to the nursing home two years ago for progressive ambulation problems and lives in the same room as Sarah. He is believed to have a mild to moderate dementia himself, in addition to being very frail physically.

Their physician, Dr. Long, is reluctant to approach Sam about Sarah's condition, because of his perceived mental and physical frailty. He feels the son, Ed, should be involved in any decisions regarding feeding tubes anyway. He feels the team has done all they can to get Sarah to eat and that it was time to call Ed to notify him of the feeding difficulties. When the physician describes the situation to Ed and suggests that a feeding tube be considered, Ed is adamantly opposed. He states that he has no specific evidence of his mother's wishes, but he cannot imagine she would want to be kept alive in a state where she recognizes no one, including her husband, and cannot speak. He also questions why the health care team would want to keep anyone alive who needs such strong pain medications for comfort. The physician tells Ed that in the nursing home all requests that tube feeding not be provided have to be referred to the ethics committee for review. He informs the son that a member of the ethics committee will be contacting him shortly.

When the ethicist on the ethics committee questions Ed further about his reasons for thinking his mother would not want a feeding tube, Ed again states that he never spoke to his mother about care issues. But he reiterates his concern that tube feeding would only prolong a painful existence, and he questions why it is even being considered. When the ethicist asks if his father might have had any discussions with the mother about these matters, Ed asks that his father not be involved in the decision. When asked why, Ed confides to the ethicist that his parents were so devoted to each other that they did not plan on having any children. When his mother became pregnant with him, she considered putting him up for adoption, but his father could not follow through with the plan. His mother made it very clear to him as a child, however, that they never intended to have him, and that if it was not for his father, he would have been "given away." Based on the closeness of the relationship, he knew his father would want everything done to keep his mother alive, regardless of her wishes.

Although the ethicist thinks Ed has a legitimate case against providing tube feeding for his mother, he is now concerned that his request could be at least partly motivated by anger toward his mother. The ethicist decides to attend the next team meeting on the nursing unit where Sam and Sarah reside. He wishes to further explore Ed's relationship with his mother, and Sam's ability to participate in the decision. With Dr. Long's permission, he asks the floor psychiatrist to visit with Sam before the meeting and address Dr. Long's concerns regarding Sam's ability to act as a surrogate for Sarah.

Assess the Team Structure

The interdisciplinary team is similar to the one in the last case. But in this case, the team culture has evolved such that the team leader is the floor social worker. She has worked on the unit the longest and represents continuity and stability to the rest of the team. The team meets weekly to discuss specific patients. Sarah's care has not been reviewed lately, and the nurse on the unit, Sarah's nursing assistant, and the physician are the only team members who are aware of the feeding issues until the ethicist is asked to come to the meeting.

Identify Patient and Family Preferences

Sarah's wishes to this point are unknown. While her son has had no conversations with her or been witness to other situations where she expressed opinions about medical care, Sarah's husband will more likely be the source of any such information. Until it is determined whether he should and can participate in this discussion, an important source of information is missing. Other chapters have referred to the "missing voice" in the health care team (McClelland and Sands 1993). Sam is the most likely person to be Sarah's voice in these deliberations. Even if he has no specific information, his views of what is in her best interest also need to be heard. By their son's own history, Sam appears to be the person closest to Sarah and most able to reflect on her values. Ed's wishes for his mother are clear.

Evaluate Quality-of-Life Issues

As previously mentioned, Sarah is no longer communicative or ambulatory. She is alert and sits in a wheelchair next to Sam. She is incontinent. She smiles when spoken to, but her response does not differ from person to person. Her response to Sam is no different from her response to anyone else who approaches her. In the past, when she was moved from bed to chair she would moan and grimace. Her husband was able to relate a long-standing history of back pain, requiring a variety of medications and intermittent physical therapy. But her pain is now managed adequately with long-acting oxycodone, as manifested by seemingly comfortable transfers. The staff are still managing to get her to swallow the medication, with much encouragement. Sam is also wheelchair bound, with some short-term memory deficits. He sits quietly next to Sarah, holding her hand. He rarely speaks unless spoken to, or to ask for something for Sarah.

Consider Contextual Factors

The physician on this unit functions autonomously. He did not discuss his decision to bypass Sam as a decision-maker with any other staff member. The staff, including the nurse and social worker, have learned that Dr. Long will usually disregard their opinions, and they rarely disagree with him. The social worker has developed a telephone relationship with Ed over business matters and knows that his actual visits with his parents are infrequent and very brief. Sam is well known by the nursing staff and the social worker and is viewed as a caring spouse and advocate for his wife. They have seen him decline physically over the two years they have been together at the home, but they consider him remarkably sharp mentally for a 93-year-old man, despite occasional memory lapses. Dr. Long takes care of both Sarah and Sam, visiting them monthly. He usually stays with them only long enough to perform the monthly physical exam.

Address Other Ethical Issues

The need for Sarah's voice to be heard has already been mentioned. The benefits and burdens of tube feeding in end-stage dementia are the topic of ongoing discussion and debate in the literature (Finucane, Christmas, and Travis 1999; Gillick 2000). What is generally accepted, however, is that whenever possible, autonomy, or patient choice, should be the guiding force in most medical decisions. When it is clear that the patient cannot decide for himself or herself, as in this case, the most appropriate surrogate must be chosen. That is the person who has the most knowledge of what the patient's wishes would have been under the circumstances. If the patient's wishes cannot be ascertained, the surrogate has the most knowledge of that person's beliefs and values. In Sarah's case, if Sam is indeed the surrogate, he must be involved in decision making to the greatest extent possible, unless Dr. Long or the psychiatrist feels the discussions would be harmful to him. When dealing with elderly patients and surrogates, decision-making capacity is often an issue. Elderly patients and their potential surrogates should be presumed to have decision-making capacity until it is clear that they do not. Even if Sam cannot make decisions, he may still provide information important to the discussion. He was bypassed as Sarah's surrogate without an adequate evaluation.

Resolve the Ethical Issues and Create the Plan

The meeting is turned over to the ethicist, after the social worker explains Sarah's situation to the staff. The ethicist explains that he is there because the son does not wish his mother to be tube fed but has not been able to provide enough information to satisfy the facility's requirement that these decisions be based on the known wishes of the patient. He further explains that Dr. Long is not comfortable going to Sam for guidance, and that the ethicist has asked the floor psychiatrist to make a determination as to whether Sam has both the mental and emotional strength to share in the discussion. The psychiatrist reports that although Sam has some short-term memory deficits, he shows no signs of depression. Sam does become tearful when speaking of Sarah, however, and the psychiatrist agrees with Ed that he may not be able to make a rational decision on her behalf. But he sees no reason to exclude Sam from the discussion. The nursing staff present, as well as the social worker, also state that they feel Sam both could and should be a part of all discussions. They acknowledge his physical frailty but also feel that no one knows Sarah as Sam does, and he will want what is best for her.

Sam is brought into the meeting and is told that they are all there to discuss Sarah's poor appetite. Sam acknowledges an awareness of her poor intake and quickly goes on to relate a conversation they had at the onset of her dementia. She was aware of her diagnosis and of the progressive nature of Alzheimer disease. Sarah asked Sam to let her die peacefully when her time came, with no "tubes or machines." He states that he loves her dearly and does not want her to die, but that she has suffered enough. He requests that she not receive a feeding tube. The team feels there is no more to add and prepares to provide her with the necessary comfort care. The ethicist states that the case still has to be reviewed by the ethics committee, according to institutional policy, but that Sam's statements are adequate to support a plan of care that will provide "comfort care only" to Sarah.

Implement the Plan

The finding and conclusions reached in the team meeting are recorded in Sarah's chart. Sam also signs a "Do Not Resuscitate" request. Sarah continues to receive oral feedings as tolerated and her pain medication. She dies peacefully in her sleep six weeks later.

Discussion

What makes the geriatric population more vulnerable to breaches in confidentiality? One reason is their high incidence of cognitive impairment. Even well-meaning others who become spokespersons for a patient may relate information in the course of care that the patient may never have wanted known by others. In addition, many older persons receive their care in institutional settings, such as in the two cases presented here. In these settings, many people are involved in the care of the patients and have legitimate access to their medical records. Furthermore, the staff in institutional settings develop relationships with friends and family members over time, who may share other types of information about the patient, in conversations totally removed from the care of the patient. Some of this information the patient would not have shared if given a choice. Philip Boyle, an ethicist and theologian, suggests in *Handbook for Nursing Home Ethics Committees* that the obligation to maintain confidentiality should extend beyond the realm of health care. He argues that on the basis of fairness, all people have an obligation to keep secrets (Boyle 1995). Those who work in a nursing home setting need to keep this in mind during the more casual interactions with family and friends.

How do we define *secrets* or *confidential information*? Ruth Purtilo (1999) states that the most commonly accepted idea of "confidential information" among the professions is "information that is harmful, shameful, or embarrassing" to the patient (150). Judith Ross adds that the word *confidential,* means "with faith." Confidential information is given "with faith or with trust that the information will not be further disclosed without permission" (Ross 1986, 82). In guiding surrogate decision makers or others involved in the lives of older persons, we have an obligation to help them distinguish what information is necessary for patient care and what is not. Conversely, though, we as health care providers owe surrogates and others the courtesy of keeping sensitive information that is inadvertently shared with us a secret.

In each of the two cases presented here, a team member had information that meets the accepted definition of *confidential.* In the first case, that information was obtained in an indefensible manner: a social worker shared a "secret" with the physician in a casual conversation that had no relevance to the patient's care. Hoffman, Boyle, and Levenson (1995) caution us that while current policies and regulations concerning confidentiality appear to condone the sharing of information within an institution, all staff within that institution must be vigilant in adhering to standards of information transfer. While the casual sharing of information is rarely done with malice, it can have a significant impact on the patient and how patients are viewed by staff (Boyle 1995). In the first case, the team reacted in a proactive manner toward Lillie and refocused the discussion more on her vulnerabilities than on how her past related to those vulnerabilities. They seemed concerned that the physician had shared information that might not even be true, much less useful to the problem at hand. The team process here both allowed for a breach of confidence, given the day-to-day closeness of most nursing home care teams, and facilitated putting the information in its proper perspective when it was shared with the larger team. The team was able to point out to Dr. Short his obligation to share only accurate information with them, as well as his ethical obligation to provide Lillie with the same representation by surrogates that other patients with impaired capacity were afforded. In a way, by allowing his information to cloud her right to family involvement, he had already stigmatized her. Her privacy had already been violated. She now needed someone present who could speak for her as that information was integrated into her care plan.

The team was less successful in convincing the social worker that Lillie and Eli's privacy was paramount. The social worker insisted that Eli's wife had the right to be told of his behaviors. While her concern for Eli's wife was understandable, there was no ethical justification for her to share Eli and Lillie's relationship with Eli's wife. As mentioned earlier, confidentiality should be breached only to protect others from serious harm. It was the team's responsibility to protect Lillie, and even Eli, as deemed necessary. It was not their responsibility to protect Eli's wife, especially at the expense of Eli's trust in his care providers, unless he posed a direct threat to her. Even though he gave consent for the transfer of information to his wife, the consequences of his action could not be judged until after the fact, at which time he could feel betrayed. There was no overriding benefit to be gained from telling the wife, especially after the fact, except to spare her the surprise of finding out on her own. Telling her something she may have never learned otherwise could have, in fact, caused undue harm to the wife and to the couple's relationship. The social worker should have been instructed to defer any questions from the wife to Eli. His relationship with his wife remained Eli's responsibility.

Because all professions share similar codes regarding confidentiality, the protection of patient secrets falls to no specific discipline. It is each team member's responsibility to be aware of confidentiality issues and to be able to identify potentially harmful information when it comes their way. This duty is unrelated to the more discipline-specific roles played by the various professions. The collective wisdom of the team is a way a safeguard to confidentiality, even after the "horse has left the barn," so to speak. This safeguard depends on a functionally intact team, however, whose members can communicate with each other. This concept is discussed elsewhere in this book. (See Chapters 10–12.)

Dr. Short and the original social worker should be commended for one aspect of Lillie's care, however: neither of them entered the information about Lillie's earlier life into the medical record such that it would be shared in the future. Good documentation of relevant history helps ensure quality care, but it is difficult to envision a situation where this information would be necessary to future decision making, medical or otherwise. Its documentation would only continue to stigmatize Lillie. Even if it was suspected, at some point in the future, that she was suffering the sequela of a sexually transmitted disease, a detailed sexual history would not be as relevant to her care as would her clinical presentation, as well as the presumption that she was sexually active at some point in her life. Both Purtilo and Siegler feel it is very important to keep information out of the medical record that is unnecessary for patient care. Purtilo (1999, 158) suggests three guidelines to follow when considering whether information should become a part of the permanent record:

1. Untrue information should not be recorded, and questionable information should be clearly labeled as questionable.

2. True information that is not relevant should not be recorded.

3. Information should be handled among health professionals with regard for the privacy and dignity of patients.

In the second case, that of Sam and Sarah, the team approach facilitated the protection of confidential information in a more indirect way, despite the fact that Dr. Long bypassed the team's involvement in the beginning. As it turned out, Sam supported the same decision for Sarah that Ed did, but for different and more significant reasons. When the team became involved in the process, Ed was removed from the role of decision maker, and the secret that he harbored regarding his mother was protected, to the benefit of all three of them. The team also preserved Sam's longtime and deeply important role as Sarah's voice and protector. The ethicist should also be given credit for not using Ed's information before it was absolutely necessary to the discussions.

Individual professional codes of ethics and confidentiality are no longer adequate to protect the privacy of individual patients. Health care teams must develop guidelines regarding the vast amount of information available to them regarding their older patients, many of whom are cognitively impaired. They need to provide guidance, too, for families and friends with whom they form relationships. There should be ongoing discussions within the team as to what information is and is not relevant to the care of the resident. This is especially important in settings such as nursing homes, where interdisciplinary care is the rule and where there is often much time over which information can be shared. Nursing home residents and their families need to be apprised on admission that information obtained from them during the admitting process and throughout the stay may be shared among a variety of caregivers. It is felt that patients do not always appreciate the extent to which this occurs (Weiss 1982). To encourage the sharing of information that could be important to the patient's care, however, patients and families need to be reassured that only clinically relevant information will be shared with others.

Where can staff start in this process of assessing what is confidential information and determining whether it should be shared? We have already reviewed Purtilo's and Ross's definitions of *confidential*. In discussing how ethics committees consider confidential information, Boyle suggests several approaches to assessing whether to share such information (Boyle 1995). The first is to ask how the information will be used and whether it is truly relevant to the decisions under discussion. Another approach is to assess the benefits and harms of breaking and not breaking the confidences. Will the information lead to potential harms such as stigmatization, or will it facilitate an appropriate decision on the patient's behalf? Another even simpler approach is to ask whether the information in question is anyone's business. These questions can be asked and discussed by any health care team.

The issue of confidentiality must permeate ongoing staff education programs and extend beyond the professional caregivers of an institution. Whenever information that meets the definition of *confidential* is shared with other members of a health care team, it should be done only with the consent of the patient or their surrogate, unless the aforementioned exceptions apply. Even when it is deemed ethically appropriate to share confidential information, doing so harms the fragile bond between the health care professional and the patient, according to Purtilo. She states it is always up to the health care professional to minimize that harm (Purtilo 1999). That remains the challenge of health care teams.

Discussion Questions

1. In the case of Lillie and Eli, can an argument be made that they should have been able to continue their relationship? How could the team have protected the privacy of their relationship, and would the inability to do so be a determining factor in deciding whether the relationship should be allowed to continue?

2. In the case of Sarah, should the ethicist or someone else from the team have confronted her son about his feelings toward his mother, or should the matter have been dropped, since there was no disagreement between him and his father regarding the use of a feeding tube? Was the health care team obligated to follow up on this sort of information, even though the son was not a resident in the nursing home?

3. With regard to confidential information, what would be a reasonable set of guidelines for health care teams to use in their day-to-day care of patients?

REFERENCES

Boyle, P. 1995. In D. E. Hoffman, P. Boyle, and S. A. Levenson, *Handbook for nursing home ethics committees.* Washington, D.C.: American Association of Homes and Services for the Aging.

Finucane, T. E., C. Christmas, and K. Travis. 1999. Tube feeding in patients with advanced dementia: A review of the evidence. *Journal of the American Medical Association* 282(14): 1365–70.

Gillick, M. R. 2000. Rethinking the role of tube feeding in patients with advanced dementia. *New England Journal of Medicine* 342(3):206–10.

Hippocrates. 1923. The oath. In *Hippocrates I,* translated by W.H.S. Jones. Loeb Classic Library. Cambridge, Mass.: Harvard University Press.

Hoffman, D. E., P. Boyle, and S. A. Levenson. 1995. *Handbook for nursing home ethics committees.* Washington, D.C.: American Association of Homes and Services for the Aging.

Jonsen, A. R., M. Siegler, and W. J. Winslade. 1998. *Clinical ethics,* 4th ed. New York: McGraw-Hill.

McClelland, M., and R. G. Sands. 1993. The missing voice in interdisciplinary communication. *Qualitative Health Research* 3(1):74–90.

Purtilo, R. 1999. *Ethical dimensions in the health professions,* 3rd ed. Philadelphia: W. B. Saunders.

Ross, J. W. 1986. *Handbook for hospital ethics committees.* Chicago: American Hospital Publishing.

Siegler, M. 1982. Confidentiality in medicine: A decrepit concept. *New England Journal of Medicine* 307(24):1518–21.

Weiss, B. D. 1982. Confidentiality, expectations of patients, physicians, and medical students. *Journal of the American Medical Association* 247(19):2695–97.

CHAPTER 7

Conflicting Interests: Dilemmas of Decision Making for Patients, Families, and Teams

Laurence B. McCullough, Ph.D.,
Nancy L. Wilson, L.M.S.W.,
Jill A. Rhymes, M.D., and
Thomas A. Teasdale, Dr.P.H.

In the bioethics literature, ethical issues in clinical practice tend to be understood and addressed within the dyadic context of a single clinician caring for a single patient. When ethical issues arise, the traditional dyadic model of clinical ethics undertakes ethical analysis and argument about the obligations of the individual clinician to his or her individual patient. The dynamics of team care and of patient-family decision making tend to be ignored by this dominant model. In the context of team care, ethical issues in geriatric medical, nursing, and social work practice take on a different character because ethical analysis and argument concern the obligations of a team of caregivers to the patient and to the patient's family. By their very nature, ethical issues in geriatric team care become more complex to understand and manage in clinical practice than in the context of the relationship between an individual clinician and an individual patient.

In both the traditional dyadic model and in the team-care model, matters become still more complex when family members become involved, or attempt to become involved, in making decisions about the patient's care. This larger scope of concern is quite common in geriatric and gerontologic ethics, especially in cases involving long-term care decision making (Arras 1995; Brakman 1995; Jecker 1995).

The case presented and discussed in this chapter involves the double complexity of team care and family involvement in clinical decision making. It involves a particularly challenging form of family involvement: an attempt to take over the decision-making role of the appropriate surrogate decision maker—a not uncommon form of intrafamilial conflict in geriatric and gerontologic clinical practice. Such family involvement in clinical decision making can become a potential source of ethical conflict for the geriatric team. It can challenge the clinical and moral cohesion of the geriatric team in ways that do not occur in the traditional dyadic clinical relationship. In the traditional dyadic model, the moral obligation and therefore task of the clinician is to clarify that his or her primary responsibilities are to the patient and to the surrogates of the patient (when the patient lacks decision-making capacity to a significant degree [Beauchamp and Childress 1994]). The individual clinician, if necessary, can simply invoke confidentiality and end communication with family members who seek inappropriate involvement or turn to more intrusive responses. But geriatric teams committed to supporting patients and their families do not have this option.

The moral obligations and tasks of the geriatric team become more complex because the team is multidisciplinary (Purtilo, Shaw, and Arnold 1998). Leadership in geriatric team work is a dynamic process, with team members of different disciplines sharing responsibility for moving the work forward or "leading" in accomplishing the task at hand, fulfilling the team's obligations to the patient. Formal organizational structures typically recognize a single team member, often the physician, as the formal leader. But well-functioning teams use the skills of all team members in performing leadership tasks. Decisions about who will provide expertise on a particular patient-care issue or who will speak for the team with other clinicians will vary. When such shifting leadership occurs, it is important to clarify both leadership roles and accountability of team members, in order to maintain the team's commitment to the patient's well-being. In responding to ethical conflict, colleagues on a geriatric team should be accountable to one another for closely coordinating their changing and shared leadership roles. Communicating with each other and keeping a clear focus on their shared moral responsibility for the patient's well being become crucial. In other words, accountability and leadership in team care create ethical issues that do not arise in the traditional dyadic model of clinical ethics.

In this chapter, we emphasize a preventive ethics approach to the ethical issues involved when a family member attempts to replace the patient's appropriate surrogate decision maker. Preventive ethics enhances geriatric team care by recognizing the potential for ethical conflict in its early stages and undertaking decisions and actions to prevent the occurrence of full-blown conflict (McCullough and Chervenak 1994). Preventive ethics draws on the conviction that ethical conflict is stressful for patients, their families, and health care teams and is therefore best avoided. Preventive ethics, we will argue, can play a useful role in developing and sustaining the moral cohesion of geriatric teams.

Case Description

Mr. Swanson was a 73-year-old man admitted to Veterans Administration Medical Center with left hip fracture after a fall. Before this admission, he lived at home with his wife and was ambulatory. His activities consisted mostly in watching television, and he was not very active physically. Mr. Swanson required assistance with most of the independent activities of daily living except toileting and eating. He married ten years ago, after he was widowed. He has a daughter from a previous marriage, Ms. Cullen. She is in her fifties and herself has suffered a stroke, leaving her unable to ambulate and reliant on a wheelchair. Ms. Cullen lives in the community with her own family. Since his marriage to Mrs. Swanson, herself a widow with two children when they married, Mr. Swanson has had little contact with his daughter, who is not pleased with her father's remarriage.

Mr. Swanson has a history of stroke eight years ago with some residual right-sided weakness, as well as mild vascular dementia, hypertension, and hyperlipidemia. He has a left hip hemiarthroplasty the day after admission and initially does well. But about three days postoperatively, he has some left arm and leg weakness. A head CT scan shows a possible new stroke. Despite this finding, Mr. Swanson is considered a candidate for physical therapy. He is thought to be too frail to do acute rehabilitation and is returned to the geriatric unit for subacute rehabilitation.

Mr. Swanson does fairly well in therapy despite some left-sided neglect. His cognitive status is impaired, inasmuch as he has trouble retaining information from day to day. Ten days after his transfer, he develops abdominal distension and vomiting. He undergoes exploratory surgery for presumed bowel obstruction. Pseudo-obstruction is found, and a decompression cecostomy is done. During his stay on the surgery service, he develops tachycardia and fever and is treated with antibiotics. After three weeks, he is transferred back to the geriatric unit.

Ten days after the transfer, Mr. Swanson has rectal bleeding and is transferred to the medical intensive care unit. He is found to have an ulcer near his cecostomy, and the cecostomy tube is pulled, with no further bleeding. Mr. Swanson is then transferred back to the geriatric unit. By this time he is considerably weaker. He does not do well in therapy, and his memory and motivation are worse than before his complications. A psychiatry consult team sees Mr. Swanson but does not think that he is depressed; still, his dementia is worse than previously.

Mr. Swanson is then noted to have an externally rotated left hip, and an X-ray shows a dislocation of the left hip prosthesis. At this point, Mr. Swanson was not ambulatory but is not in pain. He is not participating in therapy.

Mr. Swanson's wife, who has heart disease and was a rather small woman, was caring for him at home before the hospital admission. Mr. Swanson weighs 265 pounds and in the hospital requires total care by the nursing staff in all activities of daily living except eating.

The Team

Mr. Swanson's geriatric team comprises an attending geriatrician, a physician's assistant, a nurse practitioner, a social worker, a kinesiotherapist, a dietitian, a second-year medicine resident, and a physician assistant student. Each geriatric patient is assigned a medicine resident working under the supervision of the attending physician, a board-certified geriatrician. The social worker on the team routinely assesses patients' psychosocial needs and coping skills and their informal and formal support systems. The social worker uses her knowledge of financial benefits and community services to help the team identify service options for patients and their families.

The geriatric team has agreed that each team member will conduct and communicate an assessment of each geriatric patient. The team meets on a weekly basis to review progress of inpatients and develop discharge plans. Within the organizational structure of the hospital, the geriatrician is seen as the formal team leader, but the team determines who the ambassador or expert will be, depending on the nature and complexity of a problem. For example, when family meetings are needed to explore care issues or to mediate differences among family members and clinicians, the social worker often assumes a leadership role in the meeting process.

Mr. Swanson is known to the geriatric team. Prior to this admission, they were following him on an outpatient basis for clinical management of his medical problems. Advance directives have been discussed with Mr. Swanson periodically, and he has indicated that he would be comfortable with his wife making decisions for him as necessary.

Assessment of this patient's complex needs involves the contributions of several team members as well as those of other teams who are involved in the clinical management of Mr. Swanson's problems. The nurse practitioner and attending geriatrician assess his mental status. Mr. Swanson scores 11 out of 30 on the Mini-Mental State Examination (MMSE) and is judged to have significantly impaired decision-making capacity. Although he is unable to retain information from day to day, he is able to assent to decisions made by his wife when they are presented to him. Based on input from the nurse practitioner, medical resident, and physician assistant, the team's assessment is that Mrs. Swanson lacks the physical capacity to care for her husband at home and that even with home services his care needs would still exceed her physical ability to meet them adequately.

The orthopedic surgery team evaluates the patient for surgical management of his condition and finds him to be a high-risk case both perioperatively and postoperatively. They also note that he is currently not in pain and has a poor potential for rehabilitation. Their judgment is that the risks of another surgery outweigh any potential benefit and that it is probable that he would remain nonambulatory after another surgery.

The assessment by the physical therapy team (rehabilitation physician, occupational therapist, physical therapist) is that the patient has a poor potential for rehabilitation. They also note that he is not in pain at the current time. The kinesiotherapist on the geriatric team assesses Mr. Swanson's potential during rehabilitation and finds that he cannot take cueing and is not in pain. The kinesiotherapist reports to the team that going through surgery and postsurgical rehabilitation for such a patient are not likely to be successful.

The social worker on the geriatric team considers the team's assessment of Mr. Swanson's care needs and Mrs. Swanson's physical capacity to care for her husband at home even with paid support. Mr. and Mrs. Swanson lack financial resources to pay for sufficient home help and/or day care, and the twenty hours that would be provided through public benefits would be insufficient to meet his needs for twenty-four-hour standby assistance with activities of daily living (ADLs). After multiple discussions with the social worker, Mrs. Swanson agrees that she is unable to care for her husband at home, even with additional paid support. She takes the view that nursing home placement is the best, or the least worst, alternative to keeping her husband at home.

At a regular geriatric team meeting, team members discuss the differing views of the clinical management that they should take with Mr. Swanson. His daughter, Ms. Cullen, does not visit her father during his stay but, based on what she has determined by phone, she believes that he can return to full mobility without the use of the wheelchair. The social worker on the team, who is in regular phone contact with Ms. Cullen, attempts to understand and convey the daughter's viewpoint. Ms. Cullen is not open to exploring her own experiences or feelings about her prior history in the family or with health care. She remains unwilling to come to the hospital, and the social worker is therefore not able to arrange for her to visit her father there and meet with the clinicians responsible for his care. The social worker reports to the team that Mrs. Swanson has expressed fear about her stepdaughter's behavior. The social worker attempts to facilitate a family meeting, which Ms. Cullen has refused to attend. The social worker is able to recruit Mrs. Swanson's own son to support her through her husband's hospital stay.

In this case, geriatric, surgical, and physical medicine teams are all involved. When multiple teams are involved in geriatric patient care, clear leadership is crucial, both among the teams and within the geriatric team. In this case, for medical decisions with the other two teams, the geriatrician takes the leadership role within the geriatric team. But decision making within the geriatric team is shared, depending on the tasks at hand. The geriatric team bears major responsibility and accountability for the overall management of Mr. Swanson and the biopsychosocial dimensions of his clinical problems.

Mr. Swanson's care is discussed at a weekly meeting of the geriatric team. Under the leadership of the attending physician, the geriatric team reaches a consensus judgment that Mr. Swanson has significantly impaired decision-making capacity. This raises the issue of who has final decision-making authority in this case. His legally designated surrogate decision maker is his wife. Even if he had not designated her as his surrogate decision maker, as a matter of law in the this jurisdiction and the institutional policy of the hospital, she would have priority over other family members. (Different states may designate other surrogates. The reader should be familiar with relevant applicable law.) Mrs. Swanson is appropriate for this role because she has been her husband's primary caregiver at home. (Teams should counsel patients and families about the most effective way of determining and protecting the authority of surrogate decision makers.) That she is significantly limited in her physical ability to continue this care justifiably reduces her obligation to continue caring for her husband at home at this point. Such a morally justified limit on caregiving obligations in long-term care decision making by a surrogate should not, in the team's judgment, count as a potentially disabling conflict of interest. As a rule, other family members should participate in the decision-making process and support the surrogate decision maker. Whenever possible, family consensus and support should be facilitated by the team. This lessens the burden on the designated decision maker. But family participation needs to be distinguished from final decision making.

After reaching this consensus, the attending geriatrician, speaking for the team, begins the decision-making process with Mrs. Swanson by pointing out to her that further surgery, on balance, would probably increase her husband's risk of death and also the risk of survival with a much-decreased quality of life and increased pain, distress, and suffering. In addition, he expressed the team's assessment and concern that the physical demands on Mrs. Swanson to care for her husband at home would exceed her physical capacity to perform the tasks involved. He therefore not only offers but recommends nursing home placement as the best way to manage Mr. Swanson's condition and to meet his care needs, without overwhelming Mrs. Swanson in the process.

Mrs. Swanson takes some time to think about this recommendation and also speaks to other members of the team, including the nurse practitioner and the social worker, with whom she has developed a close relationship. The team's approach is to help Mrs. Swanson understand that surgery is not in her husband's health-related interests, that she can justify reasonable limits on her caregiving obligation to him, and that one such reasonable limit is the physical demands of care beyond her capacity to meet them. After considerable reflection, and many discussions with the geriatric team social worker, Mrs. Swanson agrees to nursing home placement.

Family Involvement

At this point, Ms. Cullen, Mr. Swanson's daughter and Mrs. Swanson's step-daughter, contacts the geriatric team social worker and expresses her opposition to the decision that has been made. (Mrs. Swanson has told her about it.) Ms. Cullen informs the social worker, "I would rather that my father died in the operating room than for him to leave the hospital incapacitated." She also accuses the hospital of causing her father's injury and says, "They need to repair it." She requests another orthopedic surgery consult.

In the traditional dyadic model, the social worker could simply explain to Ms. Cullen that as the patient's daughter, she lacked legal standing to act as Mr. Swanson's surrogate decision maker. She can participate in decision making, but not as the final authority. But in the context of team care, the ethical issues become more complex, and the team is obliged to maintain cohesion for the patient's benefit—a moral obligation that does not arise in the traditional dyadic model. In order for this team to fulfill its obligations to Mr. Swanson, the social worker has the moral obligation at this point to share with the team a report on her contact with Ms. Cullen. The social worker should also take leadership in developing a team response to this challenge to Mrs. Swanson's decision-making authority and in dealing effectively yet sensitively with Ms. Cullen, as well as developing a plan for identifying and addressing intrafamilial conflict.

In response to Ms. Cullen's request, the team therefore takes a preventive ethics approach, with the attending geriatrician taking the leadership role in identifying the ethical challenges to the team and determining ethically justified responses to them. In order to prevent a breakdown in communication with Ms. Cullen, to rule out the possibility of mistaken ethical and clinical judgments within the team, and to encourage confidence in the assessment of Mr. Swanson by the various teams, the attending geriatrician arranges for this second orthopedic consultation, which concurs with the initial orthopedic surgery team's evaluation. To prevent any possible confusion within the geriatric team or on the part of other teams involved in Mr. Swanson's care about legal and moral surrogate decision-making authority, the attending geriatrician, with the geriatric team's agreement, then obtains an ethics consultation, to clarify that in applicable law and institutional policy Mrs. Swanson is the legally designated surrogate decision maker. The ethics consultant agrees that medical center policy is clear: Mrs. Swanson is the sole surrogate decision maker for her husband. The use of an ethics consultation to clarify disputed decision-making authority and to support families in accepting the appropriate surrogate's authority has become more common in this hospital in the previous several years.

The geriatric team agrees that the social worker should remain the point of contact with Ms. Cullen, inasmuch as her seeking out the social worker may have indicated that she trusted the social worker more than other members of the team. The social worker conveys this information about the legal surrogate to Ms. Cullen via telephone, as she is unwilling to meet. Ms. Cullen then becomes verbally abusive of the rest of the geriatric team, especially the attending geriatrician. She asks the social worker to contact the surgeon and not to assist Mrs. Swanson with locating an appropriate nursing home. When the social worker reports Ms. Cullen's response to the geriatric team, the team accepts the social worker's interpretation that Ms. Cullen's behavior, unfortunately, appears to be an attempt to split the social worker from the rest of the team. The social worker reports that in subsequent phone calls Ms. Cullen threatens legal action and states that she does not want her father in a nursing home and wants her stepmother to continue to care for him at home as she always has. Ms. Cullen makes repeated phone calls to the surgery service requesting that her father receive surgery and stating that her opinion should prevail, as she is the "blood relative."

Case Analysis
Assess Team Structure

The geriatric team can and should maintain cohesion in the care of Mr. Swanson, so that he will continue to benefit clinically from the team's involvement in his care. The team achieves this ethically crucial goal by taking a preventive ethics approach to Ms. Cullen's attempt to split the team and to her threatened legal action. Achieving this goal requires clear communication among team members and between teams, especially about the need to respect Mrs. Swanson's decisions for her husband. This preventive ethics approach attempts to prevent ethical conflict from occurring and to use such preparation to better address ethical conflicts when they nonetheless do occur. The attending geriatrician's decision to seek an ethics consultation is an example of preventive ethics, as is the social worker's attempt to enlist Ms. Cullen's support for her stepmother's decision.

Preventive ethics in team care should be based on the concept of the team members as moral cofiduciaries of the patient. As cofiduciaries of the patient, the team members share a common obligation: to make the protection and promotion of the patient's health-related interests and the integrity of the surrogate decision-making process their primary concerns. Team cohesion must be maintained so that shared fiduciary responsibility to the patient can be routinely and effectively discharged. A major ethical issue in this case is that Ms. Cullen's attempt to split the social worker from the team threatens the team's shared fiduciary responsibility to Mr. Swanson.

Identify Patient and Family Preferences

To participate adequately in the informed consent process and thus have authority over their own care, patients need the intact cognitive capacities that are required to process information reliably. Patients need to be able to attend to, retain, absorb, and recall information; to reason from present events to their future likely consequences; to evaluate those consequences in terms of their values, beliefs, and preferences; and to express a preference that is based on this step-wise reasoning process. This process is iterative, and therefore impairments at any one step of this process can impair later steps (McCullough, Jones, and Brody 1998).

Mr. Swanson's memory loss is significant and thus impairs his decision-making capacity in the early steps of this process. It is reasonable to assess his decision-making capacity as impaired, even though he can express preferences. Even if his preferences do not express a reasoning process, they may still express his values and beliefs. Therefore, his preferences should be given weight by the geriatric team and by his wife. Mr. Swanson says that he would rather go home, but when asked to consider his wife's very limited physical abilities, he agrees that nursing home placement would be a better choice. He is not able to remember this discussion from day to day.

Mr. Swanson, however, does not possess intact decision-making capacity. Decisions should, therefore be made not *with* him but *for* him by the legally designated surrogate decision maker (Brock and Buchanan 1991). In the applicable legal jurisdiction and in hospital policy, for patients who are married, this decision maker is the patient's spouse.

Surrogate decision making is guided by two standards (Brock and Buchanan 1991). The first, called *substituted judgment,* requires the surrogate decision maker to consider the patient's express wishes from the past, as well as the patient's durable values, beliefs, and preferences, in order to make a decision for the patient that, ideally, would be the decision that the patient himself would make, were he to possess intact decision-making capacity. This judgement can be a base on explicit statements or on inferences from past behavior and expressed values and preferences. The second standard, called *best interest*, is to be used when the surrogate decision maker does not have reliable knowledge of the patient's past wishes, values, or preferences. On this standard, the surrogate should make a judgment about which courses of clinical management, on balance, best protect and promote the health-related interests of the patient.

Mrs. Swanson takes seriously the clinical judgment of the geriatric team that further surgery would not be consistent with protecting and promoting her husband's health-related interests, fulfilling the requirements of the best interest standard of surrogate decision making. Mrs. Swanson also has the advantage of knowing her husband's preferences, including his express agreement with the plan for nursing home placement, which is consistent with the substituted judgment standard. There is therefore no ethical justification for the geriatric team to question the moral reliability of Mrs. Swanson's substituted judgment about how her husband's condition should be managed in the future.

An important preventive ethics step in responding to Ms. Cullen's objections would at this point be for the social worker, the attending geriatrician, and other team members to attempt once more to gain Ms. Cullen's support by explaining the nature of surrogate decision making to her and distinguishing it from participation in decision making. She certainly has a moral right to participate in decisions, as the patient's concerned daughter, but she does not have the right to be the final authority or surrogate. The team should attempt to prevent splitting the social worker off from the team by taking the uniform view—the only ethically justified view—that Mrs. Swanson's surrogate decision for Mr. Swanson is completely consistent with the ethical and legal requirements of surrogate decision making and that the team is therefore prepared to act on this appropriate surrogate decision. This is a considerable exercise of power that does not occur in the traditional dyadic model, in which context the attending physician alone would probably deal with Ms. Cullen. When a group of health care professionals meets with a family member who does not accept the legal surrogate and when the team does so to protect the interests of the patient, the exercise of considerable power by the team is ethically justified. This power, of course, should be exercised in a sensitive and humane fashion.

If Ms. Cullen should continue to object after this meeting with the team, the next preventive ethics step would be for the team to explain to her that the moral obligation of everyone involved in her father's care is to protect and promote his health-related interests and to respect his preferences. In addition, Ms. Cullen has an obligation to respect her stepmother's well-founded judgment that she lacks the physical capacity to meet her husband's long-term care needs. The goal of this preventive ethics strategy is to undercut, justifiably, Ms. Cullen's implicit view that her primary moral relationship with her father is one of rights and the power to make decisions and to underscore that her primary relationship with her stepmother is to respect her preferences and not expect her to assume unrealistic care burdens. The goal of preventive ethics is to create common moral ground for negotiation with Ms. Cullen, in which the ethically justified conclusion is clear from the outset. This process can include health care team members helping families with differing views to work through their emotional issues and to accommodate to the ultimate outcome. To the degree that family members must deal with each other in the future, preventive ethics attempts to preserve their relationship.

Evaluate Quality-of-Life Issues

Quality of life, which originated as a concept in the social sciences, means the ability to engage in life tasks and to derive satisfaction from them. In health care ethics, a team should not have preconceived ideas about what life tasks are worth engaging in and what level of satisfaction patients should derive from doing so; these are matters for patients to decide. A team, however, does possess clinical expertise to determine when the conditions necessary for to engaging in preferred life tasks and gaining satisfaction from doing so are met. In this case quality of life is a major concern for the team's assessment of Mr. Swanson's possible surgery. Different disciplines contribute important information about different aspects of the patient's quality of life at home and in the hospital. For Mr. Swanson and all of the teams involved in his care, quality-of-life issues concern balancing the iatrogenic risks of further surgery against his remaining quality of life without surgery. The consensus judgment of the geriatric team is that surgery would in all likelihood have one of two results: Mrs. Swanson's death or his survival at a much lower functional baseline. Either outcome would leave him with a lower quality of life than that he is likely to experience without surgery, whether he returns home or is admitted to a nursing home.

Consider Contextual Factors

We have elsewhere described the problem of contested or competing realities in long-term care decision making—that is, disagreement among team members or among family members about the nature of an elder's condition and its prospects (McCullough et al. 1995). In this case, the geriatric team and Mrs. Swanson agree that the patient's condition is an unfortunate, predictable, but not negligent outcome of prior clinical management, while Ms. Cullen asserts negligence.

An important preventive ethics strategy at this point is to share with Ms. Cullen the consensus judgment of the geriatric team about Mr. Swanson's expected quality of life both with and without surgery. The team should help her to appreciate that her request for surgery would likely result only in the loss of her father's current and acceptable quality of life. Since her initial concerns were about her father's quality of life, this information will be important in her subsequent judgment and decision making. Her concerns that the surgical team and the hospital are responsible for her father's current condition and that they may have been negligent should be openly and honestly addressed. The concept of not-unexpected complications from risky surgery in a frail patient should be explained to Ms. Cullen, and she should be invited to understand in these terms her father's outcome from clinical management to date. She should be assured that concern about the effect of surgery on her father's remaining quality of life has been expressed not just by the surgical team but also by the physical therapy team. She should also be informed that everyone on the geriatric team accepts the view that surgery would not be consistent with the obligation to protect Mr. Swanson's remaining quality of life. This strategy may prevent further efforts on Ms. Cullen's part to split the social worker from the team, by empowering the social worker to repeat and reinforce the geriatric team's assessment.

Long-term care issues are important contextual concerns. We pointed out above that Mrs. Swanson is entirely justified in placing reasonable limits on her caregiving obligations to her husband at this point. Ms. Cullen is not able to provide that care herself, given that she is in a wheelchair and weakened by her own history of a stroke. Nor was Ms. Cullen willing to arrange for long-term care for her father at her own expense. Her preference that her stepmother provide such care is not realistic and also shows unjustified disrespect for Mrs. Swanson's considered ethical judgment, which is supported by the geriatric team. Indeed, Mrs. Swanson's judgment reflects the *recommendation* of the geriatric team. This recommendation is based on the well-founded judgment that an attempt by Mrs. Swanson to care for Mr. Swanson at home would not only result in his loss of health and functional status but would place Mrs. Swanson's health and functional status at risk in a lost cause. The geriatric team should take the consensus preventive ethics approach of not accepting Ms. Cullen's preference that her step-mother take her father home, and of explaining that Mrs. Swanson's decision reflects the team's recommendation and is inherently ethically justified, given her significant physical limitations.

Resolve the Ethical Issues and Create the Plan

Discharge home is not in Mr. Swanson's health-related interests and will put his remaining quality of life at unnecessary risk of serious loss. Caregiving by Mrs. Swanson at home is not ethically obligatory for her to undertake and does not reflect Mr. Swanson's own preferences. Further surgery does not pass a test of proportionality, in which benefits outweigh risks from surgery, resulting in prolonged life at an acceptable quality of life. There is no conflict within the geriatric team on these matters and no conflict between the geriatric team and other teams involved in the management of Mr. Swanson's condition.

Ms. Cullen remains unpersuaded by the attending geriatrician and social worker, and she continues to attempt to split the social worker from the team. At this point, the next preventive ethics step is for the team to review its recommendation and determine again that it is consistent with its fiduciary obligation to the patient, Mr. Swanson. The ethical principle of beneficence defines such fiduciary obligations to patients. Again, the goal is to rule out mistaken clinical and ethical judgments within the team. Such judgments are indeed ruled out. The assessments by the two surgery consultations meet the test of proportionality that is central to beneficence-based clinical judgment: the risks of another surgery outweigh potential benefits, and the patient's condition is manageable and currently pain free. His quality of life would be protected by not performing this surgery and would be jeopardized by surgical intervention (if he survived the surgery). The team should explain to Ms. Cullen that its primary and overriding concern is Mr. Swanson's welfare and not such extraneous factors as the economic cost to the hospital of the surgery.

The second preventive ethics step is for the geriatric and other teams to remain clear and unwavering, when dealing with Ms. Cullen, about the legal and moral fact that Mrs. Swanson is legally and morally the surrogate decision maker. While this is an exercise of considerable power—more than Ms. Cullen would experience in the traditional dyadic model—it is ethically justified, as pointed out above. Moreover, the ethics consultation has confirmed the final authority of Mrs. Swanson, providing important institutional backing to the team's approach to *surrogate decision making.* (This is an emerging role of ethics consultation in this hospital and perhaps elsewhere as well.) Mrs. Swanson has made a decision that protects and promotes Mr. Swanson's remaining health interests and to which he agrees.

The third preventive ethics step is to review the reasonableness of Mrs. Swanson's long-term care decision making about and for Mr. Swanson. She is making a decision that places reasonable justified limits on her caregiving obligations to her husband. Helping Mrs. Swanson see this prevents her from being whipsawed between the rock of doing everything for her husband (and jeopardizing her own health and thus his too) and the hard place of feeling selfish. This reasoning should also be explained to Ms. Cullen, and she should be invited to see that it is unreasonable and therefore inappropriate for her to insist that her stepmother take her father home from the hospital (something that Ms. Cullen is obviously unable to do herself).

The fourth preventive ethics step is to determine the weight to be given to Mr. Swanson's acceptance of his wife's decision. Even though he has experienced impaired decision-making capacity, his preference should be given serious weight, especially since it protects and promotes his health-related interests. This, too, should be explained to Ms. Cullen, and the team should explain sensitively but unambiguously that Ms. Cullen's primary moral relationship to her father is one of respect for his preferences but not the right to make decisions for him without taking his preferences into account.

The fifth preventive ethics step is to address Ms. Cullen's concerns about the hospital's responsibility for her father's condition. Her concerns should be addressed openly and without hesitation, with an explanation about known iatrogenic complications of the surgical management of her father's initial hip fracture and subsequent clinical interventions. These complications were not unforeseen and therefore not the result of negligence, an important distinction that Ms. Cullen should be helped to understand and accept.

These preventive ethics steps position the team to address a further complication that arises in the case of Mr. Swanson. On the day of Mr. Swanson's discharge to the nursing home, an attorney representing Ms. Cullen appears at the hospital and asks that, at the explicit request of his client, Mr. Swanson not be transferred to the nursing home.

The above ethical analysis fully supports the team's vigorous opposition to this attorney's request. Ms. Cullen's request is inconsistent with the team's fiduciary obligation to Mr. Swanson. Complying with the lawyer's demand would therefore be unethical on its face. Moreover, Ms. Cullen, as noted above, does not have legal standing to override her stepmother's decisions, and inasmuch as she was not Mr. Swanson's primary home caregiver before his admission, she has less moral standing as a surrogate decision maker than does Mrs. Swanson.

Given the medical decision involved (surgery), the attending geriatrician should represent the team's recommendation. Should other team members be contacted or become involved, they should also reinforce the team's integrated plan. The preventive ethics steps at this stage involve making it clear to this attorney that his client's request is inconsistent with the team's and hospital's fiduciary obligation to Mr. Swanson and is therefore unethical and should be immediately withdrawn. This attorney should be informed that Ms. Cullen has no legal or moral standing to claim the role of surrogate decision maker and that this matter has already been clarified by an ethics consultation. The attorney should therefore be informed that discharge will proceed as planned.

Conclusion

Well-founded ethical reflection and judgment, based on a geriatric team's shared fiduciary obligations to a patient, should always guide the team because every member has the same fiduciary obligation: to protect and promote the patient's health-related interests and to implement the patient's preferences in pursuit of this goal. The different disciplines involved in a geriatric team bring different clinical and scientific competencies to the clinical management of a patient's problems. Moreover, surrogate decision makers should take seriously the considered assessments and recommendations of the geriatric team, and other family members are ethically obligated to respect the surrogate's decisions when they are consistent with the substituted judgment and best interests standards of such decision making. Ethical analysis therefore teaches that in cases of conflict between the geriatric team and involved family members, there is moral common ground. This common ground can be identified, protected, and used as a basis for mutual decision making following the clinical applications of ethics in the form of strategies of preventive ethics.

Discussion Questions

1. What if the daughter's request for the management of her father had not arisen in the context of team care?

2. Could the case have been resolved more easily without the team's involvement? If it were so resolved, what insights into the ethical issues in this case would be lost?

3. What advantages did the team approach to the ethical issues in this case give to the professional ethics of the team members?

REFERENCES

Arras, J. D. 1995. Conflicting interests in long-term care decision making: Acknowledging, dissolving, and resolving conflicts. In L. B. McCullough and N. L. Wilson, eds., *Long-term care decisions: Ethical and conceptual dimensions.* Baltimore: Johns Hopkins University Press.

Beauchamp, T. L., and J. F. Childress. 1994. *Principles of biomedical ethics,* 4th ed. New York: Oxford University Press.

Brakman, S. V. 1995. Filial responsibility and long-term care decision making. In L. B. McCullough and N. L. Wilson, eds., *Long-term care decisions: Ethical and conceptual dimensions.* Baltimore: Johns Hopkins University Press.

Brock, D., and A. Buchanan. 1991. *Deciding for others.* Cambridge: Cambridge University Press.

Jecker, N. S. 1995. What do husbands and wives owe each other in old age? In L. B. McCullough and N. L. Wilson, eds., *Long-term care decisions: Ethical and conceptual dimensions.* Baltimore: Johns Hopkins University Press.

McCullough, L. B., and F. A. Chervenak. 1994. *Ethics in obstetrics and gynecology.* New York: Oxford University Press.

McCullough, L. B., J. W. Jones, and B. A. Brody. 1998. Informed consent: Autonomous decision making of the surgical patient. In L. B. McCullough, J. W. Jones, and B. A. Brody, eds., *Surgical Ethics.* New York: Oxford University Press.

McCullough, L. B., N. L. Wilson, J. A. Rhymes, and T. A. Teasdale. 1995. Managing the conceptual and ethical dimensions of long-term care decision making: A preventive ethics approach. In L. B. McCullough and N. L. Wilson, eds., *Long-term care decisions: Ethical and conceptual dimensions.* Baltimore: Johns Hopkins University Press.

Purtilo, R., B. W. Shaw, and R. Arnold. 1998. Obligations of surgeons to non-physician team members and trainees. In L. B. McCullough, J. W. Jones, and B. A. Brody, eds., *Surgical ethics.* New York: Oxford University Press.

Refusal to Comply: What to Do When the Interdisciplinary Team Plan Doesn't Work

Susan Kornblatt, M.A., Catherine Eng, M.D., and Kate O'Malley, R.N., M.S., G.N.P.

Open communication and responsible negotiations are key ingredients for a successful team-patient relationship, ensuring that quality services are provided and a good outcome for the patient is achieved. A good patient-team relationship helps create a successful treatment plan, incorporates patient preferences, and allows the patient and team to work together toward the same goals. When one partner fails to comply with treatment decisions that have been collectively agreed upon, the relationship can fray and ultimately be broken. The goals of treatment will not be met, and a good outcome may be difficult to achieve.

In a health care setting, compliance or adherence to a prescribed regimen usually implies the degree or extent to which the patient follows directions (often regarding, but not solely limited to, ingesting prescription medications) (Weintraub 1990). But compliance, like noncompliance, also includes appropriate modifications of a regimen to fit with lifestyle and to diminish adverse effects while achieving maximal benefit. As Reuben and colleagues (1996) point out, the overall rate of adherence to self-care recommendations for geriatric patients with one or more of the four target conditions (functional impairment, depression, falls, and urinary incontinence) in their study was reported as being modest to poor. Adherence by patients to self-care recommendations that are considered "major" or "most important," was found to be only "fair" because they often involve lifestyle changes which are the most difficult to follow (Shah et al. 1997). Unfortunately, these recommended lifestyle changes may present conflicts between what interdisciplinary health care teams recommend to patients and how willingly patients comply with the recommended plan. Many factors may arise to promote conflict between a patient's wish for autonomy and a health care team's efforts to implement successful interdisciplinary care plans. What is autonomy for the patient may be viewed as noncompliance by the team.

On Lok Senior Health Services in San Francisco provides community-based comprehensive medical social and rehabilitative services to frail elderly persons, integrating acute and long-term care under one health care delivery system. Service revenues are provided through capitation payments from Medicare, Medicaid, and private sources. Funds are combined into an unrestricted pool that is used to pay for all services provided to enrollees. Providing services under capitated reimbursement requires that health care teams balance risk with resources. In that balance, teams have great flexibility in decision making, which is sometimes not the case in a traditional fee-for-service reimbursement method of health care delivery. While On Lok as an organization assumes full financial risk for enrollees' care, the teams are not responsible for tracking individual costs of care for patients.

On Lok is the prototype for PACE (Program of All-Inclusive Care for the Elderly) (Eng et al. 1997). Currently there are thirty-four PACE sites in the United States serving over seven thousand frail elderly persons (National PACE Association 2001). PACE provides all care for enrollees with services including primary care, social work, restorative therapy, home care, and institutional care, in both hospital and nursing home settings. Specialty and ancillary medical services are also provided, as are long-term care services such as transportation, meals, and personal care. At the heart of the PACE model is an interdisciplinary team that manages patient care through direct service provision, continuous patient assessment, treatment planning, coordination of contract services, and monitoring of quality of care (Eng 1996). After signing an enrollment agreement, each patient is assigned to a team comprising primary care physician (and often a geriatric nurse practitioner as well), nurses, a social worker, rehabilitation staff, a dietitian, public health nurses, and geriatric aides.

Promoting patient autonomy and involvement in decision making is a guiding principle for care providers at On Lok. In formulating appropriate treatment plans, the interdisciplinary team promotes and supports each patient's capability to maintain community residence in the context of personal safety and feasible treatment options. In the case of a patient who lacks decision-making capacity due to dementia and who does not have family or an appropriate surrogate, the health care team may appropriately determine treatment goals and design a care plan to meet those goals (American Geriatrics Society 1999).

The case of Mr. William Carl illustrates the dynamics of a team-patient relationship strained by compliance issues and reveals the coping mechanisms of both parties. An analysis of the impact of this long struggling relationship on the functioning of an interdisciplinary team provides insights for improved outcomes.

The relationship between this patient and the interdisciplinary team unfolded over a two-year time frame. Rather than a single episode or circumstance, a series of actions and reactions occurred over time to highlight an ethical problem, as the team and the patient struggled with the balance between autonomy, patient preferences, compliance with the treatment plan, and safety.

Case Description

William Carl is a 71-year-old Caucasian man who enrolled with the On Lok Health Plan in April 1997. His complicated past medical history included: (1) an old right-hemispheric cerebral-vascular accident with resulting left hemiparesis; (2) cervical laminectomies, the last of which occurred three years before enrollment and was complicated by postoperative infection; (3) frequent falls as often as every day; (4) right eye blindness; and (5) alcohol abuse. Functionally, he was wheelchair dependent and needed assistance with all ADLs except feeding.

Mr. Carl lived alone in a one-bedroom wheelchair-accessible apartment. The youngest of nine children, he had no contact with family, other than occasional telephone contact with a sister-in-law who lives in another state. He never married and has no children. He received a high school education, joined the army, served in World War II and the Korean conflict, and subsequently joined the Merchant Marines. Before his disability, he was active and traveled extensively.

At the time of enrollment, Mr. Carl's health problems were chronic, and the goal of treatment was to maintain community residence and his current level of function while providing social and emotional support. The approach included medical management in the clinic, center programs for recreation and rehabilitation therapy, and one-on-one counseling with his social worker to provide support and help him achieve optimal functioning. Home care was also provided for ADL support. He attended the center five days a week. Given the flexibility of the On Lok's system, the team could vary all interventions in terms of frequency and duration to increasing levels of oversight, direct care, and supervision. If the existing treatment plan did not produce the anticipated goals, the plan could be modified at any time. On Lok has been successful in the past managing individuals with similar problems in the community; but one area of continuing challenge has been caring for the chronic alcohol abuser in a community program designed to manage frail, physically impaired elders. It was not clear at enrollment if Mr. Carl's problems with alcohol would bear on the goals for his care. Given that the goal of On Lok's services is to prevent or delay institutional placement, the intake and assessment process led to the conclusion that he could clearly benefit from the services available from On Lok. In his case, these services focused in the areas of medical management and monitoring, social support, home care, and rehabilitation therapy.

Identify Patient and Family Preferences

After enrollment, if the team does not know a participant's preferences related to resuscitation and tube feedings, team members (usually the physician) will initiate a conversation regarding end-of-life health care wishes. Information will be provided to the patient regarding the risks and benefits of various treatment options. The results of this conversation will be documented in the patient's record. When death appears imminent, primary care physicians will also raise other issues, such as use of IV antibiotics, transfers to hospitals, and other invasive or diagnostic interventions.

In conversation with his physician, Mr. Carl indicated that he did not want CPR and did not want to have any tube feedings at any time. His score on the Folstein Mini-Mental Exam was 23/30, indicating some mild cognitive impairment. But the team determined his competency was intact to make the decision to refuse CPR and tube feedings. This determination of his competency included observing his consistency over time in expressing his preferences for staying the community, staying out of a nursing home, and maintaining his lifestyle in that community despite numerous risks. He comprehended those risks and understood the consequences of his actions. This approach to determining competency is consistent with State of California competency law (State of California 1995–96), which provides that "a person may have a mental or physical disorder and still be capable of contracting, conveying, marrying, making medical decisions . . . and performing other functions. A person has the capacity to give informed consent to a proposed medical treatment if the person is able to participate knowingly and intelligently in making that decision."

The discussion of patient preferences in Mr. Carl's case ranges beyond the treatment interventions related to end-of-life care. In his case, three preferences were discussed in particular—the choice to drink excessively, the use of an electric wheelchair, and the desire to remain in the community and avoid nursing home placement.

Mr. Carl had decision-making capacity and was completely informed about the health and safety dangers of alcohol intake. Soon after enrollment, the team began to experience his unwillingness to cooperate with the treatment plan related to alcohol abuse. Geriatric home care aides reported finding liquor bottles under his sink at home, and he was falling several times a day. He received extensive counseling from the primary care physician, social worker, and nurse. He was seen by a consulting psychiatrist, who prescribed treatment for depression, as well as adjunctive therapy for his right-sided paresthesias. Counseling and support were provided continuously over many months; but the team was not successful in helping Mr. Carl stop drinking. Psychiatry and psychology appointments were made for him, and he refused to keep those appointments on many occasions. He had numerous conferences with his social worker, at times being verbally abusive toward her.

A second area of conflict between Mr. Carl and the team occurred when Mr. Carl desired to maintain his mobility and preferred the use of an electric wheelchair. All team members agreed that this was an unsafe situation where Mr. Carl was a danger to himself and others. The team met with him numerous times about the safety concerns. He refused supervision when he went out on the streets with his wheelchair and suffered several accidents. He refused to hire a personal escort or to change to a manual wheelchair, saying it was too difficult for him to maneuver. In February 1999 the social worker wrote in her progress note, "Participant is determined to maintain his 'freedom' and seems to view the team as a threat. . . . This leads to . . . contentious interactions. . . . It is frustrating to both sides. . . . Team feels he is in denial about his . . . limitations. He is noncompliant, manipulative, and . . . unreliable."

The third area of conflict between Mr. Carl and the members of the team involved the effort required to maintain community residence. Given his functional impairments, Mr. Carl needed home care services and routine center attendance to meet his ADL needs. Over time, his functional ability for self-care decreased. The occupational therapist on the care team worked on modifying Mr. Carl's apartment to adjust for his functional decline.

Mr. Carl continued to drink alcohol excessively. In early 1998 he began to exhibit sexually inappropriate behavior toward the geriatric aides assigned to provide him with personal care, such as bathing and dressing, in the center as well as in his home. He sexually harassed an aide in his home and frightened her with his advances. He verbally abused both professional and paraprofessional staff. Despite this, the team persisted in providing him the care and services he needed to stay in his apartment. He refused to have male geriatric aides provide personal care to him. The home care nurse wrote that in order to serve him at home and to protect the aides, the health plan would need to hire two geriatric aides to work simultaneously in his home. In addition to the expense of such an arrangement, it was very difficult to find staff willing to work under such conditions. Nevertheless, the plan was implemented when adequate staffing was found, and the patient exhibited no further episodes of inappropriate sexual behavior toward the workers.

Evaluate Quality-of-Life Issues

One month after enrollment, the geriatric aide found Mr. Carl lying in his bed with a plastic bag over his head. His breathing was shallow, his pulse was slow, and he was poorly responsive. He was taken by ambulance to the nearest ER, where he suddenly "awoke" and told the staff that he tried to kill himself because of his pain. After medical clearance, he was admitted to the psychiatry service, where he remained for twelve days. Evaluation concluded that the underlying problem was one of early dementia and depression with associated behavioral problems. His pain was controlled with acetaminophen and codeine every six hours around the clock. After hospital discharge, he continued to be noncompliant with medications to control his hypertension; but he made no further suicide attempts and was not rehospitalized.

Mr. Carl's major quality-of-life issues were the ability to maintain community residence, prevent major injuries, and ultimately avoid nursing home placement. Team members correctly identified that this individual who prized his freedom and autonomy would find life in a nursing home confining and un-bearable.

In late 1998 the frequency of Mr. Carl's falls at home escalated. Paramedics complained that they were receiving frequent calls to pick him up from the floor of his apartment. The building manager made numerous evening and night calls to the health plan's on-call physicians regarding the patient's falls at night. The paramedics and the building manager suggested to the care team that the patient could no longer live at home. Nursing home placement was proposed to him. He refused. On Lok sheltered community housing was also offered. He tried it for a few days, then demanded to return to his apartment. At this time, safety issues with the use of the electric wheelchair also increased.

Consider Contextual Factors

The major provider issues influencing the treatment planning process in-volved the level of authority that team members perceived they had to resolve the ethical issues. How far could the team go to respect the patient's autonomy while their treatment plan promoting safety and community residence was proving to be totally ineffective? On Lok goes to great lengths to avoid involun-tary disenrollment. Did the team have to terminate this individual's participa-tion in the program?

Resolve the Ethical Issues and Create the Plan

After almost two years of care, the team told Mr. Carl he had to go to a nursing home or the team would disenroll him from the health plan. All the team members observed his functional decline and recommended that an al-ternative living situation was imperative because a safe care plan could not be provided for him at home. The team had exhausted its care options.

Implement the Plan

In May 1999, Mr. Carl agreed to remain enrolled and to move to a nursing home under contract with the health plan. Two weeks later he attempted to stab a nurse's aide at the nursing home with scissors. He was verbally abusive to all nursing home staff. He refused to take his medications. The nursing home staff expressed a great deal of frustration managing his behavior. In June 1999 the social worker called for a volunteer from the ombudsperson's office to interview him in the nursing home. Mr. Carl complained bitterly of his confinement (he was not physically restrained) and said he could not tolerate his two roommates because they were so ill. The ombudsperson told him that he was unsafe to live in the community. But she also said that he could not be kept against his will.

Two weeks later Mr. Carl left the nursing home against medical advice, after signing disenrollment papers from the health plan. He left no forwarding address or names of possible caregivers. His case was referred to adult protective services. Two weeks following his departure, the health plan received notification from Las Vegas that the patient had been admitted to a local hospital. There has been no further follow-up from the health plan team.

Discussion

This case illustrates the ethical issues faced when individual patient autonomy conflicts with a recommended team plan of care and societal expectations of public safety and civil behavior, and when the team's commitment to beneficent care must be balanced with other ethical goals.

Several factors played a role in the conflict between this patient's wish for autonomy and the team's efforts to implement a successful interdisciplinary care plan. The efforts of professionals must be open to the empowerment of the elderly individual with disabilities, recognizing that it is he or she who must define the appropriate means and ends of care (Clark 1995). But these efforts sometimes conflict with the personal values of the patient. In this case, the team observed the patient's denial about his declining function and the fact that he often refused care.

The interdisciplinary team members (MD, RN, SW, home care RN, OT) held significant negotiations regarding best ways of maximizing the patient's ability to live alone. They struggled continuously to reach consensus in balancing a respect for the patient's autonomy with society's need for public safety and civil behavior. They expressed a moral obligation to provide beneficent care of the frail and vulnerable. Confounding their efforts were the patient's verbal and physical abusiveness toward care providers and his impulsive acts when using an electric wheelchair, which threatened the safety of other participants in the center, the nursing home, and public places. Should the team have taken more direct action in removing the electric wheelchair from the patient?

Some team members felt that they should and that the wheelchair was a threat; others saw it as enabling function and mobility for an individual who was losing these skills. The social worker's notes in the chart read, "when staff requested that the patient use a manual wheelchair while at the day health center, he adamantly refused, stating that he would rather die and that it would be taking away his independence." What may have seemed an adamant refusal and noncompliance by the patient was actually his continued effort at maintaining autonomy. As Devor et al. (1994) examined in their study, compliance is a complex phenomenon, requiring that the patient receive and comprehend recommendations, accept those recommendations, gather necessary resources, and implement the recommendations. The most common cause for noncompliance is failure to accept the recommendation. The lowest rate of compliance is with recommendations to change a living situation.

Is society, and in this case the health care team, obliged to serve an impaired patient if the patient is abusive? These issues were posed to On Lok's ethics committee in a retrospective review of this case. This eighteen-member board-level committee, formed in 1983, has community members, including nonstaff professionals with experience in healthcare, ethics, and legal aspects of care and caregivers. On Lok service providers and administrative staff also serve on this committee. Several team members involved in the care of Mr. Carl presented the case.

In their discussion, ethics committee members noted that the team took a long time to reach consensus as they struggled to balance patient autonomy with safety risks. The committee recognized that the team had a goal of wanting to provide the best care possible while maximizing patient safety. The committee questioned whether the team had taken steps to assure that the patient would experience the consequences of his actions to a degree that might have fostered behavior change or precipitated a decision to disenroll. The committee also observed that the agency has a responsibility to protect staff from abusive behavior and questioned whether the agency was making the best use of its human resources by continuing its efforts to care for this individual. Involuntary disenrollment from On Lok is a rare occurrence. The committee suggested that the team might have sought earlier intervention from administration or the involvement of the ethics committee as a forum to address such difficult issues.

Team Issues with Noncompliant Patients

How do health care teams deal with hateful, angry patients and still provide them with beneficial care? All health care providers want what is best for the patient, but they may have differing views on what that is. In Mr. Carl's case, the social worker wanted to meet his needs by providing appropriate services. The home care nurse was concerned for the safety of the patient and of the staff. This is an example of team members who share the same goal but subscribe to conflicting action steps. And these views may differ from the patient's views. Frustration can result when members of the team feel misunderstood, devalued, or villainized (Shannon 1997) by a very difficult patient.

The team acted with "ethical correctness" in trying to preserve the patient's autonomy. But "respect for autonomy cannot mean that caregivers are primarily and absolutely precluded from influencing the decisions of elders. . . . We need to acknowledge that the relationship between the receiver of care and the caregiver is far more complicated, especially in long term care, than the usual model implies" (Agich 1990). Mr. Carl, determined to maintain his freedom, at times seemed to view the care providers as a threat to his freedom. This fear led to contentious interactions and ongoing discussion about setting an appropriate care plan that frustrated both patient and team. All members of the team perceived that the patient was in denial about his functional limitations, noncompliant, manipulative, and an unreliable self-reporter, all of which put him at risk. He viewed the team as constantly trying to impose infringements on his freedom and make him do things he did not want to do. He did not trust his care providers. Hall and Berenson (1998) point out that the tests for ethical compromises should be whether they undermine the patients' willingness to participate in the care plan and comply with treatment recommendations. Were ethical compromises made that had an impact on the therapeutic plan? Were ethical compromises *not* made that should have been?

What are the limits of care for such a person? The team went to extraordinary lengths to provide compassionate care, without receiving either gratitude or decency from the patient. Is gratitude from the care recipient part of the caregiving equation? Over time, does such demanding care create stress for the team members and distract them from caring for other equally needy patients?

In the end, after a two-year struggle, the team had to let Mr. Carl go his own way, despite the knowledge that he would fail by himself. How far should the team and society extend (exhaust) its resources, both tangible and intangible (such as goodwill), in an effort to provide the best care for such a patient?

Was the Team Approach Right for This Patient?

Questions about the overall functionality of this team arise in this case. The team consisted of seven members, each of whom had been a member of the team for varying lengths of time (Table 8.1).

This conflicted patient-team relationship spanned twenty-six months. Over this period of time, the team experienced turnover in three key positions: primary care physician, social worker, and center manager/team facilitator. Consistency in setting the ground rules for behavior is crucial in caring for medically frail, noncompliant persons who exhibit socially unacceptable behavior. With personnel turnover, the team may have been neither consistent nor cohesive in monitoring the patient's behavior and implementing consequences for unacceptable behavior. Members new to the team may have had a higher threshold for tolerating bad behavior and noncompliance—a honeymoon period that can last for a number of months. While turnover may be a way of spreading the pain that a difficult patient has inflicted on caregivers, it also may just suppress, rather than reduce, the pain of the existing team members who have long tolerated the dysfunctional behavior. Over time this suppression wears away at the team's ability to make clear decisions and negotiate firmly with the patient for improvement in behavior.

The patient, who lacked self-control, perhaps did not get consistent structural support from the team. He was able to turn one team member against another. A contrasting approach might have been to provide care through a physician's office with support from a home care agency, with minimal care coordination. Had Mr. Carl's case been managed by one primary provider, there would not have been any team conflict. In cases such as his, the team approach, rather than a single-provider approach, may actually contribute to the patient's prolonged course of noncompliance. Did the team approach prolong the inevitable? As mentioned previously, the PACE model of care is based on interdisciplinary health care teams. Perhaps the PACE model was not the appropriate one for this patient.

Was the leadership of the team in this case strong enough? Although the center manager was the designated team facilitator, was she able to facilitate the decision-making process? Was the team in transition due to having a fairly

TABLE 8.1
Team Members and Their Length of Tenure

Position	Amount of time on team at beginning of case
Center manager / team facilitator	2 months
Physician	1 year
Social worker	2 years
Supervising home care nurse	5 years
Clinic nurse	5 years
Physical therapist	10 years
Occupational therapist	6 years

new facilitator? Drinka's model for interdisciplinary health care team development and maintenance (Drinka 1991) suggests phases of how team members assume leadership, pass information on to new members, continue to develop as part of a team, and strengthen the team functioning. But under pressure to perform, some teams may not follow any specific order of development. Although many on the team may have been experienced team members, and although the team appeared to be functioning well, perhaps the team had not previously been challenged by conflict or had the depth to make productive use of a major conflict (Drinka 1994a).

Was the decision-making process clear enough for all team members? In instances such as this case, having a strong leader to facilitate the team discussions and force the team to make difficult recommendations to the patient at critical points is imperative. A specific decision-making process can lead to more effective, efficient decisions (Recker, Bess, and Wellens 1996). Lacking strong leadership, the team can remain fragmented.

Did the personal values of the team members have an impact on team decision making? Professional and person values enter heavily into what one member of a health care team considers the "right" decision, and these values may interfere with the team's decision-making process of the team (Walleck 1991). Values can be a major source of conflicting and competing communication among health professionals and with the patient (Clark 1994). Without examining the personal values of each member of the team, we cannot determine if those values played a role, for example, in one team member's strong opinion that Mr. Carl should not have been allowed to use his electric wheelchair while in the center.

In this case, the team did not force an ultimatum on the patient either to behave or leave the health plan. Unable to resolve their differences, some team members wanted "administration" to intervene and disenroll the patient from the health plan. Others felt that the patient had a right to autonomy, particularly in the use of his electric wheelchair. Teams must be able to ask for support from administration at crucial decision points. Administrators, in turn, can give guidance but should not interfere with the decision-making process, unless it is apparent that the process is detrimental to the patient and to the health care team.

Conclusion

The chronic health problems of frail elders challenge care providers, whether working alone or in teams, and interdisciplinary teams themselves are complex systems in which to solve problems. Although addressing multifaceted problems in a complex system promises better, more comprehensive solutions, it also requires a large investment of time and energy. Even when the patient is motivated and cooperative, much effort is needed to consider all aspects of the situation and create, implement, and evaluate the impact of a treatment plan.

As the long struggle between the team and Mr. Carl shows, the team approach with a difficult, noncompliant patient harbors several potential complications. Numerous factors influenced the team's performance in this case. The team:

- maintained its goal to do the best job possible in providing care for this patient;
- managed the care in a day-to-day reactive way;
- lost objectivity, having invested an enormous amount into the care of the patient;
- had several members who did not know how to say no; and
- had some members with a sense of outrage at the patient's continuing behavior, while other members simply accepted it.

Perhaps this interdisciplinary team could have been more successful in working with this patient had it taken action steps to create and enforce rules related to safety and behavior. Respect for patient autonomy does not require accepting abuse and tolerating unsafe behavior. When the actions of noncompliant patients create these circumstances, the team can act to set limits, including the final step of ending the caregiving relationship.

A team process provides an ethical way to consider and balance the risks to the individual and the resources of the provider agency. But upon occasion most teams are likely to need additional resources, either administrative or consultative, to prevent the "never-ending" situations that can rob the team process of its vitality and creativity while burning out individual staff. Administrators should be watchful, especially, when a team is inexperienced or encounters significant turnover in its key members. Key considerations for team process when dealing with noncompliant patients may be noted from Drinka (1994b):

- confront conflict constructively within the team as early as possible;
- give clear and consistent orientation to new team members;
- use regularly scheduled task-focused meetings to generate solutions and encourage team solidarity, rather than meeting individually with team members to address conflict within the team;
- assure formal and informal leadership of the team has been established;
- consider using and outside facilitator or consultant to address difficult situations within the team; and
- use a team retreat/team meetings to address team problems, not just to address clinical or policy issues.

Discussion Questions

1. Does a team have the right to terminate care for a noncompliant patient?

2. Was the team approach right for this patient? Or did it prolong an inevitable outcome?

3. How can health care teams best provide beneficent care to noncompliant, angry patients while coping with conflict within the team regarding patient autonomy?

4. Were ethical compromises made, or not made, by the team that had an impact on the therapeutic plan?

5. Does demanding care necessary for the noncompliant patient create stress for team members and distract them from caring for other, equally needy patients?

REFERENCES

Agich, G. 1990. Reassessing autonomy in long-term care. *Hastings Center Report* 20(6):12–17.

American Geriatrics Society. 1999. Making treatment decisions for incapacitated elderly patients without advance directives. Position Statement. New York: American Geriatrics Society.

Clark, P. 1994. Social, professional and educational values on the interdisciplinary team: Implications for gerontological and geriatric education. *Educational Gerontology* 20:35–51.

———. 1995. Quality of life, values, and teamwork in geriatric care: Do we communicate what we mean? *Gerontologist* 35(3):402–11.

Devor, M., A. Wang, M. Renvall, D. Feigal, and J. Ramsdell. 1994. Compliance with social and safety recommendations in an outpatient comprehensive geriatric assessment program. *Journals of Gerontology* 49(4):M168–73.

Drinka, T. 1991. Development and maintenance of an interdisciplinary health care team: A case study. *Gerontology and Geriatrics Education* 12(1):111–27.

———. 1994a. Interdisciplinary geriatric teams: Approaches to conflict as indicators of potential to model teamwork. *Educational Gerontology* 20:87–103.

———. 1994b. Case studies from purgatory: Maladaptive behavior within geriatrics health care teams. *Gerontologist* 34(4):541–47.

Eng, C. 1996. The On Lok/PACE model of geriatric managed care: An interdisciplinary approach to care of the frail elderly. *Current Concepts in Geriatric Managed Care* 2(9):4–24.

Eng, C., J. Pedulla, P. Eleazer, R. McCann, and N. Fox. 1997. Program of all-inclusive care for the elderly (PACE): An innovative model of integrated geriatric care and financing. *Journal of the American Geriatrics Society* 45(2):223–32.

Hall, M., and R. A. Berenson. 1998. Ethical practice in managed care: A dose of realism. *Annals of Internal Medicine* 128(5):395–402.

National PACE Association. 2001. PACE profile: Program of all-inclusive care for the elderly, 2001: Integrated acute and long-term care and service delivery financing. Alexandria, Va.: National PACE Association.

Recker, D., C. Bess, and H. Wellens. 1996. A decision-making process in shared governance. *Nursing Management* 27(5):48A–48D.

Reuben, D., M. Maly, S. Hirsch, J. Frank, A. Oakes, A. Siu, and R. Hays. 1996. Physician implementation of and patient adherence to recommendation from comprehensive geriatric assessment. *American Journal of Medicine* 100:444–51.

Shah, P., Maly, R., Frank, J., Hirsch, S., and D. Reuben. 1997. Managing geriatric syndromes: What geriatric assessment teams recommend, what primary care physicians implement, what patients adhere to. *Journal of the American Geriatrics Society* 45:413–19.

Shannon, S. 1997. The roots of interdisciplinary conflict around ethical issues. *Critical Care Nursing Clinics of North America* 9(1):3–28.

State of California. 1995–1996. Senate Bill 730 (Mello).

Walleck, C. 1991. Building the framework for dealing with ethical issues. *AORN Journal* 53(5):1248–51.

Weintraub, M. 1990. Compliance in the elderly. *Clinical Pharmacology* 6(2):445–51.

CHAPTER 9

Protecting Patients:
The Special Case of
Elder Abuse and Neglect

Carmel B. Dyer, M.D.,
Eileen Silverman, L.S.W.,
Trang Nguyen, M.D., and
Laurence B. McCullough, Ph.D.

The Texas Elder Abuse and Mistreatment (TEAM) Institute is an alliance between two services: a geriatric interdisciplinary program and a social service agency (Dyer et al. 1999). The geriatrics program is the Baylor College of Medicine Geriatrics Program at the Harris County Hospital District, and it includes geriatricians, nurse practitioners, nurse case managers, and social workers who provide comprehensive geriatric assessment. The other arm of TEAM is the Texas Department of Protective and Regulatory Services–Adult Protective Service Division (APS), whose specialists conduct investigations of cases of alleged abuse and neglect and focus on the social and environmental aspects of client care.

In addition to TEAM's educational and research goals, this unique interdisciplinary group assesses, intervenes with, and provides care to abused and neglected elders. Once it obtains a comprehensive geriatric history, performs a physical examination, and makes an APS evaluation, the TEAM group meets to develop a plan of care. Although all members share in the mission of improving the lives of abused or neglected elders, the APS approach often differs from the traditional medical approach. The APS specialist must always respect client autonomy; the medical service also values this principle in regard to patients but recognizes that not everyone has decision-making capacity. The APS ethical perspective reflects the strong emphasis on client autonomy in the professional ethics of social work. In addition, APS acts as an agent of the state and must respect the civil rights of people. The geriatric program's ethical perspective reflects both respect for patient autonomy and beneficence as prima facie principles of health care ethics. Conflicts arise when patients without decision-making capacity need medical and social interventions. The following case illustrates how different ethical perspectives within such an interdisciplinary team create challenges to the group's cohesion and how the tools of ethics, especially preventive ethics, help to address such challenges effectively, so that the TEAM retains moral cohesion for the benefit of the patient.

Case Description

Mrs. Jean Norman is a 73-year-old German-born widow who migrated to the United States after World War II. She has been married twice and has no children. She lives in a home that she purchased before her first marriage. She has only two distant nieces, and the person closest to her is her neighbor of thirty years.

APS received a report on Mrs. Norman alleging medical and physical neglect. It made an initial investigation and found that she had multiple dogs and that there was a foul smell and fleas in the home. She did have food in the refrigerator, and all utilities were turned on. She appeared poorly groomed, her clothing was soiled, and there was no washing machine. The home was cluttered but posed no danger to her. The patient admitted to hypertension and diabetes, as well as to forgetting to take her medication. She reported a prior stroke, during which time she willed her property to her church. Since then, no church members had provided any assistance.

The APS specialist noted that the patient was oriented to person and place but not to time. She was forgetful but very clear about her desires to remain in her own home. At this point, the APS specialist asked the medical service to look for treatable causes of cognitive impairment for the expressed purpose of maintaining Mrs. Norman's autonomy and capacity for self-care and therefore keeping her own home.

A geriatrician visited Mrs. Norman's home and saw the same findings as did

APS. In addition to hypertension and diabetes, the patient admitted to some memory problems. She denied depression. Halfway through the interview, she forgot that she was speaking to a physician and had to be reminded about this fact.

Physical examination revealed a blood pressure of 220/80, a red shiny tongue, pruritic nodules all over her arms and torso, Mini-Mental State Examination score of 21/30, a Geriatric Depression score of 4/15, and a Hopkins Competency Assessment Test score was 1 out of 11 (normal score is 4 over 11). There were no focal neurologic findings.

The patient presented to clinic and was evaluated by the members of the geriatric program, who attempted to manage Mrs. Norman's blood pressure as an outpatient. Further workup revealed that the patient had (1) possible Alzheimer disease, with vitamin B_{12} deficiency, (2) flea infestation vs. scabies, (3) uncontrolled hypertension, and (4) Type II diabetes, uncontrolled with a hemoglobin A_{1C} of 11.6.

It is the APS policy to honor the wishes of its clients and to allow clients to take sometimes-considerable health risks. By contrast, the geriatric professionals were very concerned about Mrs. Norman's serious medical conditions, the ongoing poor management of which might further impair her independence and safety. The geriatric program members focused on safety as a necessary condition for independence and thus were reluctant to accept considerable health risks to the patient. They therefore felt that she could stay at home only if the following were in place: (1) provider services to administer medicines and help with activities of daily living; (2) home health services to monitor blood pressure and blood sugar values and to teach the provider how to care for the patient; (3) regular medical follow-up; (4) general clean-up of the home, including especially bedding and clothing; and (5) initiating of treatment for the above-described medical conditions. If these aspects of health maintenance and safety could not be met, the geriatric program members recommended hospitalization for acute control of medical problems and subsequent guardianship. The members of the TEAM group met, but the APS members were opposed to both hospitalization and guardianship on the grounds that these steps violated the patient's wishes, which the patient could verbalize and which were consistent with her past history. Thus, an ethical conflict arose within the TEAM group, generated by the two ethical perspectives described at the beginning of this chapter.

The patient was eventually hospitalized for accelerated hypertension after failing outpatient treatment. She did well. But some members of the geriatric program felt that guardianship was now in order. The APS members of the TEAM group did not. The APS members persuaded all members of the TEAM group that this patient should be allowed to stay in her own home, but with a guardian appointed. After a thorough investigation of the patient's neighborhood and relatives by APS, guardians of her finances and her person were appointed, and the patient is presently being well maintained in her own home.

Case Analysis

To maintain moral cohesion of the TEAM group for patient benefit in response to this conflict, we propose to take a preventive ethics approach to the management of the conflicting views of the geriatrics program and APS specialists in this case, especially concerning the conflict between safety and independence. Preventive ethics seeks to identify the potential for conflict in advance and to identify strategies for preventing such conflicts from emerging. When conflicts still do emerge, the goal is to manage them in ways that avoid deep division among those responsible for the interdisciplinary team. A preventive ethics approach responds to conflicts (i.e., either/or choices) with efforts to identify middle ground on which the parties potentially or actually in conflict may agree (McCullough and Chervenak 1994). In this way, the interests of the patient or client are advanced and, as a result, moral cohesion within the interdisciplinary team is promoted by keeping the main focus where it belongs, on the fiduciary obligation of all TEAM group members to protect and promote the interests of the patient or client. *Fiduciary obligation* means that health care professionals should make protecting and promoting the patient's health-related interests the priority consideration, with the self-interest of professionals a systematically secondary consideration. Health care professionals on the TEAM group share this obligation. The distinctive strength of the TEAM group is that the different professionals within it bring different ethical perspectives on what should count as being in the patient or client's interest. The patient or client usually benefits from this multidisciplinary approach. But this strength can also be a source of potential conflict. For example, members of the TEAM group can reasonably give different weight to beneficence-based (safety) and autonomy-based (independence) obligations to the patient or client, as they appear to be doing in this case. Preventive ethics looks for ways to harmonize the potentially competing ethical perspectives, rather than allow them to lead to unnecessary conflict, which can divide the TEAM group members and thus badly serve patients or clients.

Identify Patient and Family Preferences

Mrs. Norman was judged by APS specialists to be oriented as to person and place but not to time. She appeared very independent. When she was offered provider care services, she refused them. She was adamant about remaining in her own home. She stated that she was proud of the fact that prior to her first marriage she had worked and was able on her own earnings to purchase the home and property that she currently owned and occupied. She stated repeatedly that she wanted always to remain in her home.

On the one hand, based on the psychological evaluations described above, Mrs. Norman's decision-making capacity appeared to be impaired. As a consequence, some of her decisions (e.g., refusing provider care services) reflect diminished decision-making capacity and therefore were unwise in terms of protecting her health-related interests. On the other hand, she clearly expressed a strong preference for remaining in her home, and this preference appeared to reflect long-held, expressed values. But since individuals have the right to make unwise choices, the team had to determine if the patient both understood and accepted the consequences of her decisions.

In the discourse of bioethics, if one approached this case based on a presumption of intact decision-making capacity, then there is good reason to doubt that the presumption would apply, based on the evaluation described above. As a consequence, the patient's right to make her own decisions would be justifiably discounted. But if one approached this case on the basis of respect for Mrs. Norman as a person, because her preferences reflect lifelong values, those preferences would be given serious weight by the TEAM group. It is critical for any health care team to distinguish which patients have the capacity to participate in their decision making and which don't. Doing so avoids acts of commission as well as omission.

A preventive ethics approach emphasizes respect for the patient's values and decision making and supports those values to the greatest extent possible. While medical teams and adult protective service specialists assess capacity, only the legal profession can determine competence. Preventive ethics therefore eschews the rights-based approach and turns to legal adjudication of competence as the first response. One result of this rights-based and legal focus could be a finding of incompetence, with subsequent loss of rights. This loss would surely have imperiled Mrs. Norman's preference to stay in her home. The other result could be a finding that she was not incompetent, with full rights to refuse medical management and home supports. This, too, could have imperiled her preference to stay at home, should she become so ill that emergency hospitalization was required. Rather than seeking legal recourse, therefore, the TEAM group embraced the goal of attempting to implement Mrs. Norman's preference to stay in her home without legal review, unless this legal review became necessary later, and with needed support to maintain her health as a necessary condition for maintaining this independence.

Evaluate Quality-of-Life Issues

Without appropriate medical management, Mrs. Norman was at risk of serious loss of health and functional status. Such losses could have jeopardized her quality of life and her ability to stay at home. In the discourse of current bioethics, one way to frame the ethical issues in this case is in terms of a conflict between beneficence-based and autonomy-based obligations to Mrs. Norman (Beauchamp and Childress 1994). These two kinds of obligations originate in two possible perspectives that can be taken on the more general obligation to protect and promote Mrs. Norman's interests as a patient and client.

Beneficence is an ethical principle that translates a rigorous clinical perspective on a patient's health-related interests into clinical action guides (McCullough and Chervenak 1994). From this perspective, protecting the patient from preventable loss of health status, secondary to poorly managed blood pressure and poor living conditions, and protecting the patient from preventable loss of life, secondary to the long-term effects of poorly managed blood pressure or perhaps an unattended fall that could go undiscovered for a prolonged period of time, become paramount considerations. It is clear that in this case the medical service made its recommendations based on beneficence-based obligations to the patient; it was placing the greater emphasis on Mrs. Norman's safety.

The beneficence-based approach to understanding the obligations of clinicians to their patients has been subjected to serious criticism in the bioethics literature, because of the paternalism to which it can sometimes lead. Paternalism means restricting the autonomy of the patient on the basis of beneficence (Beauchamp and Childress 1994). Against paternalism it has been argued that patients have their own perspective on their own interests and that others should respect that perspective, creating autonomy-based obligations. Respect for autonomy means that clinicians should acknowledge and elicit the patient's or client's values and preferences and carry out those preferences. Respect for autonomy is implemented in the informed consent process and accents individual liberty and freedom, including the freedom to act in ways that others—especially clinicians and other professionals—may think are unwise or even dangerous in terms of the patient's health-related interests. Very few exceptions are allowed (e.g., life-threatening emergencies in which there is no time for consent). It is clear in this case that the APS professionals were acting on autonomy-based obligations to their client; they were placing the greater emphasis on Mrs. Norman's independence.

Bart Collopy has suggested that the perceived dichotomy between safety and independence is a false dichotomy (Collopy 1995). He takes a biopsychosocial approach to both. A biopsychosocial view treats safety and independence as complex phenomena that incorporate biological and therefore health-related factors, psychological factors, and social factors. On such a view, safety and independence should be seen not as dichotomous but as the ends of a continuum of ethical concern. Consider, first, safety. It is related not just to physical health and well-being but also to what Collopy helpfully describes as "psychological safeties." On the basis of this broader concept of safety, removing Mrs. Norman from her home would not necessarily have been a psychologically safe thing to do for or to her, because it could have deprived her of a sense of place in which she felt at home and secure in her self-identity. Moreover, violating her preference to stay in her home could have been experienced by Mrs. Norman as a severe form of psychological violence. As a consequence, she might have felt less psychologically safe away from her home, in which she took great pride of ownership.

Consider independence. It is not just related to self-image and other psychological factors but also involves physical health and well-being as necessary preconditions. On this broader concept of independence, leaving Mrs. Norman in her home without supports and leaving her medical problems unmanaged could have resulted in her losing health and functional status, and to that degree her independence as well.

When safety and independence are considered biopsychosocially, as Collopy argues, it is apparent that Mrs. Norman's health and functional status, and physical safety were necessary conditions for her psychological and social independence. The latter was a necessary condition for her psychological safety. On a preventative ethics approach, the TEAM would thus have been guided by Mrs. Norman's preference for independence and would have addressed the aspects of her physical safety that were necessary conditions for her psychosocial safety and independence. On this preventive ethics approach, the potential for conflict would have been reduced. Indeed, the goal was not just conflict resolution but management of the patient's problems in a way that protects both her safety and her independence, because protecting both is essential to implementing her preference to stay in her home.

Consider Contextual Factors

Every state has an adult protective service program, but in the absence of federal mandates, each state determines how such programs are administered. Programs differ in administrative structure, service delivery, populations served, and type of abuse reported (Goodrich 1997). Despite these differences, their ultimate goals are often the same: to provide services to their clients while maintaining the autonomy of competent older persons and to always seek the least restrictive alternative when considering dispositions.

The state of Texas has a unique model for adult protective services. The Texas Department of Protective and Regulatory Services (TDPRS) is a separate agency. APS is one of its divisions and is divided into eleven regions. The TEAM Institute is a collaboration between the TDPRS and Baylor College of Medicine Geriatrics Program at the Harris County Hospital District, but TEAM members work most closely with Region 6 APS specialists in Harris and surrounding counties. The Harris County Hospital District is supported by local property taxes and billings of insurance companies and serves the medically indigent who reside in the county.

The broad definition of elder mistreatment is that which causes unnecessary pain and suffering among elders. Self-neglect is the most common form of elder mistreatment (Fulmer and Paveza 1998; National Center on Elder Abuse 1996). The definitions of *self-neglect* differ from state to state. Self-neglect is reportable in forty-six states (Goodrich 1997). The National Association of Adult Protective Service Administrators (NAAPSA) supports the following working definition of *self-neglect*: "Self-neglect is the result of an adult's inability, due to physical and/or mental impairments or diminished capacity to perform essential self-care tasks including: providing essential food, clothing shelter, and medical care; obtaining goods or services necessary to maintain physical health, mental health, emotional well-being and general safety; and/or managing financial affairs" (National Association of Adult Protective Service Administrators 1990). The case of Mrs. Norman meets the NAAPSA definition of self-neglect.

In her case APS specialists of Region 6 conducted an initial investigation of the referral, including interviews with the client, family, and friends, and completed an overall assessment summary. There were several concerns regarding Mrs. Norman's safety and ability to remain in her own home. Some of these concerns included inability to handle her own finances, poor living conditions, poor personal hygiene, isolation, and most importantly, short-term memory problems, especially forgetfulness to take needed medications for control of diabetes and high blood pressure. In spite of these concerns, it was the opinion of APS that a nursing home placement would most likely cause the client to deteriorate rapidly both mentally and physically.

APS tried, without success, to get out-of-state family relatives to assume some legal responsibility for Mrs. Norman. The only person who appeared willing to take on some responsibility for her was a younger neighbor, who had known Mrs. Norman for many years. The realization that she was at high risk of having another stroke unless a provider could be placed in her home was, for APS, the deciding factor in agreement that a guardian be requested for Mrs. Norman.

Before her short-term memory loss, Mrs. Norman admitted that she did take her blood pressure and diabetes medications. She was aware that she was now forgetting to take them. Therefore, it could not be said that failure to take medications was a lifetime preference for Mrs. Norman. Previously, she did have a lifetime preference of using natural remedies and a healthy diet for prevention of medical problems, as opposed to conventional medical treatment. But once she was diagnosed with high blood pressure and diabetes, she did agree to take prescribed medications.

Resolve the Ethical Issues and Create the Plan

To stabilize her medical condition, Mrs. Norman agreed to be admitted to the hospital. During this period, the TEAM group decided that the required physician's statement of incapacity should be sent to the probate court, with a request by APS for a guardian of both person and finances. In addition, a letter was sent by APS indicating the findings of its investigation. Both the geriatrician's statement and the APS specialist's letter requested the court to consider allowing the client to remain in her own home.

Although the TEAM members agreed that a request for a guardian be made, there were differences in opinion among members about how Mrs. Norman's case should be managed. When she was ready for hospital discharge and prior to a guardian being appointed, some TEAM members felt strongly that she should not be returned home due to poor living conditions. Other TEAM members felt Mrs. Norman should be returned to her own home. Everyone involved was concerned that the appointed guardian might not allow her to remain in her home and might place her in either a nursing home or a personal care home, regardless of her lifetime preferences.

After Mrs. Norman was discharged to her home, the probate court appointed an *ad litem* attorney and temporary guardian of both person and finances. It was then determined that a permanent guardian would be appointed. The final decision of the permanent guardian was that Mrs. Norman should remain in her home. Her longtime friend and neighbor would become guardian of the person, and the court-appointed guardian would remain guardian of finances. The friend now sees the client daily and assures that she has personal care assistance as well as reminders to take needed medications.

APS specialists are bound by two clearly defined principles: (1) they should strive for the least restrictive environment, and (2) they must maintain the autonomy of their client. On the other hand, geriatric medical professionals have an ethical responsibility to clients that is not defined based on a single ethical principle. In addition, avoiding life-threatening illness and loss of function tend to predominate over maintaining autonomy in the minds of most medical professionals. Also, many gerontologic professionals acknowledge that in some cases the least restrictive environment may involve alternative placement other than one's home. The role of the geriatric program members in Mrs. Norman's case was to identify the medical processes at hand and correct any reversible or treatable disease. The geriatricians identified diabetes out of control, uncontrolled hypertension, scabies, possible Alzheimer disease, and vitamin B_{12} deficiency. Most of these disorders are reversible.

After these treatable medical diseases were identified, it was not clear that the treatment plan could be carried out in the patient's home. A discussion ensued at the TEAM meeting about whether a trial of care in a home with increased support was favorable over a short stay in a nursing home, where the treatments could be closely monitored. This is an example of a situation where different conclusions may be reached for precisely the same problem, based on the way the questions are framed and how vivid various alternatives are in the mind of the decider (Kane 1995). Clearly, physicians and medical staff feel more in control when the patient or client is in a health care facility. There they can call in orders and, through other health professionals, control the access to these resources and ultimately the patient/client. APS specialists more commonly project themselves into the client's position and act as protectors of patient's preferences. In this case, the specialists worked very hard to provide enough support at home that the physicians could be comfortable that attention would be paid to the medical disorders.

The APS specialist and the physician who had made the initial house call believed that the neighbor could provide the proper support. They convinced the rest of the TEAM group, and an in-home trial of therapy and support was attempted. The TEAM group then resolved the issue of how to evaluate the efficacy of the interdisciplinary care plan. At the present time, there is no easily administered litmus test for the presence of abuse and neglect. APS specialists make their determinations by follow-up visits, although there is pressure to close cases as new cases come in. Mrs. Norman's medical problems could be monitored by vitamin B_{12} levels, hemoglobin A_{1C}, the Mini-Mental State Examination, and blood pressure determinations. Home health services, critical to this process, were ordered, and the nurses were able to administer vitamin B_{12} shots and monitor the appropriate laboratory and examination parameters previously outlined. The medical service recommended that the patient be monitored every two to three months in the outpatient geriatrics clinic. The interdisciplinary team agreed to make another house call if the patient did not return to clinic.

The care plan outlined by the TEAM members was not as detailed as it would have been had the patient been in a nursing home. This plan was less likely to dictate the client's entire life since home care providers do not exert the same degree of control over the client/patient. Therefore, the TEAM had to rely on the guardian as well as the provider to ensure that the patient got the appropriate medical treatment. The geriatrics case manager would, in turn, have to oversee the whole process and make herself available to any of the related parties, should the need arise.

This case raises a number of general questions relating to the elderly and their place in society. Both agencies represented on the TEAM group were public agencies, with the support of a private medical school. In addition, the patient's hospitalization and subsequent house cleaning were all supported by public funds. Generally, Wilson notes the mismatch between the prevalence of older people for continued community residence and the public financing that has primarily funded institutional service (McCullough and Wilson 1995). In Mrs. Norman's case, a large investment of public funds was used to support her in the community. At what point should we stop investing public funds to maintain autonomy and independence of elderly people? Does that point occur when it is cheaper to live in a nursing home than in the community? Does it occur sooner if there are fewer established public service agencies than there are in a large city such as Houston? Should there be a different standard for those who are in rural versus urban areas?

There are no settled answers to these vexing questions, either in ethics or in public policy. TEAM members, therefore, must make decisions in the absence of a definitive justice-based account of appropriate resource allocation. Relevant values guide this decision-making process. Generally, most gerontologic professionals, including APS specialists, believe that it is always better to live at home than in a nursing home. Some would disagree when the patient's safety is so jeopardized that staying at home would result in a loss of function and ultimately a loss of independence. In addition, some individuals have a better quality of life in a nursing home; these are usually people who need a structured environment in order to maintain their clarity of thinking. At what point should the interdisciplinary team take into consideration the neighbors of a person who represents a hazard to the community? What if the patient is leaving food on the stove and causing fires or a gas explosion? When a patient poses a safety risk to others, what is our responsibility to the community at large, beyond our responsibility to the individual?

Conclusion

The successful team management of a complex case is similar to connecting the pieces of a puzzle. When individual team members work in separate corners, they perceive only a single piece of the puzzle. For instance, physicians are often trained in acute care settings. They rely on diagnostic techniques and data from laboratory tests, X-rays, and clinical procedures to narrow the range of options to a pathophysiological category. APS specialists, on the other hand, view a case from a psychosocial viewpoint, in which family relations, home environment, personal values and preferences, income, and availability of re-sources are considered (Wilson 2001). A geriatric program's level of success is then based on how effectively each member shares information, ideas, and perspectives, allowing their information and ethical perspective to be integrated into a coherent, fact-based account of what alternatives are in the patient's health-related interest.

In addition, the diverse cultural backgrounds, professional training, and practicing philosophies of team members shape a geriatric program's perspective. Members of any team need to recognize and appreciate these differences among the individual disciplines in order to promote the team and self-growth (Coutts and Woods 2001).

Conflict is a natural process of evolution in an interdisciplinary team (Wilson 2001). Conflicts that cannot be resolved lead to team separation and recession, whereas successful resolution of conflicts promotes team advancement. This requires, in part, the means to exchange information effectively. The geriatrics program and APS agency hold regular meetings to review APS-referred cases. During these meetings, the TEAM members identify problems, share the facts, and discuss solutions. In particular, all members work toward resolving their conflicts by focusing on a common goal. The common goal, in Mrs. Norman's case, was to act in the patient's best interests. The TEAM members agreed that several issues be emphasized. These included the patient's quality of life, personal preferences, safety, and independence.

Let's take a step back to review each service's perspective. The geriatrics program had diagnosed Mrs. Norman with possible Alzheimer disease and a vitamin B_{12} deficiency contributing to her memory loss. She was deemed incapacitated, as she could not make an informed decision regarding her health and social welfare. In addition, she had hypertension and diabetes and a history of noncompliance with her medications. This placed her at an extreme risk for further self-neglect. Mrs. Norman might experience a medical problem, such as stroke, that would further compromise her function, or she might die as a result of self-neglect of her medical problems.

Although the APS specialists' opinions differed in that they strongly preferred a home discharge versus personal care home or nursing home placement, they were able to provide crucial information pertaining to Mrs. Norman's social environment. This made a discharge to home more feasible. They had found a neighbor who had known the patient for years and who was willing to become her provider and guardian of person when none of the patient's relatives would volunteer.

The later stages of conflict resolution include accepting solutions where both parties gain, and implementing the plan (Wilson 2001). In this case, in a consensus decision, the geriatric program members and APS specialists agreed to send Mrs. Norman home on a trial of home-based care and management. This plan would preserve her independence and maintain respect for her personal preference. She was expected to fare better psychologically at home, thus improving her quality of life. APS helped initiate house cleaning and provider service. The geriatric program requested home health service for medications, blood pressure, and blood sugar monitoring, as well as provider teaching to ensure adequate health maintenance. The patient was to be closely monitored by the medical service. Should her medical or social condition worsen so as to place her at risk for medical, bodily, or psychological harm, her case would be reassessed as an interdisciplinary team, and the previous option for placement would then be reconsidered.

Discussion Questions

1. What might have happened to this patient if adult protective services alone had handled the case?

2. Would the outcome have been the same if the medical team had seen the patient without input from APS?

3. At what point might an ethics consultation have been helpful?

4. How far does the obligation of the medical professional extend to vulnerable, reclusive community dwellers?

5. What are some ways that medical teams can resolve conflict when their ethical responsibilities clash with those of another discipline or agency?

6. Who would be held accountable if the patient harmed herself or another (e.g., left the gas stove on)? Was APS or the medical service responsible for the outcome of this case?

ACKNOWLEDGMENTS

The authors would like to thank Mr. Samuel Riley for his technical assistance and the Texas Department of Protective and Regulatory Services, APS Division, especially Region 6, for their support of the TEAM Institute.

REFERENCES

Beauchamp, T. L., and J. F. Childress. 1994. *Principles of biomedical ethics,* 4th ed. New York: Oxford University Press.

Collopy, B. J. 1995. Safety and independence: Rethinking some basic concepts in long term care. In L. B. McCullough and N. L. Wilson, eds., *Long-term care decisions: Ethical and conceptual dimensions.* Baltimore: Johns Hopkins University Press.

Coutts, L., and A. Woods. 2001. Communication. In D. Long and N. L. Wilson, eds., *Geriatric interdisciplinary team training: A curriculum from the Huffington Center on Aging at Baylor College of Medicine.* New York: John A. Hartford Foundation, Inc.

Dyer, C. B., D. J. Hyman, V. Pavlik, K. P. Murphy, and M. S. Gleason. 1999. Elder neglect: A collaboration between a geriatrics assessment team and adult protective services. *Southern Medical Journal* 92(2):242–44.

Fulmer, T., and G. Paveza. 1998. Neglect in the elder patient. *Geriatric Nursing* 33(3):457–66.

Goodrich, C. S. 1997. Results of a national survey of state protective services programs: Assessing risk and defining victim outcomes. *Journal of Elder Abuse and Neglect* 9(1):69–86.

Kane, R. 1995. Decision-making care plans and life plans in long-term care: Can case managers take account of clients' values and preferences? In L. B. McCullough, and N. L. Wilson, eds., *Long-term care decisions: Ethical and conceptual dimensions.* Baltimore: Johns Hopkins University Press.

McCullough, L. B., and F. A. Chervenak. 1994. *Ethics in obstetrics and gynecology.* New York: Oxford University Press.

McCullough, L. B. , and N. L. Wilson, eds. 1995. *Long-term care decisions: Ethical and conceptual dimensions.* Baltimore: Johns Hopkins University Press.

National Association of Adult Protective Service Administrators. 1990. Position paper on self-neglect.

National Center on Elder Abuse. 1996. Homepage. www.aoa.dhhs.gov/AOA/dir/143.html.

Wilson, N. L. 2001. *Conflict management.* In D. Long and N. L. Wilson, eds., *Geriatric interdisciplinary team training: A curriculum from the Huffington Center on Aging at Baylor College of Medicine.* New York: John A. Hartford Foundation, Inc.

PART IV

Teams and How They Work
Across Health Care Settings

CHAPTER 10

Using Ethics Consultation to Resolve Team Conflict

Nancy Neveloff Dubler, LL.B.,
Kathryn Hyer, Dr.P.A., M.P.P., and
Terry T. Fulmer, R.N., Ph.D.

The number and complexity of ethical dilemmas in medicine continue to grow exponentially. Most of the problems that are encountered in clinical practice and explored in the literature relate to the appropriate care of patients in the acute care setting at the end of life. Such exploration includes analyses of the selection of surrogate decision makers for incapacitated patients, the rules and standards for end-of-life decisions, and the appropriate role for ethics consultations, risk management, and professional standards in oversight and review.

In addition to discussions of the ethical dimensions of care at the end of life, dilemmas about the coverage or benefit package of managed care plans, about the costs and distributive justice of allocating scarce health care resources, and about conflicts of interest between providers and their patients have infused the ambulatory setting. These inquiries even engage potential patients before illness when, as consumers, they must make choices about which plan and what set of benefits most closely fits their anticipated needs.

Ethical discussions and analyses must now address a range of interconnected ethical, financial, and professional decision points. In 1999 the ethics consultation service at Montefiore Medical Center noted that the fastest-growing category of consultation requests had come from the clinical care coordinators on the hospital floors, predominantly nurses and social workers whose primary responsibilities included monitoring length of stay and planning for and expediting discharge. Time in the hospital rather than time to death is rapidly emerging as the decision issue that triggers discussions of rights, duties, and obligations.

The "business" of doing ethics has also changed remarkably over the last decade. The term *informed consent* first appeared in a law case in 1957 (*Salgo* v. *Leland Stanford Jr. University Board of Trustees* 1957) that explored the allocation of decision-making authority between the patient and the physician. Somewhat later the dialogue was enlarged to encompass discussions among the patient, family members, and the health care team (Beauchamp and Childress 1994). Concurrently in the scholarly ethical, religious, and clinical literature, a multidisciplinary dialogue developed that identified the rights and interests of all of the parties involved in a medical encounter in the context of race, class, gender, and ethnicity.

Many of these analyses were used by an increasing number of bioethics consultants to help practitioners, patients, and families reach decisions that made sense in the context of the needs, wants, desires, and interests of the patient in the larger context of the family and quality of life. Along the way, however, and in a development that is promising, ethics moved out of the realm of the sacred and into the profane reality of medical care and practice. Doctors, nurses, and social workers began to note that there were ethical issues in the cases that they were managing, and they began to grapple with them, with greater or lesser degrees of success. The job of ethics consultants was to conduct an ethical analysis of the situation, lead the discussions, and train the trainers so that they, too, could address the issues comfortably when they came up in the context of medical care (Veatch 1997).

Finally, in this rather brief overview of the history of the integration of bioethics into the medical arena, the Joint Commission on Accreditation of Healthcare Organizations (JCAHO) required that all hospitals demonstrate the capacity to address ethical issues both as they relate to patient care and as they emerge from the larger world of organizational and institutional commitments. In this maelstrom, one of the few stable points for consideration and serious contemplation of the patient in the context of medical care is the team.

The ability of professionals to work together to create an integrated plan and coordinate care over time and place is frequently a function of how well these professionals operate as an interdisciplinary team. When multiple specialists separately coordinate care, services can be at odds with each other and patients can suffer. This "layering" of orders, one upon another, is multidisciplinary care. Multidisciplinary care contrasts sharply with interdisciplinary care—integrated care developed by skilled clinicians who jointly agree to prioritize care activities, work together to implement the plan of care, and hold each other accountable for that care.

Well-articulated and coordinated patient-centered interdisciplinary care does not just happen. It requires the establishment of team norms, operating standards and agreement across disciplines, ongoing communication, and shared decision-making processes. Sometimes when teams agree to a standardized approach for handling a complex patient, the cross-disciplinary agreements can be formalized through the use of protocols. Thus, the team requires little ongoing communication as long as the patient remains stable and the care proceeds as expected.

Conflict can emerge, however, when the patient's values are at odds with the team's standard operating procedures. To arrive at an acceptable plan of care, the team will need to determine the appropriate way to analyze the facts and reconcile them with the patient's wishes and preferences. The focus on the patient requires that the team members work to reach consensus on the goals of care, set priorities for treatment, and develop a plan for monitoring and evaluating the outcome. Without a full and sometimes heated discussion of the patient's needs, there may not be adequate recognition of the tradeoffs inherent in the plan of care, and the benefit of team care may not be realized. Effective teamwork in health care requires agreement on the team's plan of care or on the outcome of the team process by all members of the team. Furthermore, all members must contribute to the implementation of the care plan, and each must accept accountability for the plan.

Teams can offer an important advantage in the resolution of clinical dilemmas by creating a forum for a full discussion of the patient's values, including the patient's right to refuse care. The group discussion ensures that all perspectives are taken into account and that the plan developed has a good probability of being accepted by the patient and family. Some forms of teams discussed elsewhere in this book (see Chapter 3) assume that the patient is the center of the team and an integral member of the team process. But when a patient refuses to participate, disagrees with the plan of care, or has values that are at odds with the values of the clinical team members, ethical dilemmas are bound to arise that challenge the ability of the team to function effectively. In such circumstances, the team must be supportive of each member so as to maintain the larger cohesiveness of the group and the appropriate functioning of the team for the sake of other patients cared for by the team. (See Chapter 8.)

Becoming a team requires work. Tuckman (1965) has identified the four stages of team development as forming, storming, norming, and performing. (See Chapter 2 for a more thorough discussion of these stages.) Such ethical dilemmas as a patient's refusal to participate in planning care can cause roadblocks for appropriate team functioning. On the other hand, ethical dilemmas and their subsequent in-team controversy can help identify circumstances in which teams believe they are "performing" but may not actually be doing so. When ethical dilemmas do inhibit the full functioning of the team, members may request adjudication by an outside body, such as an ethics consultation service or committee. If consultation is used to assist the team in ensuring that all perspectives are taken into account and that the plan of care has a good probability of being accepted and adhered to by the patient and family, ethics consultation may be an appropriate enhancement. But the primary care team must take precautions not to abdicate its decision-making function and responsibility for managing the patient by transferring that role to the ethics consultant. When a team refuses to resolve issues at the primary care team level, it may not only reduce the quality of the conversation but also actually defer the care of the patient to someone who may be less capable of ensuring that the patient's values are included in the discussion and who has no ongoing responsibility for implementing the plan.

Teams and team members must also be aware that within the overall institution, not all teams may be considered equal. If another team, such as an ethics committee, is deemed superior to the primary care team, the perspectives of the members of the primary care team may be considered less valuable than the values of the ethics committee members. Teams must not only avoid the groupthink that comes from performing as a well-functioning team (see Chapter 11) but recognize what aspects of the institutional context might inhibit their ability to perform as a team.

Finally, team members must always walk a fine line between their personal values and beliefs, their identity as a member of their own profession (nursing, social work, medicine, etc.), and their identity as a member of the team within their institution (discharge planning team, ethics team, etc.) (Drinka and Clark 2000). Team members must recognize the values and professional roles of the other members of the team, as well as the role each person plays in the larger organizational context. For instance, if the care plan agreed to by the other members of a team appears, in the opinion of one team member, to conflict with her legal obligations as a member of her profession, the team must recognize this dilemma and include the issue in the overall discussion of the plan of care. Helping the individual professional reconcile his or her responsibility as a solo professional while recognizing that the team is also responsible for care can be a positive aspect of being on a team and an important support to the professional. Ultimately, an awareness of the larger context in which teams work may be essential to understanding some of the ethical dilemmas that are posed by caring for older patients with complex care needs.

At Montefiore Medical Center, one of the teams that has had the most experience with ethical issues is the geriatric team, which comes together each week in rounds to consider the care of a particular patient in the geriatric service. Founded in the late 1970s, the team continues to meet weekly. The team is composed of the main members of and consultants to the geriatric practice. Ongoing participants include geriatric physicians, social workers and nurses who work on the acute care service, and the allied professionals in the long-term care step-down unit or the ambulatory care practice. Experts who are not normally members of the primary care geriatric team are invited to provide additional expertise at the request of the team. As patient or family needs dictate, invitees to team meetings may include consulting physicians from gastroenterology, orthopedics, ophthalmology, cardiology, or other subspecialties, as well as nutrition, home care, rehabilitation, neurology, psychiatry, and bioethics. In some cases, home care administrators and community social workers are also present. Members of the city agencies involved in protecting abused elderly persons have also been invited to act as legal representatives for some elderly patients.

The format, the accepted ground rules for behavior, and the protocol for the rounds are always the same and provide the predictable context within which the team process of an open, full discussion can occur (Hyer 2000). Experts and members of the team discussing the case join the geriatrician at the front of the room. The presenting physician prepares, in advance, a written summary of the medical events in the case. One of the geriatricians will present the case in the agreed-upon format for this meeting: history, medical conditions, social support, and summary of the problem to be discussed at the meeting. Experts offer their analysis and references, and a discussion follows. In certain cases, the patient will be invited into the room, and the geriatric psychiatrist will interview the patient to provide additional information for the assembled group. The ethics expert sometimes sits among the team members and sometimes, when the ethical issues are the most prominent, among the panel for the day. On the day in question for the following case, the ethics resource person sat with the team.

We present here one case that was discussed in the ethics rounds using the format suggested by Jonsen, Siegler, and Winslade (1998). Names and circumstances have been changed as necessary to protect the anonymity of the participants while maintaining the integrity of the circumstances at issue.

Case Description

Mr. Leon Telly was a 73-year-old African American who had become legally blind as a result of poorly controlled diabetes. He had severe retinopathy with neuropathy and hypertension. He had been admitted to the hospital eight months earlier due to a change in mental status and what initially seemed to be some temporary ambulatory problems related to a slight stroke that apparently had occurred several days before the admission. When questioned about the delay in seeking medical assistance, the home health aide who accompanied him to the emergency room complained that Mr. Telly refused to go to the hospital earlier.

Mr. Telly's long stay in the institution began with admission to an inpatient unit, where he had a second stroke, followed by a transfer to a subacute care unit within the institution for rehabilitation. After the subacute admission, approximately three months after the initial admission, he was transferred to the long-term care facility, where it became apparent that Mr. Telly needed medical care to stabilize his diabetes. After stabilizing his diabetes, the physician decided to try to change from injectable insulin to an oral agent despite his history of insulin dependence. Approximately three months later, the oral agent, along with diabetes education, seemed to be working.

His prehospitalization history was unremarkable except for his stable pattern of neglecting his medical needs. He was treated in the community for his diabetes but regularly let his medications lapse and would go for months on end without insulin. When his eyesight had deteriorated, his physician tried to get him to accept the services of a visiting nurse so he could receive insulin injections. He agreed to receive services but then refused to admit the visiting nurse or any other ancillary service provider, other than his personal care attendant, into his home. At the time of admission to the hospital, Mr. Telly admitted that he was not able to read his insulin bottle or see the level of insulin in his needle. His injection practice was, at best, inadequate. If his diabetes and hypertension could be managed, his prognosis was quite good, as he had no other life-threatening illnesses. There were no signs of physical neglect—he was clean and well nourished—but clear signs of medical neglect. The patient denied that he was blind as the result of his neglected diabetes and assured the team that he had injected his insulin adequately for years. He also denied hypertension or any other medical problem.

Mr. Telly had lived alone in the same apartment building for over a decade. He had no close friends and had never married. He had one brother, who appeared to be concerned about his care and who had even offered to have him placed in a nursing home nearby so that he could help him. The patient dismissed this offer and explained that the reason his brother wanted him nearer was to steal his money. Since the patient was on Medicaid, the medical staff assumed that there was little to steal. He explained that if there were any problems in the home, he contacted the superintendent in the building, who had helped him in the past and would be expected to continue to help him when he returned to his apartment.

The patient's aide, who was paid by Medicaid, was quite attached to him. Some of the staff felt that the attachment was not appropriate to the role of a paid worker. The aide did the patient's bidding, continued to visit frequently even after he was in the hospital for months, and at one point attempted to take him home against medical advice. Security was called, and the patient was prevented from leaving the subacute unit. The aide's behavior was of concern to many of the staff because she was his only constant visitor. On several occasions the nursing and social work staff were certain that the aide was intoxicated and speculated that the alcohol contributed to her combative attitude about helping Mr. Telly to go home. Yet when asked if she was willing to serve as the patient "proxy" and learn to give insulin injections to Mr. Telly so he could be discharged, she refused. She stated, "I don't want that responsibility," and recognized that giving injections was well beyond her customary Medicaid personal care attendant role.

Mr. Telly had an admittedly difficult personality that sometimes made him a problematic patient for all the staff who dealt with him. The social worker on the subacute unit expected that he would be a permanent resident and did little to expedite the discharge to home when the physician or patient asked for it. But Mr. Telly continually asked when he could go home and finally began demanding to be released.

The Team Conference

At the time of the conference, the physician was in the process of weaning Mr. Telly from injected insulin and expected to stabilize him on an oral agent. Once the patient was stabilized, the physician expected no problem with his return to home. But the physician and the social worker clashed on two questions: (1) was Mr. Telly capable of making the decision to return home? and (2) did the arrangements constitute a "safe discharge plan" as detailed in the language of the state governing statute? The social worker was convinced that the patient was not competent and, furthermore, that it was irresponsible to discharge him to his home.

The geriatric team requested an ethics case conference because there was disagreement about the patient's competence. The assembled "experts" were the director of the Division of Geriatric Psychiatry, the director of the Division of Bioethics, the home care administrator, the geriatrician caring for Mr. Telly, the social worker assigned to the subacute level, and the primary nurse.

The geriatric physician presented the case. She portrayed Mr. Telly as an isolated patient who was mistrustful of professionals and family but for one person—his home health aide. He trusted her and was quite dependent. The physician described the medical course of the patient and his shift from injected insulin to an oral agent. She stated that the patient had consistently and repeatedly requested to go home over the six-month stay in the hospital and long-term care and was, in her judgment, able to do so in his present state. Since he was now capable of controlling his diabetes with an oral agent, he could be discharged to his home safely.

The geriatric psychiatrist discussed the issue of the patient's capacity. He stated that he, and most others at this point, used a notion of "decision-specific" capacity when responding to the query of whether a patient was capable of making a decision—in this case, a decision about the discharge plan. He explained that the patient had some isolationist tendencies but did not qualify as afflicted with paranoid delusional disorder or paranoid personality. There was no clear indication that the patient was psychotic—difficult, isolationist, intimidating, and unpleasant, but probably not psychotic. Therefore, the question of forcing antipsychotic medications was problematic, and since the patient was not willing to take medication, only a court order would permit forced administration. The psychiatrist certainly believed any court action would be counterproductive. He acknowledged the patient's problematic relationship with the family and the unclear motives of the home health aide. Nonetheless, the patient was clear about his wish to return to his apartment and aware of the limited social supports available to him.

After interviewing the patient, who was, understandably, not asked to come in to talk to the entire team, the psychiatrist offered the opinion that Mr. Telly was capable of deciding. While he possessed the negative characteristics described by others, he was nonetheless capable of making the decision to return home with some support from visiting nurse services and the support of his home health aide; Mr. Telly was not a candidate for decision making by others.

The ethics consultant presented the ethical issues in the context of the patient's medical, social, and individual history. This patient had worked as a baker until such time as his deteriorating eyesight forced him to stop working and accept Social Security disability. He was fiercely independent and valued his independence and even his isolation over connectedness and relatedness. He was a loner determined to go home alone. His values were clear and consistent—independence was the most important characteristic of his personal existence. Whether or not others would opt for this isolation, the patient clearly did and did so with articulate support for his position and for his choice. He explained that he could reach the second floor of his apartment house and could get help if he needed it. He was confident that his aide could provide all of the assistance that he needed.

The ethics consultant detailed the history of individual patient decision making in the context of feasible alternatives. If the team agreed that the patient was competent to make this decision, he should be allowed to return home even though the team felt that this was not the best option medically. But if Mr. Telly was determined to lack decisional competence and was incapable of understanding the issues, applying his values and preferences, and communicating his wishes, several other options became available for the consideration of the team members. These included: empowering the agent or proxy who had been appointed by Mr. Telly when he was capable of making decisions; relying informally on Mr. Telly's brother, who appeared to be the only family member involved in his care and decisions; permitting the caregiving team to act in what they deemed to be Mr. Telly's best interest; creating a hiatus in the decision process and proceeding with the plan last chosen by Mr. Telly; or petition-ing the court to appoint a guardian to make decisions for Mr. Telly, specifically decisions about medical care and discharge plans. None of these, she argued, was a particularly appealing option, particularly in the light of the psychiatrist's evaluation of Mr. Telly's capacity.

Whereas there was some controversy about Mr. Telly's capacity, the weight of the opinion deemed him capable of making decisions. All agreed that his judgment was poor, but it had likely been poor for much of his adult life, and this crisis was not designed to sharpen previously dulled faculties. Patterns of behavior honed in calmer times are not likely to evolve positively in moments of crisis. This was a man who had regularly disregarded and neglected his health for much of the previous decade. He would not be moved to remedy this pat-tern by rational argument or cogent logic. Patterns of character, as much as consciously adopted value schemes, often determine the choices that people make.

Patients, the ethics consultant argued, have the right to refuse care and treat-ment and the right to refuse "caring." The plan that some of the team advo-cated—discharge to a sheltered setting or to a nursing home—was anathema to this patient; he had the right to choose wrongly even if such a choice might cause him suffering in the future or actually shorten his life. His translation of "Eat, drink and be merry" was simple: go home to a life of isolation and inde-pendence—a strange vision of the personal good but one that was well estab-lished and settled in this particular patient's life course. Our task as care pro-viders, she argued, was not to structure the reality that we thought was best but to place our notions of the good life in the context of the patient's ideas and try to reconcile the patient's expectations with our own professional judgments. In many cases this is precisely the process that occurs; in this case the patient's fixed and rigid ideas remained unreconstructed by the process of discussion and dialogue.

When questioned by the psychiatrist, the nurses caring for Mr. Telly on the long-term care floor stated that he was difficult, angry, uncooperative, and oc-casionally threatening when he did not want to take his insulin. But there was no problem with his accepting treatment that he wanted if he did not feel forced to comply.

The issue that remained on the agenda arose from the reaction of the social worker to this patient and to the plan to discharge him to his home. She felt that he was not capable and that sending him home abandoned him to the worst of his own instincts and patterns of behavior. She was furious with the team and intimated that they were planning this discharge as an exercise in bedside rationing and not in response to the patient's real needs. There had clearly been a clash between the social worker and Mr. Telly, but the psychiatrist stated that this might be a factor intrinsic to that particular relationship and not necessarily characteristic of all of the patient's interactions.

The social worker had contacted the office of risk management and raised the issue of whether the hospital courted possible future liability by sending Mr. Telly home to what might be a less than optimal outcome. She felt that there was no question that Mr. Telly needed to go to a relative, a supervised group setting, or a nursing home. She argued that if Mr. Telly did not agree, he should be forced by family, team, or court to accept this plan. She stated that by acceding to this wish, which she thought was mistakenly categorized as respecting the patient's autonomy, the team was actually reneging on its ethical commitment to notions of professional obligation.

Team Dynamic

During the course of the team's meeting, the ethical issue under discussion shifted subtly from the patient's capacity to choose to the team's ethical responsibility to the needs of the patient. The social worker expressed her opinion that the team was being unethically and unprofessionally swayed by the long length of stay of this patient (made bearable to the hospital by the shift of the patient to the associated long-term care facility) and the difficult and expensive course that the hospital would have to take to override his consistent expressed wishes. Most of the team felt that these "spoken choices" actually reflected the patient's values, preferences, and settled character. But a minority steadfastly held that these statements reflected Mr. Telly's lack of decisional capacity. Were these staff members correct, then, that honoring the patient's spoken position would be the moral equivalent of abandoning him?

This team had met together for years. They respected each other and valued the different perspectives that the various voices brought to the discussion of a complex patient's decision-making ability. These long-standing relationships, however, also permitted the establishment of an intellectual and power hierarchy. Some members of the team were more articulate and focused more consistently on the decision-making ability of the patient and valued the principled positions that framed and constrained the analysis of capacity. In this case, the bioethics consultant and the geriatric psychiatrist were the most comfortable with the language and concepts that were critical to the resolution of the case. They were also senior attending physicians with extensive experience working in the hospital and lecturing in outside forums. They had sections of lectures and chapters at their beck and call that supported their positions eloquently. They were not, however, persons who needed to take responsibility for the discharge plan. That person was the social worker.

And what about her position? She was clearly at odds with this patient. The patient himself was quite disagreeable. He had, at one point in his stay, convinced his aide to get him dressed and take him home. It had fallen to the social worker to call the security office and ask them to physically bar his exit. It may also have been true that a level of countertransference in this case heightened the social worker's resolve not to discharge this patient to what she felt was not a safe plan.

Patients' rights can never be protected by vote. The fact that the majority of the team favored discharge to the patient's home might not have been the most supportable decision ethically. There is no question that the increasingly commodified nature of medicine affects how professionals think about patient needs and the risk/benefit ratio of professional action. There are good and bad reasons for sending a patient home in a timely fashion. The hospital makes money; the patient escapes the danger of nosocomial infection; the insurer is insulated from disputes over coverage for an extended hospital stay; and the health care system (if one were to exist) acts rationally to maximize the equitable distribution of scarce resources. But if the discharge is unsafe and the patient returns "quicker and sicker," professional standards have been violated at the expense of the patient.

There is always the concern, whenever a team is composed of very different sorts of people with different status in the organization, that those with more power and authority will determine the outcome. That concern is exemplified by this case. It was the social work staff who insisted that the patient was not safe at home, and they persisted in that opinion despite the articulate support for patient choice offered by the psychiatrist, geriatrician, and ethics consultant. This conflict raised a substantial ethical concern. The concern was not only in representing the patient's interest but also in processing the case. The team meeting was a method of processing a disagreement among team members, but in the end the social worker remained unconvinced about the experts' views on the team because they did not agree with her. Despite the team elements that would permit a full discussion of the facts—respectful dialogue, careful explanation of facts, and identification of issues—the social worker continued to oppose the discharge plan.

"Doing Ethics" as a Team: Benefits and Burdens

In the last years the goal of ethics professionals has been to integrate identified principles and analyses into the provision of medical care. This is a substantial challenge. One could argue that there is nothing new that needs to be written about the notion of informed consent. We have a wealth of case studies, articles, data-driven analyses, principled discussions, and practical guidelines about the idea and the reality of informed consent. The task before us is to turn these abstractions into the realities of patient/provider communication.

Teams are one very important way of accomplishing this goal. The team, in this case the geriatric team, has its own dynamic, agenda, processes for doing business, and ability to highlight issues for discussion. It also, at its best, has a collegial approach to surfacing, exploring, and critiquing issues in the context of the realities of caring for a particular patient. A bioethics consultant has been a part of the Montefiore geriatric team for the past two decades and highlights the value issues inherent in discussions about individual choice, patient competency, and the religious and social context of medical decision making. At most team meetings, the social worker, the psychiatrist, the physician, and sometimes other members of the team will all have concerns about the patient's understanding or perceptions about the patient's values that will help to enrich the conversation. When one member of the team is missing, others will take up the individual professional agenda. So it is common for a member of the team to say at a conference at which the bioethics consultant is absent: If bioethics were here, they would ask: "Who has engaged this patient in a discussion about future care? How do we know that the position the patient has presented really reflects her values and has not been unduly influenced by the staff or family? How do we know that the patient understands the risks, benefits, and alternatives?" These and other questions have become so much a part of the discussion that, in the absence of the "expert," the other members of the team will assume the responsibility for stating the questions and ferreting out the answers.

In a coherent team the ethical agenda of exploring and understanding statements, values, wishes, needs, cultural and religious contexts, and decisional capacity becomes part of case analysis and patient care rather than the arcane tool of one subspecialty. Such standard practice is as it should be. The question of decisional capacity is a matter of central importance for most of the members of a team. The fact that the bioethics consultant often explores these questions does not mean that over time they will not become part of the general knowledge base sought by all of the members of the team. In a team whose members begin to learn from each other, the ethical issues that surround care should become part of the comfortable material that all team members can incorporate into patient history, examination, and care planning.

This absorption of allied skills is the real strength of the team. All team conferences are really exercises in education, problem solving, and protocol development. Each time the team meets, it uses its combined intellectual strengths in diagnosis, prognosis, patient communication, and best practices to focus on the situation of one patient and arrive at a newly formulated care plan. Each time the team engages in this process, it helps the care providers for one patient while, at the same time, providing an integrated methodology for complex geriatric assessment and care planning. As ethics becomes part of the intellectual infrastructure, it has an impact not only on the particular case under discussion but also on all similar cases that members of the team will deal with in the future.

In a sense, a team is a setting for the "casuist" process, which learns from the instant case and applies the lessons in like cases in the future. This case-based learning is one of the most effective methodologies for integrating new information into practitioner practice. By making the process of doing ethics part of the team's regular approach, the questions and issues that surface become part of the comfortable routine of many members of the team.

Sometimes the regular questioning will not suffice to explore a particularly difficult case, and the case cited in this chapter is a good example. In the case of Mr. Telly, members of the team questioned his decisional capacity. His refusal to face his disease and its consequences, his insistence on returning home to a situation that had led to neglect of his medical needs, his rejection of family, his attachment to an aide of uncertain skills and unknown power over him and his welfare, his isolated habits and preferences all combined to make some of the staff members question his capacity. These are hard calls that require experience, skill, wisdom, judgment, comfort with the ideas in play, and the willingness to take a position, based on the best evidence, that may be wrong. This case required the participation of senior people. This patient might have represented either the "right of a competent patient to make a bad decision" or the need for an incapacitated patient to be protected from harm. The benefit of the team process was that it included the possibility of drawing together all of the experts and forcing them to take responsibility for their interpretations of the case as well as the ultimate decision.

The danger in the team process is that it uses the experts as "heavies" to set aside the discomfort and contrary opinions of other members of the staff. Certainly, in this case, it could be argued that the bioethics and psychiatry experts imposed their view of the patient on the other members of the health care team. But there is one final but important aspect to this case—the concerns of the social worker. One member of the team was tremendously concerned about the state statute that required the discharge planner to arrange a "safe" discharge plan, and she felt that this mandate fell directly on her shoulders. In addition, she had been the staff person to see Mr. Telly's inebriated aide and was the one who had called security when the aide had tried to leave the hospital with the patient. Her database was different from all of the other members of the team; her notion of individual responsibility was heightened because of her position and her perceptions of the situation.

The team was able to shoulder some of the responsibility for this staff person, who had felt very alone. But in so acting, it also overpowered her perceptions and her personal sense of responsibility. A team is a powerful advocate for its own beliefs and can ride roughshod over the objections of some of its members. Majority rule does not provide equal status for the opinions of the minority in teams—just as it does not in government (see Chapter 11).

The situation was even further complicated by the conflicts of interest that have been inherent in medicine for years but that have recently become more prominent. This was a patient who had been in and out of the acute care hospital for over six weeks and who stayed in the long-term care facility for four months. During the acute care days, the hospital lost money; in the time in the nursing home, the hospital probably earned a bit but not enough to want the patient maintained in that setting. Furthermore, the great benefit of the long-term care setting is that it provides a pressure valve for patients with expected or actual longtime stays who become hospital liabilities. The pressure to discharge patients is enormous; having professionals who are willing to stand up and contest this juggernaut is critical.

Conclusion: Implementing the Plan

While Mr. Telly was medically stable and able to be discharged, it took another month to attend to the details of the community discharge. The social worker had to process Medicaid forms to allow him to receive community-based services rather than nursing home services. Furthermore, the home care agency had to be assured that Mr. Telly would be safe if they were responsible for the home care plan. About five weeks after the conference, Mr. Telly was discharged home with a visiting nurse from the hospital home care. Within two weeks of discharge, he dismissed the home care nurse, stating that he no longer needed services. He did not show up for his follow-up appointments with the geriatrician, nor did he return to the hospital's outpatient clinics. When phoned by the physician, he said he was fine and didn't need any more help.

The geriatrics team continued to work together, and the relationship between the social worker and the physician thawed after a period of time. A second social worker, assigned to the case when the first one refused to help, stated, in an interview with an outside person, that "the team is good. I felt lucky dealing with special people and people who want the patient to be healthy and happy. The patient was the one who was least able to understand the problems. I got annoyed with the brother who wouldn't or couldn't help Mr. Telly go home. . . . Mr. Telly was strong willed and I admired him. He stuck to his guns. I'm glad he was able to be happy and to go home."

Teams are helpful in identifying and promoting the values and preferences of the patient. Yet, sometimes even what appears to be a fairly well-functioning team can fail to incorporate the patient's preferences or adjudicate among conflicting views of team members. In such cases, the team may seek an alternative communicative forum, as was requested here of the ethics team by the geriatric team. Yet, while both teams had the possibility to broaden the perspectives discussed and promote the patient's wishes, team dynamics of power and authority also serve to create possibly unidentified ethical dilemmas that do influence the outcome of team decision making. In an environment that is often more supportive of team members with power and authority or those who follow and support the rules of fiscal thrift, ethical dilemmas become more subtle and difficult to identify and separate from the standard practice of care. Even one of the highest values of clinical practice, support for patient autonomy, becomes more difficult.

Teaching students and professionals how to process disagreements appropriately and guard against groupthink must be the first line of defense against such dilemmas (see also Chapter 9). Furthermore, we must continue to be vigilant in our socialization of students into the profession. We must help them to identify not only the standards and norms of their profession but also the standards and norms of the other professionals with whom they work, so as to enable them to recognize ethical dilemmas before they occur and prevent them from creating barriers to good clinical care.

Discussion Questions

1. In the ethical analysis of this case, was the patient's seeming indifference to his medical problems different from a situation in which a client decides not to undergo an onerous medical procedure? Why or why not?

2. When you, as a professional, realize that you have done everything you can to articulate your concerns and you are unable to convince your team members to agree with your position, how do you continue to work with them? Or do you?

3. Imagine you are the social worker who did not want Mr. Telly discharged, and you learn that Mr. Telly died one week after discharge. What would you say to your team members? Would your reaction change if he died six months after the discharge? How would the time frame change your ethical analysis?

4. The relationship between the paid aide and the patient caused concern among the team. Even though the caregiver was paid, she obviously cared about Mr. Telly, visiting him without compensation. Does the payment to the aide affect your view of the appropriate way for her to care for him? What are Mr. Telly's rights in this matter?

REFERENCES

Beauchamp, T. L., and J. F. Childress. 1994. Respect for autonomy. In *Principles of biomedical ethics*, 4th ed. New York: Oxford University Press.
Drinka, T. J. K., and P. Clark. 2000. *Health care teamwork: Interdisciplinary practice and teaching.* Westport, Conn.: Auburn House.
Hyer, K. 2000. Teams and teamwork. In M. Mezey, ed. *Encyclopedia on aging.* New York: Springer.
Jonsen, A. R., M. Siegler, and W. J. Winslade. 1998. *Clinical ethics*, 4th ed. New York: McGraw-Hill.

Salgo v. Leland Stanford Jr. University Board of Trustees. 1957. (154 Cal. App.2d 560, 317 P.2d 170).

Tuckman, B. W. 1965. Developmental sequences in small groups. *Psychological Bulletin* 63:384–99.

Veatch, R. M. 1997. Hospital ethics committees: Is there a role? In N. S. Jecker, A. R. Jonsen, and R. A. Pearlman, eds., *Bioethics: An introduction to the history, methods and practice.* Boston: Jones and Bartlett.

CHAPTER 11

Avoiding the Dark Side
of Geriatric Teamwork

Rosalie A. Kane, M.S.W., Ph.D.

About Geriatric Teams
Definition and Variation

The multidisciplinary team is an enduring organizational feature and meta-phor in health care and human services. Although teams vary enormously in their composition, function, size, duration, leadership style, and way of work-ing together, by definition they have in common the following: a group pur-pose, differential roles or contributions, and a system of communication among team members (Kane 1975).

When the elements of this definition are probed, its variability is revealed. First, the team purposes may be vague and general, on the one hand, or highly specific, on the other; the common purpose may be measurable (e.g., a home care team aspiring to delay or postpone nursing home placements for clients) or expressed at the level of slogan (e.g., maximum health and well-being). All the team members may subscribe to and be willing to be evaluated by the same general overall or client-specific purpose, or they may hold specific measurable purposes of their own. For example, the overall purpose of a stroke rehabilitation team may be to bring the client to maximum functional ability and help him or her compensate for remaining disability, but the physical therapist's goal may be expressed in terms of range of motion and ambulation, the occupational therapist's in terms of ability to prepare meals, and the social worker's in terms of the client's and family member's adjustment to the disability status.

The roles and contributions may be distinctly allocated by professional discipline or considerable overlap may occur; and the communication patterns may be infrequent and formal (via memo and formal team meeting) or informal and almost constant. A team may come together as an ad hoc group for a particular patient or family (such as is common with teams assembled in medical and surgical hospital units) or it may also be constituted as a staff of a particular organization, such as a falls clinic, a rehabilitation unit, or even the management staff of a nursing home. The team metaphor is also used when the "team" includes members who work for and are paid by separate organizations; in that instance the team is interorganizational as well as interdisciplinary. Some teams are hierarchical in nature (consider the operating room team), and some aspire to a democratic, participatory, group decision-making ideal. Some teams, particularly those that serve elderly people needing long-term care, attempt to include on the team frontline paraprofessional workers such as nurse's aides, personal care workers, or home health aides. In such cases the well-known power disparities in health teams, most notably between physicians and other team members, are multiplied. It is indeed perplexing to consider how to sustain a democratic model of decision making in teams where some members have direct supervisory authority over others.

Why Have Teams?

The team is constantly being rediscovered as a hypothetically superior way of providing services to people with complex and often enduring problems. From a client-centered perspective, the justifications for teamwork are that the client will benefit from the considered contributions of a group whose members have different backgrounds and skills and that the client cannot know how to and should not be required to assemble the team members separately or coordinate their activities. Evaluation of any team's effectiveness is made difficult by the problem of finding a proper comparison group. For example, a physician acting alone in an outpatient setting may be compared to a team approach whereby additional personnel are brought into the picture (say, a dietitian, a social worker, and a pharmacist). In contrast, a variety of professionals may already be on hand in an outpatient or inpatient setting, and the difference that the team brings about is that it works on behalf of particular clients together instead of in tandem. Or, to take another example, an organization such as a nursing home, previously organized into disciplinary departments, may be transformed into functional teams based on, say, a particular section or unit of the nursing home, where a designated group of nurses joins with an activities professional, a social worker, a dietitian, and a rehabilitation specialist to form a team. In that instance, the effectiveness of this new structure of teams reporting to top management would be compared to the original departmental structure. In all these examples, presumably the most important rationale is a disinterested one of generating better service and better outcomes for the individual client or the collectivity of clientele. It may also be believed that the team will create an efficiency that permits serving more people for the same amount of money, which, once again, potentially brings better service and outcomes to more clients.

But other reasons for advancing teamwork are less purely disinterested. In the 1970s, teams were advanced as a way to mitigate the authority of the physician (Wise, Beckhard, Rubin, and Kyte 1974). Although such health teams arguably could provide fuller care to patients with the likelihood of better results, they also had the goal of enhancing the power of the less advantaged and less powerful disciplines, possibly giving them access to clientele and enhancing their visibility, respect, and self-respect. As new programs serving older people became established and older ones more refined in policy, statute, and organizational practice, professional associations have found it in their interest to advocate for teamwork and for their own established place on, say, a hospice team, or a rehabilitation team, or a home health team. A cynic might even note a certain self-interested etiquette in place that requires leaders in various professions to call for teamwork and embrace the inclusion of many species of professionals on the team rather than blatantly argue for inclusion of themselves.

Teams in Geriatrics

It is a truism but also true that many very old people live with multiple interacting health problems that also have psychological and social dimensions.

Even in narrow terms, the health care group needed to diagnose such a person or to provide ongoing care may include a primary care provider and several medical specialists; it may also include a nurse specialist who has a role in coordinating all the health-related efforts. To more fully identify the problems and meet the needs of the client, others, including physical, occupational and speech therapists, social workers, psychologists, pharmacists, dentists, recreational therapists, could be included.

Comprehensive, multidimensional geriatric assessment has become a hallmark of geriatric medicine (Rubenstein, Weiland, and Bernabei 1995), emblematic of what a geriatrician can provide that differs from other specialists. Some of the attention to teams in geriatric medicine is a result of the development and testing of geriatric assessment programs. For example, the Interdisciplinary Team Training in Geriatrics (ITTG) Programs, funded in a dozen Veterans Administration Medical Centers in the 1980s, were designed to improve communication across disciplines and, therefore, the effectiveness of multidisciplinary work, developed in parallel with the Geriatric Assessment and Evaluation Units (GEUs), short-term inpatient units dedicated to improving the functioning of older patients whose acute illnesses were stabilized through careful assessment and short-term therapeutic trials (Oriol 1985). Another impetus for teamwork has been the recognition that long-term care, especially in group residential settings, can have an enormous impact for better or worse on a client's quality of life; this recognition in turn, led to a convention for including a full panoply of disciplines in the care planning process in nursing homes and similar settings. One of the best-articulated models for teamwork in geriatrics and long-term care grew out of San Francisco's On Lok program, an entity at financial risk for providing the full range of Medicare and Medicaid acute care and long-term care services to a low-income, functionally impaired group of older people. The program, now replicated all over the country as Programs of All-Inclusive Care for the Elderly (PACE), was originally build around an adult day center where seniors came for health maintenance and rehabilitation as well as socialization; salaried physicians interacted with a wide range of other personnel in a highly participatory model of team management (Kane, Illston, and Miller 1992).

Not all multidimensional assessment requires a team, and not all interdisciplinary communication on behalf of a patient requires teamwork in the strict sense of the word. In terms of assessment, multidimensional assessment tools can and have been designed with the input of persons of many disciplines but are administered by a single individual, perhaps a nurse or social worker. Arguably, the singular administration of an assessment tool is efficient and considerate of the client, as long as various professionals viewing the results can bring themselves to trust information collected by someone else. (This is not solely an issue of cross-disciplinary trust, because organizations and even new personnel in the same organization have a tendency to repeat each other's assessment work.) In terms of ongoing care, a role known variously as care coordinator or case manager has sprung up to help coordinate and rationalize services to older people across time and organizations. Case managers, be they nurses or social workers, may be entrusted to make referrals and gather input from disciplinary experts as needed, which leads to a model that differs from the team management of the PACE program mentioned above. Possibly a case management model may be more efficient or more effective in some instances than a team model.

Ethics and the Dark Side of Teams

An ethical issue, put simply, arises when it is unclear what is right or fair to do from a moral perspective. Typically ethical issues arise when competing interests or values can be identified (e.g., between an older person and a family member or among family members) or when the older persons themselves and the people providing care can discern multiple but conflicting desirable goals for the older person. Geriatric care, and especially long-term care, is a minefield of ethical issues, regardless of whether teams are involved (Kane 1994a). Often the dilemmas center on whether a course of action preferred by the client and recognized by the professional as having advantages is sufficiently safe to be pursued in good conscience, a type of dilemma exacerbated when the client has fluctuating and limited decision-making ability because of cognitive impairment. On the level of organizational ethics, a variety of issues arise about the rights and obligations of the frontline workers in long-term care to the clients and the obligations of the employer to these individuals, who themselves may be underpaid, disadvantaged, and forced into disagreeable or even unsafe situations. Finally at the policy and programmatic levels, a large number of ethical issues arise around the best and fairest way to distribute resources. None of these organizational or policy issues are necessarily team issues.

Because team care entails a group of individuals who each have their own personal and professional ethics related to the client but who also have a commitment to working together on the client's behalf, a variety of ethical issues arise concerning the right way to behave toward a team member from a moral perspective. Many such examples are analyzed in the cases in this book. This chapter sets the stage by considering some of the systemic ethical problems that can arise with teams regardless of how necessary or important the teamwork is. Some of these problems arise because more weight is given to the goal of a well-functioning team and the well-being of team members than to the clients being served. Some arise from the perils of group functioning, especially because a smoothly functioning, cohesive group is a legitimate process goal in teamwork. The darkest side of teamwork from an ethics perspective is that problems may fail to rise to consciousness as ethical dilemmas on the part of the team.

Some key ethical problems on the dark side of teamwork are summarized below; each is then discussed separately, with brief case examples.

- Outnumbering and overwhelming the client
- Making the client part of the team
- Squelching individual team members
- Lack of accountability
- Team process trumping client outcome
- Orthodoxy and groupthink
- Overemphasis on health and safety goals
- Squandering resources

Ethical dilemmas arising for teams will rarely be couched in these terms. Rather, they will concern the safety of the care plan for an individual or the problem of resolving disagreements among team members in a respectful way. The problems just listed relate to the ethical foundations of the whole endeavor rather than puzzles involving specific clients.

For the detailed analysis of specific cases, most contributors to this book use a common framework, entailing seven major action steps: (1) gathering clinical information; (2) identifying patient and family preferences; (3) evaluating quality-of-life issues; (4) considering contextual and team-related issues; (5) resolving the ethical issues, setting priorities, and creating a plan; and (6) implementing a plan, and (7) evaluating the plan after it is implemented (Jonsen, Siegler, and Winslade 1998). That systematic way of proceeding is pertinent and appropriate to teamwork, and yet following such a framework hardly protects against the dark side of teams. Steps 1 to 3 can proceed without a thorough examination of problems in the way the team gathers clinical information, identifies consumer and family preferences, and conceptualizes and evaluates quality of life. Step 4 requires review of a useful laundry list of considerations (e.g., provider concerns, financial and economic issues, clinical research issues, legal complexities, institutional conflicts of interest, and the like). But the team issues may be so embedded in the team's philosophy that they never are reconsidered as creating an ethical problem. Finally, the devil is in the details of step 5, identifying and resolving ethical issues and setting priorities. The snippets of case vignettes included in this chapter are not examined according to the seven-step sequence, since providing a rich case analysis is beside the point of these illustrations. Nonetheless, these issues and case vignettes were prepared with the framework as a clear backdrop, and at times the text alludes to one or another step.

Outnumbering and Overwhelming the Client

The team metaphor immediately evokes an athletic team. Extending the metaphor, the team members know the rules of the game, and the client does not. If the perceptions of the older client and the team diverge, the client is outnumbered and the match is unfair.

• Mrs. Ellison has been worked up by an outpatient geriatric team to which she was referred by her daughter, who is worried about her mother's increasing forgetfulness, her anxiety living alone, and her seeming inability to manage her diabetes and multiple medications. Over the course of three weeks, Mrs. Ellison undergoes a series of interviews, lab tests, and other assessments of physical capability and endurance. The core team, consisting of a physician, nurse, social worker, and physical therapist as well as a behavioral psychologist called into the case, meets to review their findings. The social worker reports that Mrs. Ellison's daughter is near the breaking point with worry over her mother and with the stress of responding to frequent demands. As a group, the team considers options such as relocating Mrs. Ellison to assisted living, simplifying the drug regimen, and facilitating her attendance at an adult day center. The team determines that an adult day center might be optimal for Mrs. Ellison because socialization can be combined with monitoring of medications and of changing mental status.

• Mrs. Ellison and her daughter meet the team in the conference room, and each team member presents his or her findings, leading to a coherent and consistent statement of the problems and the recommendations. The cognitive assessment is presented as in normal range. The recommendations included a hearing evaluation, changed medications (including an antianxiety drug), and day care twice a week. When team members turn to Mrs. Ellison for her reaction, they are greeted by nervous silence. Finally, Mrs. Ellison asks if she is losing her memory. The psychologist reassures her that her memory is in normal range, but reiterates that she seems sad, anxious, and lonely. Mrs. Ellison expresses some hesitation about whether she would enjoy adult day care since she thinks a lot of the people who attend are confused; she is assured that she would love the program. Mrs. Ellison lapses into silence.

It is a common and perhaps laudable practice for assessment teams to discuss cases and recommendations before they interpret their findings to the client. Such discussion and rehearsal may serve to get all ideas on the table and spare the client the confusion of listing to diverse opinions of team members. But too often the client is simply outnumbered and hesitant to express concerns. The stylized presentation that respectfully gave all team members a voice failed to clearly address Mrs. Ellison's major concern: was she losing her memory? The recommendation for day care seemed to come out of the blue to Mrs. Ellison. Perhaps she was unaware that the team's recommendations would extend this far. One gets the sense that despite the extensive work on gathering clinical information through wide-ranging assessments, the team failed to examine Mrs. Ellison's own preferences for how she spends her day (Degenholtz, Kane, and Kivnick 1997; Kane, Degenholtz, and Kane 1999). And if Mrs. Ellison's preferences were assessed in a general way (step 3 of the team model), apparently no effort was made to ascertain her preferences for the scope and nature of the team consultation.

An ethical issue related to limiting client autonomy surely arises when a client is unable to assert herself against a team. But this case vignette is not offered as a classic autonomy dilemma (e.g., will Mrs. Ellison's health and safety be sufficiently addressed if she stays at home as she prefers rather than attends day care? Does Mrs. Ellison's daughter's anxiety and desire for some free unworried time have any weight on the choices of Mrs. Ellison herself? Is Mrs. Ellison capable of making an informed, autonomous choice?). These are all ethical issues that may be worthy of discussion, but the systemic issue is the possibility that Mrs. Ellison and other clients are unable to reach autonomous decisions because of the very way the team collects and reports its views.

How can a team guard against exerting subtle pressure on a client? How can a team meeting be made less of a formidable ordeal? How can the team be sure it is hearing the voice of the client as it makes its way through its own routines? There is no certain formula, but the following idea may be helpful. The team should assure that someone has come to know Mrs. Ellison as an individual and has an idea of her preferences as well as her views about what is to be gained from the consultation. It may be helpful to designate one team member to perform that task. The team meeting needs to be examined to ensure that it is conducive to dialogue with the client. It may be that everyone does not need to be present for such a meeting. Perhaps more time with fewer people would permit the client a fuller, freer discussion.

Making the Client Part of the Team

• When Miss Applebee is diagnosed with inoperable late-stage cancer and is told she will live about six months, she decides to receive palliative care at home. Her main hope is to die at home in her own apartment in her own bed, and she asks not to be hospitalized. The team includes a geriatric physician, a consulting oncologist, several nurses, a case manager (a social worker who arranges for personal attendant services from a different agency), and an environmental specialist who advises about and arranges for medical equipment. Early in her acquaintance with this group, Miss Applebee meets with the physician, care manager, and nurse, who explain to her that they viewed her as an important member of the team. They leave written materials with Miss Applebee that reiterate that she, along with her close family members (in her case, an out-of-town daughter and an out-of-town son and their spouses and an elderly sister living down the street), are all members of the team and that their views are as important as anyone's. At first Miss Applebee likes that idea, but as she thinks it over, she finds it less comforting than she did at first. How many votes will she get, as a member of the team? she wonders. What are her obligations? What if everyone else on the team thinks that she should be in the hospital? Will she have to go? What if she feels she needs more pain medicine than the rest of the team? Anyway, Miss Applebee is too tired to use her precious energy being a team member. She merely wants to have a good health care group working for her.

The concept that the patient is a member of the team is meant to be inclusive and is certainly an enduring idea in the teamwork literature. The concept recognizes that treatment plans for chronic illness cannot succeed without the patient's concurrence and that the patient is the most concerned about the outcome. But Miss Applebee was right to note a problem in this formulation. When used inappropriately, putting the patient on the team is akin to the previously discussed problem of outnumbering the client. To characterize clients as team members diminishes their importance and authority. The team works for and on behalf of the patient. The patient, or his or her agent, may wish to change the team when that is plausible. If a general contractor told a homeowner that he or she is an important part of the renovation team whose views will be taken seriously, the homeowner may express a preference to advise, guide, and evaluate the team rather than join it. Because metaphors are potent, it is prudent to consider whether construing the client as a member of the team is the optimal way of saying that the client's preferences, views, and evaluations of performance are paramount to the endeavor. Step 4 of the analytic framework calls for considering the context of the team in relation to identifying ethical issues, but teams rarely consider the implications of their own cherished rhetoric.

Squelching Individual Team Members

Often the team subscribes to the ground rule that everyone's input is equal, but various team members, by dint of their verbal and persuasive powers or their ascribed power due to their role, typically have more input than others. Moreover, teams develop their own standard approaches to service, and it takes a strong team member to go against the force of the group. Paraprofessionals who are ostensibly on a team may be too timid to actually volunteer an opinion, or they may feel that their opinion is unlikely to be technically correct.

• At Trailblazer Convalescent Center, care planning is done quarterly, as is required by law, and more often if seen as necessary. The team consists of the unit manager, who is a nurse; the charge nurses; a social worker, who is assigned to this unit and one other; an activities person; a dietary technician; and a therapist. The team is convened by the minimum data set (MDS) coordinator, whose job it is to ensure that mandatory assessments are completed on schedule and that care planning meetings take place.

• A special meeting of the team has been convened because one client, Mrs. Thompson, has become a management problem. She has become demanding and combative. She is negative about attending activities. She refuses assistance with bathing regularly, and other residents are complaining about her appearance and behavior. She sleeps poorly and disturbs others at night. The team discusses Mrs. Thompson from all perspectives and determines that she may be a good candidate for the dementia pull-out program in the facility, where she can engage in activities more suited to her cognitive abilities. Changes in medication are also determined.

• Dottie Smith, the day LPN, has her own ideas about the problem. She thinks that Mrs. Thompson is bored, and she has noticed that she still maintains an interest in gardening. She has also noticed that Mrs. Thompson has formed a sort of a friendship with a housekeeper who is assigned to her room and that she misses her when she is gone. She also knows that Mrs. Thompson asks for wine in the evenings, but the decision had been made not to add that additional stimulant. Dottie does not think Mrs. Thompson should be in the pull-out dementia program, since she functions at a higher level than those participants. Dottie is considering suggesting that Mrs. Thompson be encouraged to begin a pot garden in her room, that the housekeeper be called upon when Mrs. Thompson is most difficult to manage, and that she be served wine and cocktails when she asks for them, which might also help her sleep. But the activities director has mentioned nothing about gardening, and the dietary department has mentioned nothing about cocktails, so Dottie decides to keep her mouth shut.

As in the previous example, the ethical problems, if any, raised directly in this case vignette have little to do with the dark side of teamwork. It is possible that ethical problems may be articulated about the rights of Mrs. Thompson compared to those of the group, or the amount of resources she has a right to command. There may be an ethical issue around the use of alcohol, if the team decides to further explore that strategy. But the problem that Dottie Smith has relevant but unexpressed observations is not noted at all. In the interests of beneficence—that is, doing the best for Mrs. Thompson—the team needs input from all those in a position to know. An L.P.N. on the floor or even more likely a housekeeper (who was not even invited to the team meeting) might hold a key to solving the problem.

How does one guard against this particular systemic problem in teamwork? Speaking up in a group may not be what comes naturally to a given team member, particularly to one with a low position in the hierarchy and low education and salary. Moreover, Dottie reports to the unit coordinator, who has already expressed her view. The likelihood that some team member will be intimidated must be anticipated. Team leadership includes drawing out each team member and incorporating each person's contribution to the summary of the issue. Training exercises for teams and problem solving related to communication could be incorporated into staff development and might help team members develop the skill to assert themselves. Eventually the team may be able to model how it takes seriously and acts upon minority views. Individual team members must also consult their own moral compass and be encouraged to state when they think an action is wrong from a moral perspective, or is wrong technically or strategically.

The issue of the individual team member against the collective transcends the problems of nonprofessionals with limited prestige. One example written up in the literature concerns a nurse who went against an entire interdisciplinary team in an HMO context (Kane, Freda, and Heikoff 2000). The case involved a morbidly overweight woman in her forties who had not left her home for years and who managed her family from her bed. The team concluded that she could never diet successfully enough to get down to 400 pounds, where she would be a candidate for surgery. Her condition was life-threatening, and after the home health physician made a visit, hospice was proposed. One nurse, herself somewhat overweight, was outraged by this decision and worked relentlessly—and for a time covertly—with the patient on a weight-loss plan that eventually succeeded to the point where the patient had surgery a year later.

Lack of Accountability

There is safety in numbers. A side advantage of teamwork is that the team members can cushion each other from a sense of responsibility for difficult, sometimes heart-wrenching decisions. Nobody needs to feel alone in responsibility. But the downside of this advantage occurs when the client cannot get a clear sense of who is responsible for their case.

• Mr. Jackson, a widower, had a stroke that has left him with residual problems in the use of his right arm and leg. He lives in an assisted living setting with an in-house medical clinic; the assisted living setting is part of a large geriatric complex that includes, on the same campus, a nursing home and a rehabilitation center. His daughter Emily is concerned because her father called her three weeks ago to describe his plan for solving world hunger, which required in part that he set aside a portion of each meal as an example of philanthropy. Mr. Jackson has a history of bipolar disorder and has been hospitalized many times because of this condition; he takes lithium. After his stroke, he received rehabilitation from the rehabilitation unit affiliated with his assisted living center. Emily has noted for many months that the stroke rehabilitation team, the mental health team, and the geriatric team seem to be at cross-purposes in planning her father's medications, even though they are all part of the same health care group. Emily mentions her current concern that the bipolar illness is out of control to the attending geriatrician, who indicates that he will bring the issue to the care planning team. Emily attends that care planning meeting a week later, when the collective decision is reached to refer Mr. Jackson back to the mental health group and to coordinate their recommendations. Another week later, no appointment has been made. Emily is uncertain to whom she should speak next. That night her father arrives in a taxi at her home twenty-five miles away, having assured the taxi driver that his daughter is expecting him on important business; the taxi driver required $120 in cash. When Emily speaks to the wellness nurse at the assisted living center, the latter says she thought the social worker had implemented the referral to the mental health clinic long ago. The next day the social worker expresses surprise that the nurse has not followed through with the referral.

The problem described here is one where, continuing the team analogy, the ball got dropped. That can happen quite easily in a team context, especially, as in this case, when interlocking teams are involved and the health issues concern stroke care as well as mental health. Other variations on lack of accountability occur when nobody feels authorized to give information to the client. An approach to avoiding or solving such problems includes clear assignment of follow-through for various actions determined by the team. From a consumer's viewpoint, however, it may be even better to have one individual to whom he or she can go with questions and problems.

Team Process Trumping Client Outcome

• The falls prevention team has been operating for a year as a specialized clinic in a health maintenance organization. The team consists of a geriatrician, a bioengineer with expertise in gait, several nurses, an occupational therapist, a physical therapist, a social worker, and an environmental specialist. On the anniversary of the team's existence, the group meets to set in motion an evaluation of their effectiveness. The ideas generated included: questionnaires to be completed by team members regarding their satisfaction with the team; and questionnaires completed by referring agents regarding their satisfaction with the team. They also consider having an ethnographic researcher examine the effectiveness of team meetings. The engineer is uncomfortable with the plans since he thought that they should be evaluating the frequency of first falls and repeat falls and the extent to which fear of falling negatively affects clients' lives. The rest of the team tells him that he is missing the point—this is an evaluation of teamwork itself.

It is common for teams to emphasize their own process and their own satisfaction over and above the outcomes for which they have come into existence. Some might argue that a team needs to enjoy a certain amount of satisfaction among its members to achieve good results, itself an empirical question. But even if this is true and evidence of a smooth, enjoyable process is necessary, it is hardly sufficient. No matter how much the team is enjoyed and appreciated by its members, if it is not achieving its goals, it cannot be said to be effective.

Orthodoxy and Groupthink

Groupthink is a term coined by Irving Janis (1983) to refer to a phenomenon of insularity and imperviousness to new ideas that occurs in cohesive groups. Janis first studied this phenomenon in policy-making groups. He noted that if the composition of a group is constant and its members are characterized by high mutual respect, the deliberations can become characterized by high levels of agreement and inability to critique one's own work. Sometimes even obvious problems or solutions are overlooked, and certainly the group is unlikely to be refreshed by new ideas about the problems or how to deal with them. In the policy arena, groupthink has led to overlooking the obvious as well as an inability to take in new ideas or evidence, and, ultimately, policy fiascos.

• A team on a special care unit (SCU) for Alzheimer disease is particularly proud of its performance, and indeed the group has worked hard together to achieve a common understanding of how best to meet the needs of people with moderate dementia in a residential setting. The team was formed two years ago and the physical space was renovated to accommodate twenty residents with dementia who were not flourishing in the facility as a whole. All team members volunteered for this unit, and they set out together to educate themselves as a group. They eventually evolved a frame of reference that included a view that frequent short activities are optimal for the attention span of the person with dementia and that stimulation should be subdued to avoid overexcitement and catastrophic reactions. Family members are discouraged from making frequent unannounced visits so as to avoid confusing residents further, but regular events are scheduled three times a week that involve family. Although the SCU seems to work well, as measured by behavior problems, sleep patterns, and absence of overt distress, over the years several residents have not seemed to flourish under this regimen. When these cases are reviewed, the team attempts to determine how they can help that individual by simplifying his or her routines and removing stressful stimulation. Occasionally family members suggest a different tack for their relative, such as frequent use of familiar music and surrounding the resident with objects from home. The team educates the family member about the dangers of overstimulation. Although the team has a literature club to keep up to date with innovations in dementia care, somehow they have failed to review any literature that reflects additional viewpoints about dementia care. Whenever a team member resigns, such as when the social worker leaves the labor force to have children, the team interviews replacements to ensure compatibility with the team's philosophy.

This kind of scenario is frequently found in teams that grow up together and become committed to a particular theoretical framework. In mental health teams, the view might be toward the therapeutic community. In alcohol treatment teams, the view might be to promote abstinence and emphasize twelve-step programs (or conversely but less frequently, to promote responsible social drinking). In a nursing home, the team may become "Edenized"—that is, committed to William Thomas's formula of combatting loneliness, boredom, and helplessness with plants, animals, and children (Thomas 1994, 1999). If the team is highly cohesive and monolithic in its approach, the members are more likely to talk largely to each other and to like-minded people. Even if the original driving theory is largely correct, the team is poorly positioned to evolve that theory to its next steps or to recognize and deal with exceptions. However comforting the presence of animals may be in nursing homes, for example, some individuals experience cats and birds negatively. However valuable the concept of creating a community in a nursing home may be, some people will flourish better with a chance to avoid groups and express individualism.

In a multidisciplinary team, groupthink may be minimized if the various team members maintain ties to their original professional group and through this contact and other means have independent ways of refreshing their own intellectual base. Another approach calls for deliberately inviting new information in the form of guest lecturers, attendance at outside seminars, and the like.

Overemphasis on Health and Safety Goals

Multidisciplinary teams in aging, and particularly in long-term care, have been constituted to take into account "the whole person." Typically several team members (for example, a social worker, a recreational therapist, an occupational therapist, a pastoral counselor) specialize in the social and psychological side of the patient's well-being. Other disciplines, such as nursing, lay claim to a rounded view of individual well-being, and physicians who select themselves to be active on teams also tend to take a broader view of well-being than morbidity and mortality. Yet multidisciplinary teams, however broadly they envisage well-being, arise largely in the health sector and tend to order their goals to put health and safety first. The ethics literature in long-term care is replete with specific cases where the goals and priorities of the providers differ from those of the client (Kane and Caplan 1990, 1993), and more case examples are found in this book. The case vignette below, therefore, deals with no particular case but a team deliberating on its own conduct.

• The Home and Community Based Waiver program in a particular city has contracted with Helping Hands Home Care to provide services to its nursing home–eligible clientele. The organization is divided into regional teams that include nurses, therapists, a social worker, a respiratory therapist, and a medical director, who meets monthly with the group in sessions the consider general policies as well as cases. The state is initiating a "client-directed home care program" to permit up to twelve hours daily of attendant service to older people who live alone, and the team is considering whether it should participate. It would require reconfiguring its services to allow clients to more directly supervise those who give care. The home care agency would do an initial assessment, provide backup care in emergencies, directly provide occasional technical services, and teach and generally do the work of the attendant. From a client perspective, this program would allow for more hours of services in a week with more direct input from the client about how helpers should spend their time.

• The team has a spirited discussion to consider who, among the present clients, might benefit from such a service. Several clients are identified who might "abuse" the service by persuading attendants to take them out to restaurants and sporting events, and other clients were identified as having insufficient judgment to have oversight over an attendant. The discussion turns to whether the goal of staying at home is appropriate for people with heavy care needs who live alone. Several nurses and the physical therapist express concern about the likelihood of falls at night. They talk briefly about Mr. Bruce, a gentleman with advanced Parkinson's disease, who falls regularly and needs help with toileting; although cognitively intact, Mr. Bruce has great difficulty communicating. The team reviews its own goals and reaffirms that it is particularly focused on achieving the best possible quality of life for older people that is consistent with their health and safety. The social worker remarks that people living alone, including Mr. Bruce, often have inadequate socialization and that moving to more protected settings can be a win-win situation. The team concludes that it would compromise its own client-centered values to participate in a program that would lead to less oversight of health conditions and more unsafe community situations. Several current clients with high needs who cannot be cared for cost-effectively under the waivers would be candidates for the program, but the team really thinks these individuals should face the reality that they need heavier care than should be provided at home.

Helping Hands Home Care is blessed with a team that emphasizes quality of life and that brings many disciplines to bear on how it achieves that state. It prides itself on its desire to arrange and foster the best quality of life possible consistent with health and safety. But team members, even those in the more socially oriented disciplines, are placing their view of health and safety first. Mr. Bruce and others in the caseload may prefer to stay in their familiar settings and neighborhoods. How different the goal would be if the team aspired to provide the safest situation and achieve the best health outcomes possible that are consistent with the client's quality of life! The fact that "quality of life" is treated as a slogan rather than specified as a goal just adds to the problem.

Differing views of safety and its importance are at the root of ethical conflicts in long-term care (Kane and Levin 1998). Implementing a plan that meets a client's preferences typically involves making tradeoffs since, like professionals, clients hold conflicting values relevant to their care. The problem is that health care providers often consider some values related to safety to be nonnegotiable. If the provider is an entire team of providers, the verdict is harder to fight, and the client has less chance of escape. At Helping Hands, as far as we can tell, the team encourages out-of-home placement for people with heavy care needs living alone, but it has no evidence that these placements have worked to the client's advantage in terms of health or safety let alone other values. When the social worker advocates the socialization that might occur in a group living situation, she probably has no firsthand experience of the nature of those social activities and whether they would be more stimulating and enjoyable for

Mr. Bruce than what he musters at home. A meaningful social life cannot be readily constructed through a variety of therapies and scheduled activities. It is likely that even teams ideologically highly committed to quality-of-life outcomes do so in a context that puts health outcomes first and fails to take into account the enormity of what clients are asked to give up for that possible improved safety. A lack of follow-up by the team that makes the protective recommendation adds to the problem, yet is highly likely because of segmentation in services for seniors. This problem, I emphasize, is not particular to teams, but teams do provide an illusion that the whole person is well considered even when the team has its own clear guidelines that emphasize safety and protection.

Too easily professionals take for granted that the client understands and accepts the role of the team. But the far-reaching tentacles of the team can be quite mysterious to the client. The late Janet Tulloch (1995), a longtime nursing home resident and advocate, wrote that a care plan can be "an instrument of terror" to a nursing home resident who begins to comprehend the power that that plan will have over his or her daily life. To avoid medicalizing everyday life, the team needs to explicitly consider social, psychological, and spiritual well-being, but even more importantly, it should probably refrain from prescribing anything at all for areas of life that are purely personal. Simply adopting a framework that holds, as its fourth step, considering the consumer's quality of life provides little assurance that the consideration will be sufficient in the face of other values that health teams hold more dear, or even correct (if a narrow view of quality of life is used).

Squandering Resources

Teams are expensive. A one-hour team meeting of eight people entails a day's worth of collective labor. If the team also requires a great deal of maintenance for its smooth functioning, that also bears a cost. Therefore, one could argue that teams should be put in place only when they are necessary, so that more resources will be available for the client or for all clients. Just as a full-blown multidimensional assessment is unnecessary for each senior who calls a help line to arrange home-delivered meals or transportation, it is also unnecessary to have a full team plan and work with every senior. Furthermore, when a team is necessary, it need not include every discipline known to health and human services. The motto should be to limit team involvement to those who clearly benefit by it, and to limit the size of teams in the interest of using resources well.

• Mr. and Mrs. Elliott, both in their early eighties, have a great many health problems between them. Mr. Elliott has chronic obstructive pulmonary disease, which is exacerbated on muggy days. He needs to rest frequently, gets tired from walking across the house, and is often gasping for breath. Mrs. Elliott is legally blind because of macular degeneration, and her osteoarthritis causes her considerable pain. The couple owns a condominium that they bought when they downsized their house, and their income from their investments yields $70,000 a year. Their expenses for medications are high, and as they add help, they anticipate eventually needing to sell some assets, which, of course, would lower their monthly income. Both the Elliotts are seen by the same geriatric clinic based in their local medical school. Mr. Elliott is briefly in the hospital, and afterward the geriatric team assesses them. The team recommends a team home care program that includes weekly nursing visits to set up medications and extensive coverage of a home health aide. They recommend that OT, PT, and a respiratory specialist visit the home to make recommendations for modifications. They put the Elliotts in touch with a shopping service and advise purchase of an emergency alarm system. When all the parts of the plan are put together, the costs are $400 a week or more than $20,000 a year, plus $1,000 in initial costs. The Elliotts feel this is a high proportion of income to pay for services and wonder if a less expensive solution is possible. The team points out that if the Elliotts' funds were exhausted, they would be eligible for Medicaid programs. The care coordinator on the team indicates that too often they must come up with very inexpensive plans because of what Medicaid allows, and that it is a delight in this case not to have to skimp on the best plan.

It is ethically incumbent on a team to consider the cost of a plan that it puts in place, whether those costs are borne by Medicaid, other third-party payer, or the clients themselves. The team might have provided a variety of options to Mr. and Mrs. Elliott with different price tags, including a lean plan similar to those covered under Medicaid. For example, it may not be necessary for three individuals to visit the home to suggest modifications. The hours of the home health aide might be reduced. The consideration that once their money is spent, Medicaid eligibility will kick in, is hardly reassuring to Mr. and Mrs. Elliott and seems to reflect inadequate stewardship of both private and public resources.

Lightening the Dark Side: A Final Comment

This chapter is not meant to be antiteam. It is clear that collaboration must occur in geriatric care, and that it takes place within disciplines and roles, across disciplines and roles, and across organizations. The complexity of collaboration increases as multiple professions and multiple organizations are involved. Yet given the complexity of needs of geriatric clientele and the complexity of service delivery, interprofessional teamwork is often necessary. If we did not have it, we would be inventing it.

When a team works well together, when it is imbued with a common sense of purpose and an appreciation of each member's contributions, and when it develops an effective way of communicating its business, it becomes a formidable force. Many of the issues discussed in this chapter are a by-product of that force. The views of a quieter, dissenting member may be repressed even if what that person has to say comes from a unique disciplinary expertise that others on the team lack. The team may be arrayed against the client in an intimidating way and not even be aware that this intimidation occurs. The team may also lose sight of its main purpose and embrace the secondary goal of happy team members, which is surely at best a means to an end. The team may become such a cohesive working unit that groupthink sets in.

Training team members to anticipate these problems would be part of a preventive strategy. Early detection of problems is also necessary. This may require a certain amount of group introspection around selected cases, asking questions such as: Did this client's voice get heard? Did all team members express an opinion? Has accountability for the actions of the team been clear? Have there been unnecessary delays? Does this client know how to get access to the team or to individual team members? Does the team appreciate the goals of the client?

Most of all the team must remain self-critical and refrain from becoming its own cheerleading group. Although they are harder to discern than questions about what is right to do in a single case, ethical issues related to autonomy, beneficence, and justice are embedded in these questions about how teams function or malfunction. As individual ethical issues arise, it would be worthwhile to raise the question: Is there anything in the way this team is designed or in the way it thinks that helps create this individual dilemma or interferes with its solution?

REFERENCES

Degenholtz, H. D., R. A. Kane, and H. Q. Kivnick. 1997. Care-related preferences and values of elderly community based long-term care consumers: Can case managers learn what's important to clients? *Gerontologist* 37:767–76.

Janis, I. L. 1983. Groupthink: Psychological studies of policy decisions and fiascoes. Boston: Houghton Mifflin.

Jonsen, A. R., M. Siegler, and W. J. Winslade. 1998. *Clinical ethics*, 4th ed. New York: McGraw-Hill.

Kane, R. A. 1975. *Interprofessional teamwork.* Social Work Manpower Monograph no. 8. Syracuse, N.Y.: Syracuse University School of Social Work.

———. 1994a. Ethics and long-term care: Everyday considerations. *Clinics in Geriatric Medicine* 10(3):489–99.

———. 1994b. Ethics and the frontline caregiver: Mapping the subject. *Generations* 18(3): 71–74.

Kane, R. A., and A. L. Caplan, eds. 1990. *Everyday ethics: Resolving dilemmas in nursing home life.* New York: Springer.

———. 1993. *Ethical conflict in the management of home care: The case manager's dilemma.* New York: Springer.

Kane, R. A, H. B. Degenholtz, and R. L. Kane. 1999. Adding values: An experiment in systematic attention to values and preferences of community long-term care clients. *Journal of Gerontology: Social Sciences* 54B(2):S109–19.

Kane, R. A., K. Freda, and L. Heikoff. 2000. Ethics, power and case management. In R. Applebaum, and M. White, eds., *Key issues in case management across the globe.* San Francisco: American Society on Aging.

Kane, R. A., and C. A. Levin. 1998. Who's safe? Who's sorry? The duty to protect the safety of clients in home-and community-based care. *Generations* 22(3):76–81.

Kane, R. L., L. H. Illston, and N. N. Miller. 1992. Qualitative analysis of the Program of All-Inclusive Care for the Elderly (PACE). *Gerontologist* 32:771–80.

Oriol, W. 1985. *The complex cube of long-term care.* Washington, D.C.: American Health Planning Association.

Rubenstein, L. V., D. Weiland, and R. Bernabei, eds. 1995. *Geriatric assessment technology: The state of the art.* Milan, Italy: Editrice Kurtis.

Thomas, W. H. 1994. *The Eden alternative: Nature, hope, and nursing homes.* Sherburne, N.Y.: Eden Alternative Foundation.

———. 1999. *The Eden alternative handbook: The art of building human habitats.* Summer Hill.

Tulloch, J. 1995. A resident's view of autonomy. In L. Gamroth, J. Semradek, and E. Tornquist, eds., *Enhancing autonomy in long-term care: Concepts and strategies.* New York: Springer.

Wise, H., R. Beckhard, I. Rubin, and A. Kyte. 1974. *Making health teams work.* Cambridge, Mass.: Ballinger.

Exploring Responsibility, Accountability, and Authority in Geriatric Team Performance

Phillip G. Clark, Sc.D., and
Theresa J. K. Drinka, M.S.S.W., Ph.D.

Responsibility, accountability, and authority in geriatric clinical practice are complex, interrelated, poorly defined, and shifting concepts that are heavily influenced by historical patterns and current modes of health care. More important, these concepts are also influenced by newly emerging models of teamwork; the expanding role of managers and insurers in health care decisions; and personal, professional, and social values and norms. These concepts promise to play an increasingly central role in the debates over health care costs, systems, and management, because it is at the interface between them and decision making at the clinical level that many of the current conflicts in the delivery of health care arise.

The once simple, dyadic relationship between the physician and the patient has given way to more complex, multidimensional relationships between the patient and various health care team members, between the team members themselves, and between providers and corporate managers. Traditional biomedical ethics that was based on this simple dyadic relationship is no longer adequate to deal with the more complex issues of teams and organizations in the delivery of health care. For example, a major set of recommendations has supported interdisciplinary geriatric team training for medical residents, though nowhere does this report explore the implications of this joint responsibility for the actual preparation of health care professionals for working on teams (Counsell et al. 1999).

Similarly, in geriatrics the concept of authority is not often discussed, but implicitly it figures prominently in everyday matters of clinical practice, system management, and reimbursement. For example, individual health care professionals and teams of professionals may assume *responsibility* for patient care without having the *authority* to implement certain types of treatment. An organization may have *authority* to make decisions concerning health care services but not assume the *responsibility* for making or implementing them.

The ethical dimensions of issues involving responsibility, accountability, and authority have been explored in general terms in the past (Agich 1982; Erde 1981; Kapp 1987; Newton 1982). Kaufman's (1995) overall observation that geriatric practice is fraught with ambiguities, tensions, and contrasting interpretations and lines of responsibility and authority applies especially to geriatric teamwork. Dilemmas arise in conflicts involving competing personal, professional, and organizational values, and they deal with principles of autonomy, beneficence, paternalism, and distributive justice.

In exploring these issues, this chapter has three major objectives. First, we develop a conceptual framework for thinking about issues of geriatric team responsibility, accountability, and authority, encompassing different levels and axes in the creation of a three-dimensional model. Second, we explore two different cases involving geriatric teams—one in a nursing home, the other in the community—that embody the intersecting issues between teamwork and ethics that characterize this discussion. Third, and finally, we develop some general observations and recommendations on how to think about and act in dilemmas involving responsibility, accountability, and authority in geriatric practice.

A Framework for Exploring Responsibility, Accountability, and Authority in Geriatric Teamwork

In exploring these issues and imposing some structure on our discussion, we must first consider definitions of these concepts and the development of a framework for thinking about the levels and dimensions of responsibility, accountability, and authority in geriatric practice.

Definitions

Responsibility. The initial need in this discussion is for terminological clarity around the concept of responsibility and its different dimensions. Following Green (1988), we can trace the term back to its Latin root, *respondere,* meaning "to answer an accusation, to answer for, to be answerable to." These two senses of the term are captured in the words *accountable* and *liable.* To answer an accusation involves being *liable for* the consequences of your actions and *accountable to* someone for those consequences. Traditionally, the discussion of responsibility has focused on individuals—not on groups or teams—as moral agents. Recently, however, arguments have been made that collectives can also be held accountable when that term is used to refer to a specific type of group—one whose members are unified or integrated in a particular manner.

This argument for collective accountability also hinges critically on the level of definition, function, and development of the team. For example, the defined roles of different health care professions on the geriatric team must be related to the patient care problem(s) at issue, as when the expertise of various health professionals is required to address the multifaceted needs of older persons. This relationship may vary among different patients and over time for the same patient. In addition, the level of integrated functioning of the geriatric team is critical for it to be termed a "collectivity." A multidisciplinary team—in which different professions offer their contributions in parallel or serial fashion—would not be considered a collective in the same sense that an interdisciplinary team would because of its capacity for integrated dialogue (Clark 1993; Drinka and Clark 2000).

But even if the team serves as a collectivity and is jointly responsible for the outcomes of its actions (or inactions), individuals can still be held responsible individually for their behavior as members of the team. As French (1982) said, "But team members do not hang together so as to avoid hanging separately. They hang together and they may also hang separately for their failures as individuals to perform their team or role tasks" (83).

Authority. Notions of responsibility and accountability also raise questions about authority, its basis, and who has it. *Authority* can be defined as the power to influence or command thought, opinion, or behavior. In Greek, one of the meanings of authority is "doer." In English, the meaning of authority (the right and power to command) originates from the creator of a work of art or craft having the power to make decisions about it (Senge et al. 1994). Senge and colleagues also discuss the notion of *shared authority,* meaning to be mutually responsible for the same effects, with or without explicit shared decision making. This interpretation fits with the nature of decision making and responsibility in interdisciplinary teamwork, where issues of what sharing and mutuality mean come to the forefront in discussions and disputes involving ethics.

We can further distinguish between two types of authority: formal and informal. Formal authority is based on governmental, legal, or structural factors within a group or organization. Informal authority is founded on less overt and more intrinsic factors, such as personality, leadership ability and style, moral suasion, and the like. Both of these types of authority are important in health care settings, where they may be related to the different levels of organization in the system.

Even though members of an interdisciplinary geriatric team do not all have formal power to influence decision making, they should all have some power to influence it. For the purposes of this chapter, we are concerned with three interrelated dimensions of authority that are relevant for team decision making: organizational, professional, and moral. The health care organization creates an ethical mission ("patient welfare") that establishes its organizational authority and guides its employees to act in accord with this mission. But exceptions and complexities related to patients can place qualifiers on the organization's mission. For example, if a physician confronts an exception in patient care that appears to go against the mission of the organization, that physician might attempt to make a decision using professional authority that could supersede the authority of the organization. A third dimension—moral authority—encompasses the values and ethical behavior of organizational members, team members, and patients. This can play out in moral argument or discourse and eventually in a decision based on that discourse.

All authority in relation to a team's work must be informed authority. By this we mean that it is the responsibility of the organization and the team's members to understand the mission of the organization and the team, the values of each profession, and the values of the patient. This obligation for being informed is correlated with the different levels of responsibility and authority in health care: organizational, professional, and individual.

Levels of Responsibility and Authority

The concept of geriatric team responsibility also takes its place within a broader context of personal, professional, and organizational responsibility and authority in health care, which corresponds roughly to periods of historical development when a different level was predominant (Rodwin 1998).

Personal. This is the initial period in the evolution of the health care system, from colonial times to the mid-1800s, when each physician made clinical choices individually and was responsible for them. The physician had clear authority, based on presumed knowledge and social convention, in the domain of health care. Patients deferred to this authority and were expected to follow doctor's orders. Traditional medical ethics tends to rely on this level of personal provider responsibility and authority.

Professional. From the mid-1800s until the early 1970s, personal responsibility and authority and traditional medical ethics were bolstered by the norms and practice standards of groups and associations. Organizational ethical codes and guidelines—which set forth the standards of conduct for different professions—became more important. Greater authority was vested in these organizations, due to their association with increased professional status and visibility. Though government gave legal authority in patient care decision making to the provider—through licensure and certification processes—professional associations helped to establish these requirements and had a vested interest in promoting the further development of the profession in both economic and political senses. Importantly, the physician still assumed the top position in the hierarchy of health care providers.

Team. With the advent of organized health care teams in the 1940s and '50s, a new form of collaboration among different professions emerged: the health care team. Teamwork introduces increased scrutiny of clinical practice by different health care professions outside one's own field of practice. Issues of authority arise on the team with regard to such questions as "Who is the team leader?" Initially, physicians—because of their historically preeminent position in the health care system—assumed the roles of leader and authority on the team. This role was bolstered by the presumed ultimate legal responsibility of the physician for the patient. But in recent times the role of team leader has been increasingly assumed by other professions like nursing and social work.

Organizational. In the 1970s, managed care organizations, purchasing cooperatives, and hospital systems started using their control of funds to set practice standards and expectations for health care providers. Importantly, this level of responsibility may challenge the ethical frameworks of personal and professional responsibility by introducing control on clinical decision making by personnel from outside the traditional health care professions. In addition, growing authority—due to the control of financial resources—has become vested in the organization and its management.

For example, individual health care providers may still have a responsibility toward the patient, but increasingly their authority to make independent professional decisions about treatment options is constrained by organizational guidelines and standards. Physicians may be penalized by the organization if their clinical decisions and associated costs fall outside a certain expected range, based on the extent of testing or days of hospitalization. Alternatively, the health care organization may have the authority to make certain types of decisions about health care services, but it is not willing to take the responsibility for acting on that authority. For example, in the case of costly mental health services, many managed care organizations are severely limiting access to them by the patients for whom they are responsible. Similarly, a health care team may feel that it is responsible for the well-being of the patients for whom it cares, but the organization within which it works is unwilling to give the team the authority to act on this responsibility in the case of really controlling resources and making decisions about their allocation.

Horizontal and Vertical Responsibility

Downie (1982) notes that collective responsibility for health care exhibits both "horizontal" and "vertical" dimensions. The current coexistence of differing levels of authority, responsibility, and accountability creates a set of multidirectional lines that can similarly be conceptualized as horizontal and vertical (see Figure 12.1). The disk in Figure 12.1 can be construed as a table where the members of the health care team have horizontal authority, responsibility, and accountability to each other as members of the same unit or group—tasks that are shaped by their own personal values, professional training, and organizational standards for conduct. Additionally, members of a team also have vertical responsibility and accountability toward, on the one hand, the organizational structure within which they work; and, on the other, toward the patient and the family, whose interests and needs they serve by virtue of being health care professionals.

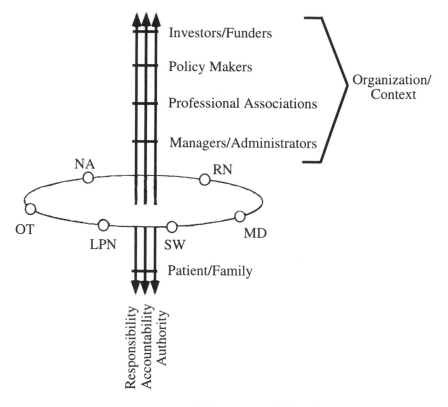

FIGURE 12.1 Responsibility, accountability and authority:
vertical and horizontal integration

Importantly, the organizational structure includes "sublevels" of managers/administrators, professional associations, policy makers, and investors/funders. Those individuals representing the organizational levels usually exercise their vertical responsibility and authority downward and expect accountability upward from the team. They often ignore downward accountability and seldom see the horizontal responsibilities they also have to the other members of the vertical structure, including the patient and the team. It is essential that members of the organizational structure also come regularly to the table to dialogue with the team and the patient system, to learn from them so they are able to understand their needs and incorporate them into a structure that is both vertically and horizontally dynamic.

This bidirectional model captures the complexity of the overall network of responsibilities that surrounds the geriatric health care professional and reiterates the complicated nature of responsibility, accountability, and authority in the health care system. In addition, it positions the team as a buffer or interpreter between the patient and the family on the one hand, and the health care system on the other.

Against this backdrop of conceptual complexity, we will examine the nature of the ethical and team-related issues of responsibility, accountability, and authority using two case studies: one on institutional (nursing home) care, and one on community care. These complex cases and recommendations about how to deal with them involve issues of factual knowledge, values and ethical conflicts, behavioral assumptions, and conflicting personal and professional loyalties—which are related particularly to the axes of responsibility and accountability we previously explored (Potter 1973). These issues are frequently interrelated; for example, the definition of a clinical "problem" encompasses factual and value-based dimensions, and this definition leads us toward a particular set of solutions to it.

The application of the analytic framework for "unpacking" the cases helps to clarify the ethical issues relating to responsibility, accountability, and authority on the teams. The second case, representing a community-based example, raises different issues from the first one.

Case Description

Mrs. Josephine La Rue was a 74-year-old nursing home resident with chronic obstructive lung disease from smoking a pack of cigarettes a day for sixty years. She also had osteoarthritis and mild dementia of unknown etiology, although she was not judged incompetent. Mrs. La Rue's daughter lived in another city and visited her mother three or four times a year. She said that she often felt guilty that she could not visit as often as she would like. Mrs. La Rue's daughter told the social worker that she was visiting nursing homes in her area so she could move her mother closer with the hope of visiting her every day. But the social worker did not feel that the daughter was sincere in this desire. The social worker also did not feel a responsibility to help the daughter find another nursing home, as the administrator had informed the staff that they needed to do everything they could to keep private pay residents happy so they stayed at the nursing home.

Mrs. La Rue had been treated at a local hospital for pneumonia and was returned to the nursing home (in which she had spent the last year as a private-pay resident) with a prognosis of "probable recovery." The physician who treated her in the hospital was the same physician who cared for her in the nursing home. But he had been extremely hard to reach, as he was carrying an extra caseload for another physician who was on maternity leave.

Mrs. La Rue's condition started to deteriorate during the two days after her readmission to the nursing home. She developed a slight fever (99.7) and she seemed more lethargic. The team discussed Mrs. La Rue's case at the weekly team meeting, two days after her discharge from the hospital. The RN, LPN, and social worker on the floor were regular attendees at the weekly meeting. But the RN who attended this meeting was called to a family emergency during the meeting and was not present for the discussion of Mrs. La Rue's condition. The nursing assistant who was assigned to care for her had mentioned several times to the LPN that, since her return, Mrs. La Rue had expressed a wish to die.

The discussion at the meeting centered on Mrs. La Rue's condition. The RN felt that her current status was a remnant of the infection and had planned to inform the physician of significant changes in her condition if the fever increased or if her physical status deteriorated further. The RN said that she wanted the staff to closely monitor Mrs. La Rue's vital signs and to alert her if anything changed. After the RN left, the LPN mentioned several times that Mrs. La Rue had expressed her wishes to the staff for no extraordinary measures and that she did not want to be resuscitated. Mrs. La Rue died that night in her sleep.

Mrs. La Rue's daughter informed the state nursing home survey office of her mother's "untimely death." Following an investigation, a state surveyor noted that "the facility did not immediately inform the physician of significant changes in the resident's condition, creating a substantial probability for the resident's death." One staff member, the LPN, who was asked to explain the notification delay, told surveyors that Mrs. La Rue had an advance directive indicating that she did not want to be resuscitated.

Gather the Clinical Information

The "knowledge" dimensions of this case set the stage for the real dynamic of how the issues of responsibility, accountability, and authority were played out within the nursing home. For example, we know that Mrs. La Rue had recently been treated for an acute condition, pneumonia, before returning to the nursing home, where she was expected to recover. But shortly after returning to the institution, she developed a slight fever and seemed more lethargic. She was not treated, nor were plans made to return her to the hospital. Importantly, and as discussed in more detail in the next section, there was substantial "factual confusion" over whether Mrs. La Rue had, indeed, expressed a wish to die and whether this "fact" had been substantiated in a written document. Related to this problem, there was confusion over what constitutes an advance directive and what it actually means for patient care decision making.

Identify Patient and Family Preferences

The nursing assistant in the facility reported that Mrs. La Rue had expressed a wish to die several times since returning from the hospital. The LPN also said that Mrs. La Rue had shared her wishes with the staff for "no extraordinary measures" and that she did not want to be resuscitated. Following the resident's death, the LPN reported that Mrs. La Rue had an advance directive indicating that she did not want to be resuscitated. But it was difficult to ascertain the validity of these statements, because Mrs. La Rue had dementia or possibly a delirium caused by the fever, and there seemed to be conflicting interpretations among the health care providers in this case about precisely what the patient really wanted. Moreover, her daughter appeared not to visit her mother very often and apparently wanted her to be kept alive—perhaps motivated by guilt that she did not visit more often—though she apparently had not informed the nursing home of this wish. Further evidence of her conflicted feelings revolved around her (presumed) attempts to move her mother to a nursing home nearby.

This case seems to represent a breakdown in the clear determination by the facility and its staff of the wishes of the patient and the family—an expectation grounded in the nursing home's organizational responsibility. Such a determination would have supported the value of autonomy, expressed in this case by the exercise of control over decisions affecting one's own life. In this regard, the "vertical" responsibility of the professional staff toward the patient seems to have been ignored, as was the responsibility of the nursing home for educating its entire staff about the autonomy-enhancing requirements of the Patient Self-Determination Act (PSDA) for informing residents and their families about their options for advance directives (Clark 1996; High 1991). These breakdowns in legal and moral responsibility resulted in undermining the value of autonomy—a concern of major proportions in geriatric clinical practice, especially in long-term care settings (Hofland 1988). The various interpretations of the (presumed) wishes of the patient and the family by the staff were also colored by their own personal and professional values and assumptions about quality-of-life issues.

Evaluate Quality-of-Life Issues

Based on their professional training and socialization as health care providers, different professions have varying value assumptions—frequently not explored or overtly communicated—about the quality of life (Clark 1995, 1997; Drinka and Clark 2000). These assumptions are based on the differential weighting of factors considered important to quality of life, including physical, psychological, and social dimensions; and they can lead to ethical conflicts on teams in determining the "right" course of action. These differences were seemingly never discussed by the nurses and social worker at the weekly team meetings, meetings that the physician apparently did not attend—so his "voice" was missing from the discussion of this case. This probably resulted in a clinical decision being made that was different from what would have been the outcome had he been present (McClelland and Sands 1993). It is obvious that the different members of the team interpreted the meaning of the patient's comments about "wanting to die" differently, each from their own perspective and background, due in part to their assumptions about Mrs. La Rue's quality of life. The fact that these assumptions or interpretations were never openly addressed and discussed is linked to the suboptimal level of team functioning.

Consider Contextual Factors

This category includes both the team and the organizational factors that bear on this case. Here, issues of responsibility and accountability were related to the horizontal responsibilities of the team members to communicate clearly among themselves, and to the vertical responsibility of the nursing home (organization) to provide an adequate setting in which the team can function.

In the case of the former issue, the level of team functioning seems to have been problematic, with the physician not present at team meetings and with the RN leaving a team meeting early due to a personal emergency. This raises the question of whether the team was a truly interdisciplinary one that was functioning at the level of a true collectivity (as discussed earlier), or whether it was simply a loosely organized collection of individual health care providers. Regardless, it still failed the patient and the family by not effectively addressing important clinical decision-making issues as a team. Its members did not adequately report to each other what was happening to the patient and her family, due to workload and personal/family issues. For example, issues related to the daughter's wish to move her mother to another facility were not shared with the team by the social worker, presumably due to the pressure from the nursing home administrator to keep private pay patients. Similarly, the RN, LPN, and CNA did not communicate adequately with each other and with the MD regarding the patient's medical condition and her (presumed) preferences for care. This failure in team communication once again resulted in the lack of recognition of values central to the quality of care. The low level of team functioning may have led to a situation where "because everyone was responsible for recognizing important values, no one was responsible" for doing so.

Additionally, we can question the level of knowledge about the nature and requirements of advance directives, particularly on the part of the social worker. Perhaps, as is the case in many states, this person had no formal training in social work and simply worked as the "social worker designee." In such a case, should not this individual have been responsible for getting more knowledge and training, if necessary, in the legal and clinical requirements for the use of advance directives? At the very least, we can say that the individuals did not fulfill their responsibility to each other as team members; nor did they fulfill their responsibility to the patient and the family to correctly ascertain their wishes.

With regard to the latter organizational issue, the nursing home had apparently failed to adequately educate its staff on understanding advance directives and their application. By its failing to establish a common ground of understanding of these issues, it left the door open to individual biases, misunderstanding, and haphazard decision making. We can speculate that perhaps pressures from the owners of the nursing home—especially if it was a proprietary facility—kept resources for staff training at a minimum. This is further evidence of the impact that the vertical dimensions of organizational responsibility can have on patient care and a substantiation of the importance of distributive justice considerations (how resources are allocated) in the context for geriatric teamwork. At the end of the case, we see the nursing home itself being held accountable to the state regulators for the apparent lapses in communication and training that led to Mrs. La Rue's "untimely" death.

If this nursing home had had an institutional ethics committee, it might have been possible to involve this group in reviewing such cases as this. But in our experience it is unlikely that an "official" committee of this sort would have been called upon for advice or consultation. This is so because the ethical issues are likely to be obscured by the team communication and dynamics problems, which are part of the very fiber of clinical practice in this case. The interprofessional and interpersonal conflicts and coordination issues prevented the recognition of the significant moral dimensions in this patient's care. Even if this case was brought before an ethics committee, it is likely that the LPN and the CNA would not be expected to participate.

The nursing home itself would have had an organizational responsibility to use an institutional ethics committee, if it existed. This committee would provide, minimally, an educative and sensitizing function for staff and team members on how ethics and teamwork issues need to be considered as interrelated in geriatric practice.

Resolve the Ethical Issues and Create the Plan

Due to unclear lines of responsibility within the team itself (e.g., who was the team leader? was someone on the team responsible for the team's actions? were all the team members responsible as individuals?), no specific plan seems to have been developed. Indeed, one of the criticisms of team accountability, as Green (1988) points out, is that "where all are responsible, no one is responsible, thus we tend to lapse into a state of moral indifference or acquiescence" (40). This seems to have been the case in this instance.

Arguably, the physician had the ultimate responsibility for the patient, at least in a legal sense, but he had failed to use his professional authority properly to pull the team together to discharge its responsibility toward the patient and the family. Individual team members also had their own responsibilities toward the patient and the family, but they failed to act effectively on them, perhaps because they felt they had no authority in the informal sense. As mentioned above, they failed to act out of a sense of moral indifference—the "where all are responsible, no one is responsible" moral trap. Similarly, the nursing home itself had both organizational responsibility and formal authority—as vested in it by law—to guard patient well-being, but it failed on both counts when it did not provide adequate training to all its staff in advance directives and also did not develop adequate guidelines for the care team with regard to lines of responsibility and authority. This created a situation in which patient welfare was openly threatened by a lack of procedural safeguards on how the team made care plan decisions.

In this case, then, we see an instance of how poor team functioning and inadequate organizational responsibility can undercut the ability of individual health care professionals to recognize and adequately incorporate the important value of patient autonomy into their collective decision making. Thus, the voices of the patient and the family were ignored or at least muted, leading to a breakdown in the communication of important wishes about care.

Case Description

Mrs. Gertrude Camebo is an 82-year-old, divorced female with Type II insulin-dependent diabetes, hypertension, vascular dementia, prior cerebrovascular accident with left-sided weakness, angina, and a history of falls. She has prescriptions for six medications that require a complex dosing regimen. Mrs. Camebo has an income from Social Security and her former husband's pension that puts her above the income limit for support services. She lives in her own home with her only child, a daughter, and the daughter's husband and their teenage son. Mrs. Camebo has told them that they can live in her house as long as they help her get by. The daughter works part time as a grocery store bagger and the son-in-law is looking for work. Although the daughter appears fond of her mother, she seems unable to comprehend her mother's disabilities. For example, the daughter expects her mother to do her own laundry, which is in the basement of her home. Mrs. Camebo has fallen numerous times in the past year—once down the basement stairs. She was treated for a concussion and hospitalized briefly for observation after she fell and sustained multiple abrasions.

After her most recent fall, Mrs. Camebo is referred for a competency hearing at which the judge rules her mentally competent. She reiterates to the social worker that she wants to live at home. Although the daughter says that she understands her mother's medication regimen, medication reviews and blood glucose levels indicate poor compliance. A community-based home health care team that provides Mrs. Camebo's care suspects that her falls may be due in part to the noncompliance. Also, the house needs extensive repairs, inside and out, and it could use railings on both sides of the stairways. The home health social worker has found a repair service that would install the railings at cost.

But the daughter says that they do not have the money. The team has evaluated Mrs. Camebo's activities of daily living (ADLs) and also her instrumental activities of daily living (IADLs). She appears to be independent in most of her ADLs. But she needs help with many of her IADLs, like shopping, cleaning, money management, home repair, medication management, meal preparation, and transportation.

Mrs. Camebo's son-in-law drinks heavily and has difficulty holding a job. He is home alone with her during the day when his wife is at work. All of the falls have occurred when the daughter is at work. The nurse on the team suspects that the son-in-law may be responsible for several falls. But the social worker notes that the team has absolutely no proof that there has been any abuse. Although she appears somewhat depressed, Mrs. Camebo's medical conditions are currently stable. Because of this, Medicare guidelines will not support continued home visits.

At the weekly team meeting, there is considerable discussion about Mrs. Camebo's safety at home and whether abuse or neglect is occurring in the household. The physician favors a more aggressive approach to the situation and recommends reporting the current circumstances to the state authorities for an investigation. She also admits that she has been "liberal in documenting disabilities" to permit continued monitoring by home care. The registered nurse on the team, who is a close friend of the agency's administrator, accuses the doctor of Medicare fraud, saying that the doctor is being irresponsible in her behavior, and she threatens to report the MD. The social worker is shocked. He feels that the nurse is behaving in a heartless manner and tells her that he does not think it is a good idea to report anyone. The rest of the team's members (occupational therapy assistant, nursing assistant, and licensed practical nurse) are silent.

Gather the Clinical Information

In summary, Mrs. Camebo has a litany of chronic health problems—including insulin-dependent diabetes, cardiovascular disease, vascular dementia, and a history of falling—including a recent hospitalization following a fall. Her medical conditions require a number of medications, with complex dosing requirements. It appears that she does not have the judgment to handle her medication regimen, and her family members are either incapable or unwilling to help her. Mrs. Camebo does not have dementia that is serious enough for her to be judged legally incompetent. Although her medical conditions appear stable, there seem to be major questions about her safety at home and possible abuse or neglect. There is also a question of whether Mrs. Camebo's family should be held responsible and accountable for her care, especially for her twice daily insulin injections.

Although some team members may think that Mrs. Camebo's family is responsible for her, others may disagree. Policy makers do not currently hold themselves or family members accountable for the welfare of elderly parents. Some disciplines like social work may feel professional responsibility for viewing the entire family as the client, while others like occupational therapy do not. Also, some physicians may feel pressure to "do no harm" (beneficence) and thus be unwilling to let go of a case like this. This sense of responsibility is not, however, held by funding sources like Medicare.

Identify Patient and Family Preferences

Mrs. Camebo's family has a vested interest in remaining in her home, but it is not known whether they desire to or are able to care for her. There do not appear to have been expressions by the individual or the family regarding type and extent of treatment. But the presumed noncompliance with the current medication regimen suggests that the patient and her family are not able to cooperate fully in the treatment plan. Her statement to the social worker that she wants to live at home is Mrs. Camebo's only explicit communication about these issues with the health care team or its members. Additionally, the family issues suggest a pattern of neglect or perhaps even exploitation, which complicates the treatment decisions and, indeed, makes attempts to keep her at home problematic.

Evaluate Quality-of-Life Issues

While her overall medical conditions at present appear stable, Mrs. Camebo's quality of life seems at risk, with the danger that a fall at any time or neglect could place her in the hospital and subsequently in a nursing home. Despite the fact that she has the legal authority to determine where she wants to live, we do not know if she is mentally capable of assuming this risk to stay at home. One is left with the feeling that this case may be an example of the "classic" geriatric ethical conflict between individual autonomy on the part of the patient and the team's professional concerns about her safety—a tension between the ethical principles of autonomy and beneficence (Kaufman 1995). There is no clear-cut resolution to this conflict, which is tied to the shifting contexts and levels of personal care ability, family caregiving and support, and service delivery from the health care system. This team seems to lack the level of integrated communication necessary to effectively resolve this dilemma.

Funders and health care policy makers do not define quality of life for geriatric patients who live at home. Most health care professionals tend to define quality of life in terms of safety. But each team member ultimately defines it in terms of his or her professional and personal experiences. It is the team members' collective responsibility to openly discuss their individual perceptions of quality of life with the team and to arrive at some agreement regarding the team's approach to quality-of-life issues. The team must act as a buffer and an interpreter between the patient, the family system, and the organizational entities that set rules for when care is and is not appropriate.

Consider Contextual Factors

From the perspective of horizontal responsibility, the level of functional integration of the differing perspectives or professions on the team seems problematic. The physician and the other team members seem to disagree about how aggressively to move ahead on the concerns about suspected abuse or neglect. This question of the "pace of team activity" may reveal a deeper division among the team members (Qualls and Czirr 1988). Moreover, the family and the health care team have not discussed these issues together, presumably because the team members misunderstand their team roles and tasks in regard to patient assessment. While some team members have assumed individual professional responsibility for their discipline's assessment of the patient, the team has not assumed collective responsibility for patient assessment and treatment. Focusing on collective team responsibility would mean arriving at an integrated problem list for the patient and an array of interdisciplinary solutions that address the integrated problems.

In addition, the thinly veiled dispute over authority between the nurse and physician members of the team suggests conflicting bases of authority. The physician is assuming that she has the formal authority as presumed team leader and legally as the doctor to make decisions about care needs and their appropriate documentation. The nurse, however, is asserting moral authority in questioning this assumption and suggesting that the physician is lying to Medicare about the level of need for home care services. In addition, the way in which the nurse accused the physician indicates a fundamental lack of trust within the team. This may reveal a problem with team development and function.

We must also address the issue of accountability. The funding sources and policy makers do not appear to feel accountable for the welfare of a geriatric home care patient who is too stable for Medicare and has too much money to qualify for Medicaid and not enough money for private insurance. The professions have not developed a collective accountability for such patients. Administrators ultimately look at a patient's ability to pay for a service. This again leaves the geriatric team as a buffer and interpreter between the patient and the other organizational entities. It is helpful if the team can understand its position and use that knowledge to unite in its approach to this type of ethical dilemma.

Examining the same issues from the perspective of vertical professional responsibilities, we can ask: Is the physician acting responsibly by perhaps overstating the patient's level of disability in order to keep her on home care? Should the nurse "blow the whistle" on the physician, or should she simply acquiesce since it is the physician's responsibility to document and defend program eligibility requirements? Such "gaming of the system" is not an uncommon practice among clinicians, but it raises an important ethical issue over conflicting lines of responsibility between loyalty to the patient and her welfare on the one hand (the value of beneficence), and responsibility for honesty to the governmental funding source (the value of truth telling) on the other.

Thus, broken lines of accountability, conflicting lines of responsibility, and different types of authority are embedded in this clinical case—which play out in a resultant ethical dilemma or value conflict. It is to be hoped that an understanding of these complex dimensions can suggest an avenue for resolution and moving forward on developing an interdisciplinary care plan.

Resolve the Ethical Issues and Create the Plan

The development of an interdisciplinary care plan for the patient would be dependent on the ability of the team to address the issues of conflict that threaten to split it apart. Hopefully, the recognition that it needs to keep its focus on the goal of patient welfare will help to overcome the divisions that seem to be appearing. This is, in turn, dependent on the team members' ability to communicate more openly with each other around issues of professional responsibility. In this sense, the team needs to reassert the importance of the members' horizontal responsibility to the team in coming up with a good plan of action and, ultimately, its vertical responsibility to the patient in putting her welfare first.

Every member of an interdisciplinary geriatric team is accountable for the actions of the team. As such, each team has the responsibility to develop a formal or informal understanding that the team as a whole will discuss ethical dilemmas. The team also must decide on structures and processes for handling ethical dilemmas relating to collective and professional authority.

For any team, the entire team has responsibility for discussing and resolving conflicts. But in this case, the social worker may have an obligation to play a more active role in bringing the physician and the nurse together. Professionally, social work is one of the disciplines that best prepares and trains its members to deal with process analysis of a team's dynamics (Clark 1997; Drinka and Streim 1994). But paradoxically, a social worker's ability to communicate on an interdisciplinary team may be impaired by his or her socialization and professional orientation toward patient advocacy (Kane 1975). This suggests a conflict in lines of responsibility for a team's social worker: on the one hand, allegiance toward the patient and raising his or her "voice" in the discussion; on the other, loyalty toward the other team members and the team as a whole (Mailick and Ashley 1981).

It might be argued, as in the previous case, that an institutional ethics committee or consultant could play a role in identifying and resolving the significant moral conflicts here. But a community-based clinical team of this type is unlikely to have access to such a resource—unless it is sponsored by a hospital or part of a larger health care network. Moreover, as mentioned earlier, such conflicts over professional values and practice are likely to go unrecognized as moral dilemmas and are more likely to be characterized as simply interprofessional or interpersonal conflicts.

In this case, a recognition that different bases for authority are at stake, both from within and from without the team, may help to clarify the nature of the conflicts facing it. Currently, the nurse and the physician both seem to be trying to "trump" each other's authority, using different sources of legitimation. In the meantime, the team is distracted from its primary mission of patient welfare. An agreement by team members to set aside time to work on issues of team trust and problem solving would undoubtedly be helpful in handling future ethical dilemmas.

It is likely that the team nurse will report this incident to management. Management has responsibility and accountability to the funding sources. But it also has responsibility and authority for the development and maintenance of the team. Management may have to assume the responsibility for helping the team repair its divisions by helping it focus on the ethical dilemmas that are part of this case and by applying subsequent learning to future cases. In sum, however, this case once again represents a situation where problems in team functioning serve to obscure values important to patient well-being and to reduce the team's ability to respond appropriately to a moral conflict among responsibility, autonomy, and authority.

Conclusion

Lines of responsibility and accountability, and bases of authority, have become more complex as the health care system has become more complicated. The old, simple dyadic relationship between provider and patient has been replaced with a network of conflicting and confusing lines of responsibility toward different players at differing levels of the system. New sources of authority, frequently linked to organizational factors such as payment structure, have emerged as the dominant players in the health care system.

New ethical concerns will emerge as these changes unfold. Conceptualizing issues of responsibility, accountability, and authority as horizontal and vertical, with different levels and players at each level, enhances both our understanding of them and our appreciation of their complexity. At the heart of these concerns is the ability to assess accurately a geriatric patient's well-being and the ever-shifting capabilities and responsibilities of the patient and his or her family. The responsibilities of the professionals, the team, and the organization need to mesh with their accountability and authority in each case. Ethical analysis is at the heart of these issues, as individuals as moral agents increasingly work together in the collectivities we call teams within larger health care organizations. Interdisciplinary teamwork can serve to enhance and promote our understanding of ethical dilemmas, or it can obscure them and undercut our ability to act in a responsible manner toward resolving them.

As is the case in much of teamwork, understanding and clarity can facilitate concrete action in bringing about changes that improve teamwork, quality of care for patients, and—hopefully—their quality of life as well. It has been the goal of this chapter to examine the weblike lines of responsibility and accountability, as well as the different dimensions of authority, that are at stake in these cases. By doing so, we have attempted to point the way toward resolving both the ethical and the teamwork issues at their heart. Building on an earlier suggestion by Moody (1988), perhaps we should consider adopting the "three C's of a communicative ethic" for negotiating the shifting shoals of responsibility, accountability, and authority in geriatric practice. We need open *communication* about all three issues, *clarification* of the areas of conflict and dispute, and *collaboration* in the development of a plan of care that meets the needs of the patient and incorporates the unique contributions and strengths of all the members of the team. This ethic is more akin to a template for understanding and resolving than a machine for producing simple solutions.

Discussion Questions

1. How are the traditional interpretations of responsibility, accountability, and authority changing in the face of new forces at work in the health care system? How do these changes affect the geriatric team?

2. Do you think that a highly functioning and effective team should always have collective responsibility for all its actions? Why or why not? How do individual team members continue to exercise their responsibilities as health care professionals?

3. Which values are most likely to come into conflict on geriatric teams when lines of responsibility and accountability are not clear? How can teams deal effectively with these moral dilemmas?

4. How can a geriatric team insure a high level of communication among its members with respect to issues of responsibility and accountability?

REFERENCES

Agich, G. J., ed. 1982. *Responsibility in health care.* Dordrecht, Holland: D. Reidel.
Clark, P. G. 1993. A typology of interdisciplinary education in gerontology and geriatrics: Are we really doing what we say we are? *Journal of Interprofessional Care* 7:217–27.
———. 1995. Quality of life, values, and teamwork in geriatric care: Do we communicate what we mean? *Gerontologist* 35:402–11.
———. 1996. Communication between provider and patient: Values, biography, and empowerment in clinical practice. *Ageing and Society* 16:747–74.

————. 1997. Values in health care professional socialization: Implications for geriatric education in interdisciplinary teamwork. *Gerontologist* 37:441–51.

Counsell, S. R., R. D. Kennedy, P. Szwabo, N. S. Wadsworth, and C. Wohlgemuth. 1999. Curriculum recommendations for resident training in geriatrics interdisciplinary team care. *Journal of the American Geriatrics Society* 47:1145–48.

Downie, R. S. 1982. Collective responsibility in health care. *Journal of Medicine and Philosophy* 7:43–56.

Drinka, T. J. K., and P. G. Clark. 2000. *Health care teamwork: Interdisciplinary practice and teaching.* Westport, Conn.: Auburn House.

Drinka, T. J. K., and J. E. Streim. 1994. Case studies from purgatory: Maladaptive behavior within geriatrics health care teams. *Gerontologist* 34:541–47.

Erde, E. L. 1981. Notions of teams and team talk in health care: Implications for responsibilities. *Law, Medicine, and Health Care* 9:26–28.

French, P. A. 1982. Collective responsibility and the practice of medicine. *Journal of Medicine and Philosophy* 7:65–85.

Green, W. P. 1988. Accountability and team care. *Theoretical Medicine* 9:33–44.

High, D. M. 1991. A new myth about families of older people? *Gerontologist* 31:611–18.

Hofland, B. F. 1988. Autonomy in long-term care: Background issues and a programmatic response. *Gerontologist* 28(Suppl.):3–9.

Kane, R. A. 1975. *Interprofessional teamwork.* Social Work Manpower Monograph no. 8. Syracuse, N.Y.: Syracuse University School of Social Work.

Kapp, M. B. 1987. Interprofessional relationships in geriatrics: Ethical and legal considerations. *Gerontologist* 27:547–52.

Kaufman, S. R. 1995. Decision making, responsibility, and advocacy in geriatric medicine: Physician dilemmas with elderly in the community. *Gerontologist* 35:481–88.

Mailick, M. D., and A. A. Ashley. 1981. Politics of interprofessional collaboration: Challenge to advocacy. *Social Casework* 62:131–37.

McClelland, M., and R. G. Sands. 1993. The missing voice in interdisciplinary communication. *Qualitative Health Research* 3:74–90.

Moody, H. R. 1988. From informed consent to negotiated consent. *Gerontologist* 28(Suppl.): 64–70.

Newton, L. H. 1982. Collective responsibility in health care. *Journal of Medicine and Philosophy* 7:11–21.

Potter, R. B. 1973. *War and moral discourse.* Richmond, Va.: John Knox Press.

Qualls, S. H., and R. Czirr. 1988. Geriatric health teams: Classifying models of professional and team functioning. *Gerontologist* 28:372–76.

Rodwin, M. A. 1998. Conflicts of interest and accountability in managed care: The aging of medical ethics. *Journal of the American Geriatrics Society* 46:338–41.

Senge, P., A. Kleiner, C. Roberts, R. B. Ross, and B. J. Smith. 1994. *The fifth discipline fieldbook: Strategies and tools for building a learning organization.* New York: Doubleday.

13 CHAPTER

The Locus of Care and
Its Effect on the Presentation
of Ethical Conundrums

Steven K. Rothschild, M.D., and Russell Burck, Ph.D.

He who would do good to another must do it in minute particulars.

WILLIAM BLAKE

In this casebook, discussions draw on Jonsen, Siegler, and Winslade's (JSW) Clinical Workup Model of ethics, focusing on the clinical facts of a case, patient and family preferences, quality-of-life factors, and contextual features (Jonsen, Siegler, and Winslade 1998). This chapter considers one contextual feature, the clinical setting, and examines its impact on the ethical commitments, issues, conundrums, and dilemmas facing interdisciplinary teams.

Ethics of Place

At first blush, the reader might wish to challenge the premise that the location in which a team works should in any way affect the ethical analysis. Certainly, one of the most important characteristics of a case, the clinical facts, would not seem to be directly affected by the location in which the team and patient are interacting. Some would go so far as to argue that giving attention to the locus of care can only distract from a thoughtful concern for patient preferences, rights, and quality of life. It is our experience, however, that attention to the locus of care contributes to our understanding of patient and family preferences; makes us more sensitive to the patient's assessment of her/his quality of life; can enhance the interaction among patients, family members, and health care providers; and even indicates what goals of care or treatment the team considers feasible. Accordingly, our thesis is that attention to place has an important role in the ethics of health care.

If we look at the etymology of the word that gives us *ethics*, we see an odd definition in the derivation portion of the dictionary: "dwelling" (*Webster's* 1961). Most of our students do a double take when we tell them that ethics is related to dwellings. The link seems less forced when we ask them to consider the legal requirements (which ethics has helped shape) for the amount of space that a day care center needs to provide for each adult. In a recent lecture at the University of Illinois, Kenneth Vaux made a point of distinguishing utopias from eutopias and dystopias. Utopias are imagined ideals and are also literally "nowheres": places that do not exist in the real world. Eutopias are good places, like a comfortable retirement village that offers full services and many activities. Dystopias are "bad" or "not so good" places, like nursing homes that ignore smells or do just enough to keep their licenses or a physician's waiting room filled with coughing and sneezing patients.

A "thought exercise" can help illuminate these points. Close your eyes for a moment and visualize yourself in a hospital room. What do you see? What does this place sound like? Are there smells you associate with this setting? What emotions do these sensations trigger? Take several minutes to review the full experience of being in a hospital room. Now repeat this exercise with a room in your current home. How are the sights, sounds, smells, and feelings different? How do these differences affect your emotional state? How might these differences influence your decision making?

In considering the setting of care in the case of Mrs. Lucy Gomez, we faced a choice. We could accompany her sequentially through episodes in which her health care needs required services in different settings. Her health care could start anywhere—for example, in the doctor's office—then shift to a hospital, then to a nursing home, and then back to home care. Such a sequential approach would necessitate introducing changes in the clinical facts of the case, as Mrs. Gomez's history unfolded over time. Examining the case at different points in the patient's life, however, would distract us from the central task of examining the impact of locus of care on the ethical problems facing the team. As much as we plausibly could, we have therefore controlled all variables other than setting.

The case of Mrs. Gomez will be examined in four parallel settings: her home, the outpatient clinic, the hospital, and the nursing home. The clinical information and the composition of the team will be roughly the same in each setting, with only enough variations to make it consistent with the locus of care. Although minor clinical details will be changed, we will repeat the entire case in each section; this will allow the reader to use any of the four sections of the chapter separately or in another sequence.

After presenting the facts of the case, we will outline the dilemmas that Mrs. Gomez presents to the team. Then, each section will review the same four discussion points:

- "Power of place" for the patient
- Impact of the locus of care on team goals, leadership, and processes
- Interaction of the patient and team
- External factors

The chapter ends with a series of trigger questions that may be used to develop classroom discussion or further personal exploration of the case in each setting.

Case Description: Home

Lucy Gomez is an 85-year-old widowed Hispanic woman who lives alone in a ramshackle apartment (in the view of team members who have been there) in an inner city neighborhood. For the past five years she has received care from a primary health care team, which provides services in her home. Members of the team include a GNP, physician, SW, OT, and chaplain.

Mrs. Gomez has been fairly independent in her self-care, although she does not go out very often. She pays a neighbor to pick up her medicines and groceries. Her medical problems include hypertension and diabetes; both of these have been fairly well controlled with medications. She has had very mild dementia (a Mini-Mental State Examination score of 22 out of 30) for the past two years, without identified reversible causes.

The nurse practitioner comes to see Mrs. Gomez after she receives a call from the patient's niece, who lives across town. The niece is upset because Mrs. Gomez has fallen five times in the past two weeks. Recently when she stopped to visit, she found her aunt sitting on the floor in the bathroom, unable to get up without extensive help from the niece.

She is found to have lost fifteen pounds since the prior visit three months ago. A small abrasion that she had on her left shin is now a Stage III ulcer, with poor healing. Mrs. Gomez appears disheveled and dehydrated. She is very deconditioned and cannot stand without full assistance of two people.

Mrs. Gomez refuses to go to the hospital. She is given one liter of intravenous fluids at home, and blood tests are performed. Social work arranges for four hours of a home health aide, five times a week, from the city department of aging. PT and OT begin to work with the patient, coming to her home several times a week. No new pathology is found after a thorough workup.

Two weeks later, her condition is unchanged. More frustrating to clinicians is the nurse practitioner's report of Mrs. Gomez's poor effort and follow-through on exercises and oral intake. She refuses to have any family move in with her because she believes they will steal from her. The team is concerned for her safety if she remains in the home by herself. Despite her dementia, however, she appears to understand her situation and refuses to go to a nursing home: "I know you all are trying to help me and are worried about me and all. I'm worried about falling too. I'd like to have help, but I'm afraid they would steal from me. My niece says I can come live with her, but this place means so much—and I don't really trust her either. No, the only way I am leaving this house is going to be in a box."

In this scenario, and those that follow, the team must address the problem of a patient who is falling at home and at times may be unable to get up or ask for help. The clinical facts are that she is deconditioned and is dehydrated and may be malnourished, but she refuses to go to a hospital. She needs closer supervision, but she refuses either having family move in with her or moving to a nursing home. Mrs. Gomez has a responsibility to exercise and to eat enough, but she is not doing so. She apparently wishes to be considered a decision-making member of the health care team and, with reasonable accuracy, is able to tell clinicians the nature and consequences of her decisions. At the same time, these decisions continue to harm her, and she behaves more like a recipient of care than an actor on her own behalf.

"Power of Place" for the Patient

In considering the effects of the home on the dilemmas posed by Mrs. Gomez's case, one can begin by examining "the power of place." From two points of view, the professionals on the team have an ethical responsibility to try to understand the meaning of home to Mrs. Gomez. First, a goal of medicine is to educate patients; and second, patient education is not just telling patients about their situations and their options but also involves hearing and learning the patients' perspectives: how patients see their situations, their options, their life choices. If we ask about Mrs. Gomez's perspectives, we are not just asking about what she prefers. We are asking about her story—specifically, what does her home mean for her?

In ethics, options form a continuum from obligation through permissibility to prohibition (see Figure 13.1). On this continuum, professional members of the team have an absolute responsibility to learn from Mrs. Gomez how she thinks about her living situation. On the surface, her situation looks like a garden-variety conflict between beneficence and respect for patient autonomy. At the very least, however, respect for autonomy entails a commitment to search out the particulars of Mrs. Gomez's desire to stay in her home. Katherine Montgomery Hunter writes that such "particulars . . . may represent what is most valued in a life or a history. Narrative remains mired in the particulars of human experience" (Hunter 1995). Thus, the team must begin by seeking to understand the cost to Mrs. Gomez's integrity, to her life story, if she is forced to move from her home. We call this the "narrative cost" to the patient.

For Mrs. Gomez, the power of place derives from having lived in the same home for many years. Each room, each piece of furniture is associated with dozens of memories. She recalls when she and her husband picked out the couch in the living room; thirty years later she remembers intimate details of the fight they had about what color to paint the kitchen. Her home is her history, especially her history with her late husband. Home is a repository, perhaps a sanctuary, of memory. This sanctuary may become progressively more important to her as she becomes more frail or if her memory begins to fail. Although it may be difficult for Mrs. Gomez to put these points into words, it is critical that a team member be responsible for exploring the power of place with the patient and her family.

What the team *does* know already is that Mrs. Gomez is emphatic about remaining at home. We have quite a bit of her story about why she wants to

Obligation		Permissibility		Prohibition	
Absolute	Stringent	More Preferable	Less Preferable	Stringent	Absolute

FIGURE 13.1 The continuum

Source: Burck 1996, 243. NCP 11: 244, 1996. Reprinted with permission American Society for Parenteral and Enteral Nutrition.

remain there, but part of the professionals' responsibility is to be alert for new pieces of this narrative. Perhaps staying there affords her autonomy. She can control, even if only to a limited degree, who comes and goes, what she eats, when she gets up, and when she goes to bed, in a manner that she could not achieve in her niece's home or a nursing home. Again, the team needs to hear from her not only the importance of remaining at home but also *why*.

Impact of Locus of Care on Team Goals, Leadership, and Processes

The first rule of effective interdisciplinary team care requires that team members have a shared purpose and work together to establish and achieve explicitly stated goals for patient care. We do not have this team's charter, but we can infer from its model of providing care in the patient's home that one of their goals is to help older patients remain at home as long as possible and to facilitate a move when remaining at home is inconsistent with safety. While a worthwhile goal, it may not always be the patient's goal, and it may conflict with another team goal. In this case, other team goals such as maximizing functional status or preventing avoidable morbidity and mortality seem in direct conflict with the goal of keeping Mrs. Gomez at home. In addition, motivations besides beneficence may be at work; for a Medicare HMO, the decision to keep her at home may be based on an analysis showing a greater cost of care in a hospital or nursing home. The team must not only explore Mrs. Gomez's goals and their meaning but must also be open about their own team goals.

By providing care in Mrs. Gomez's home, this team gains an advantage that is not available to teams working in other settings: direct observation of the context in which the patient cares for herself or receives care. In the clinic or hospital, professionals are limited to making observations of a patient's functional status and then extrapolating to predict the patient's ability to perform

ADLs and IADLs. In the home, this team can readily observe Mrs. Gomez's performance of her daily activities and safety. This information should help them consider her needs and tailor recommendations to her context.

The team should, however, be sensitive to the "power of place" in its own professional development; because clinicians are trained primarily in the hospital or outpatient clinic, they may misinterpret their perceptions in the home as if they were hospital or clinic data. For example, if health professionals observe boxes and cans of food left out on Mrs. Gomez's kitchen counter and table, they may conclude that Mrs. Gomez is behaving inappropriately or is cognitively impaired. For Mrs. Gomez, however, this may be a deliberate adaptive strategy in response to falls that occurred when she bent over to reach food in low cabinets or stretched to reach high cabinets. When crossing the boundaries between institutions and home, health care teams must be extremely careful not to fall into the clinical trap of interpreting observed behaviors only as clues to pathology.

Interaction of the Patient and Team

The patient's clinical setting affects the interaction among professional and patient/family members in the area of leadership. In the home, some patients behave more like consumers or passive recipients of health care services. If asked about their role on the health care team, they would either not understand the question or say that they are being served or treated. Other patients may feel honored that professionals come to their home but still do not think of themselves as team members. Still others are clearly intentional, alert participants in their own plan and care. Whether involved or not, in the home setting, the patient often controls the agenda. Unlike the hospital or nursing home setting, the patient can choose whether to adhere (or comply) to the treatment plan; the patient has passive veto power over most interventions and recommendations of the clinicians.

Family therapists have long noted that the power relationships between therapist and family vary, depending on whether the therapy is occurring in the office or in the family's home. The risk or probability that the therapist will be "inducted" into the family increases when therapy occurs in the home. In home care, some clinicians might adopt an idealistic, and overly simplistic, view of their team: "The patient is always the team leader." This may be true, but does Mrs. Gomez understand this role? Does she wish to have this role? Is "team leader" an accurate description of her role, or is it a rhetorical trope? The team needs to examine this issue carefully. Mrs. Gomez may be a *member* of the team and is certainly the *focus* of most of its attention. For certain functions, she may in fact be the team leader. But although she bears some responsibility for the formulation of the treatment plan and its implementation, she cannot be seen as the sole bearer of these responsibilities, even when the locus of care is in the home. The team cannot ethically defer all judgments to respecting her autonomy simply because they are working in her home.

The home setting introduces other contextual differences. For example, time spent with the patient in the home differs significantly from time spent in other settings. In a hospital, clinicians may interact with a patient for only a few minutes at a time over the course of several days; in an outpatient office, professional team members will see a patient for a few minutes too, but the next encounter may be weeks or months later. At home, at least one health care provider has seen Mrs. Gomez for about an hour at a time, and has done so every one to four weeks for the past few years. The professional members of the team have had the experience of seeing problems arise and be resolved over long periods and thus may be more willing to allow for the passage of time to resolve a conflict rather than force a decision.

Decision theory is an analytic approach to understanding how people weigh alternatives in a given situation. One critical variable in decision making is risk and the willingness to accept risk. Institutional settings are typically risk averse; thus, in a classic conflict between patient preferences and contextual features of cases, hospitals and nursing homes have historically preferred to subject older adults to the humiliation of restraints rather than assume the relatively small risk of falling and sustaining an injury. One form of decision theory, called game theory, would describe this as an application of the max-min rule: taking an action in which the worst possible outcome is equal to or better than the best outcome of not taking the action. Hospitals choose to use restraints because their analysis suggests that the worst possible outcome of restraint use (incontinence, depression, skin breakdown) is equal to or better than the best possible consequence of not using restraints (there will still be some patients who fall, leading to injury and possible litigation).

Team members who have worked with patients over longer periods will both perceive and weigh risks differently. Knowing how Mrs. Gomez has coped with prior health challenges may lead the team to conclude that the risk of her dehydration and falling is not as severe as it seems. One or more team members may observe, "Lucy has had bad times like this before, when we all thought she was going to die." More important, knowing that a degree of obstinacy has been her coping style for many years may cause the team to conclude that violating her wishes, and disrupting her deliberate life narrative by moving her out of her home, poses an even greater risk to Mrs. Gomez.

External Factors

Health professionals and patients face a wide range of external constraints on their actions regardless of the locus of care. Each setting is governed by unique legislative and regulatory issues. In addition, payment structures for services will differ between settings. Home care agencies are largely regulated by Medicare through the Health Care Financing Agency; some are also reviewed by the Joint Commission for the Accreditation of Health Care Organizations. Unlike professionals working in hospitals or nursing homes, the home care team does not have full control over the security and safety of the patient's home and thus cannot be held directly responsible for these conditions. Health workers will vary in their responses to this different degree of control. Some may feel that professionalism requires the same sense of responsibility for conditions in the home as in the hospital. Others will feel freer to pursue the goals preferred by Mrs. Gomez than they would in an institutional setting.

Finally, it is critical that the team consider the impact of finances in the home setting. American elderly persons pay over 50 percent of their health care costs out of their own pockets. Mrs. Gomez's desire to remain at home may well be the result of a careful, if unspoken, economic comparison of the costs of remaining in a fully paid-off house versus the daily costs of a nursing home or assisted living facility. She may well have concluded that moving to her niece's home or to a facility does not add enough value to offset the economic and narrative costs of leaving her own home. The professionals will need to consider the relative economic costs of various scenarios and discuss these with her, along with the other issues outlined above.

Case Description: The Outpatient Clinic

Lucy Gomez is an 85-year-old widowed Hispanic woman who lives alone in a ramshackle apartment in an inner city neighborhood. For the past five years she has received care at a nearby community health center. This outpatient clinic uses a team of clinicians to care for frail elderly, including a GNP, physician, SW, OT, and chaplain.

Mrs. Gomez has been fairly independent in her self-care, although she does not go out very often. She pays a neighbor to pick up her medicines, and groceries. Her medical problems include hypertension and diabetes; both of these have been fairly well controlled with medications. She has had very mild dementia (MMSE of 22 out of 30) for the past two years, without identified reversible causes.

Mrs. Gomez has come to the outpatient clinic for her regular follow-up appointment, brought in by her niece, who lives across town. The niece is upset because Mrs. Gomez has fallen five times in the past two weeks. Recently when she stopped to visit, she found her aunt sitting on the floor in the bathroom, unable to get up without extensive help from the niece. When asked about this directly, Mrs. Gomez denies having a problem, saying, "Everybody slips once in a while; it's not so bad."

She is found to have lost fifteen pounds since the prior visit three months ago. A small abrasion that she had on her left shin is now a Stage III ulcer, with poor healing. Mrs. Gomez appears disheveled and dehydrated. She is very deconditioned and cannot stand without full assistance of two people.

Mrs. Gomez refuses to go to the hospital. She is given intravenous fluids in the clinic, and blood tests are performed. Social work arranges for four hours of a home health aide, five times a week, from the city department of aging. PT and OT begin to work with the patient, coming to her home several times a week. No new pathology is found after a thorough workup.

Two weeks later, her condition is unchanged. More frustrating to the team is her poor effort and follow-through on exercises and oral intake. She also refuses to have any family move in with her because she believes they will steal from her. The team is concerned for her safety if she remains at home by herself. Despite her dementia, however, she appears to understand her situation and refuses to go to a nursing home: "I know you all are trying to help me and are worried about me and all. I'm worried about falling too. I'd like to have help, but I'm afraid they would steal from me. My niece says I can come live with her, but this place means so much—and I don't really trust her either. No, the only way I am leaving this house is going to be in a box."

"Power of Place" for the Patient

How is the team's work altered if Mrs. Gomez consults its professionals in an outpatient clinic rather than in her home? Whereas at home Mrs. Gomez had the undivided attention of the care team, in the clinic she must sign in and wait with other patients in the reception area. Her perception may be that the staff has no particular investment in her, that she is just another patient; this may have a profound impact on her relationship to the team and her response to care.

Although the team perceives risk in the patient's home, for Mrs. Gomez and many other patients the clinic symbolizes grave personal risk: a place where painful tests may be inflicted and where incurable diseases may be diagnosed. This anxiety may lead some patients to make greater use of denial as a coping mechanism; some will also be more rigid and unwilling to negotiate options than they might be in an environment perceived to be safe, such as their home.

Impact of Locus of Care on Team Goals, Leadership, and Processes

In contrast to Mrs. Gomez, team members find that the clinic represents a familiar, comfortable, and safe environment. This feeling may lead some professional team members to have a false sense of confidence. This is, after all, their milieu, in which they may fully express their expertise. Working in "their own home," the team's language and appearance differ as well. Whereas the team working in the patient's home may be less burdened by professional jargon, in the clinic setting their language may become formal, technical, and obtuse. Physical reassurances, such as touching a hand or shoulder, hand holding, or even hugging the patient, may be frowned on as unprofessional or even explicitly prohibited by policy. The addition of a starched white lab coat adds still another potential barrier.

Although the team members are unchanged from the first case, the team as a whole is subtly altered. In the first case discussion, the professional portion of the team was explicitly formed to provide home-based services. In the outpatient clinic, the formation of the professional portion of the team is more likely to be implicit: multiple members of disciplines working side by side in the office gradually develop formal and informal processes of collaboration. If the latter is the case, the team may not have established clear goals and values for itself. Working with a patient like Mrs. Gomez, it may be hindered by lack of a clear vision and purpose.

The flow of data is different in the outpatient clinic than in the patient's home. In the home, each team member can directly observe the patient's functional status and the context of her living, and the patient can demonstrate her own abilities. In the clinic, by contrast, the team receives data from secondary sources: the patient, her niece, the physical therapist, and the occupational therapist who go to the home. Coupled with these data, team members can only extrapolate what they believe Mrs. Gomez's functional status to be, based on their clinical observations. Thus, the team's own biases may have a greater impact on their decisions in the clinic setting. Teams in the clinic setting must be aware of the impact of using secondary sources of clinical data.

Team meetings may also differ in the clinic. In contrast to the home team sitting around Mrs. Gomez's kitchen table, sipping coffee she has made herself expressly for them, the clinic team retreats to a conference room to discuss their findings. After a period of discussion, the door will be opened and Mrs. Gomez invited in for her input. Although patient and team may have the exact same conversation in both settings, in the clinic she is more of an outsider to the process of her own care. Each of these factors—professional milieu, lack of explicit team charter, the need to extrapolate functional status, and separate team meetings—all introduce a distance between the patient and team that will influence their interactions and choices and suggest to Mrs. Gomez that the professionals do not consider her part of the team.

Interaction of the Patient and Team

As illustrated in the above description of the team meeting, the patient's role on the team changes in the clinic setting. Although the observations point to a shift in power from the patient to the professionals, this shift is not altogether one sided. In coming to the clinic, Mrs. Gomez herself needed to take some action: either to ask her niece to bring her to the clinic or at least to not oppose the niece in bringing her in. This in turn moves her from a recipient of services to a consumer or purchaser. It may be as good a choice as she knew at the time, or the least bad option, or an acceptance of medical attention without acceptance of recommendations and treatment, or implicit acceptance of the professional portion of the team and its care. For whatever reason, she has chosen to come to this clinic at this time, and she has herself made the choice to consult the team.

Mrs. Gomez also continues to retain the choice of whether to follow the team's recommendations. As in the home, the patient in the outpatient clinic ultimately has more veto power over the treatments recommended by the team than she does in the hospital or nursing home. This option is clearly exercised by Mrs. Gomez in her nonparticipation in the rehab program. Thus, while she no longer controls the team agenda to the degree that she did at home, she retains more control than she would in a hospital or nursing home setting.

How will these factors play out in the process of resolving the conflicts about Mrs. Gomez's care? Unfortunately, the clinic setting is rarely designed to solve this type of problem. Rather, outpatient and inpatient medical facilities focus on the problem of making decisions and obtaining further data when data are insufficient. The problems are familiar ones: a patient complains of a sore throat—is it a viral infection or a streptococcal infection? Another patient reports having chest pain—is it gastritis or a heart attack? In this framework, the tools of the outpatient clinic are generally designed to provide diagnostic data: a throat culture, a blood test, an electrocardiogram, an X-ray. These are the tools that a primary care team based in an outpatient clinic will have at hand and thus are the ones that the team will be most likely to use. Mark Twain's well-known adage "If your only tool is a hammer, every problem tends to look like a nail" is applicable here.

Unfortunately, further diagnostic testing is unlikely to be of use to this team. The team's effectiveness in finding an ethical resolution to the issues this patient poses will come only from their ability to use a different set of tools from those usually associated with medical care. Empathy is needed for them to hear and understand Mrs. Gomez's feelings, especially about her home. They must be imaginative in their ability to ask about and to visualize her living space. They must also use negotiation skills to ask what is involved in assuring her safety and well-being at home, and what kind of help she will and will not accept.

External Factors

Working in the outpatient clinic, some members of the health care team may be more concerned about liability issues than they would in the patient's home. Physicians in particular may raise issues of risk related to decisions that support Mrs. Gomez's decision to remain at home. The presence of Mrs. Gomez's "upset" niece may heighten a physician's fear of potential litigation; if Mrs. Gomez breaks her hip at home, will the niece sue the physician for failing to take more definitive action? The physician's fear, in turn, may put pressure on the team to take action. Where the team working in the context of the home may be more prone to errors of omission, the clinic team may be more inclined to errors of commission: overtesting, overprescribing, or perhaps more disturbingly, overriding patient autonomy.

Cost is a reality that increasingly concerns all actors in the health care field. In managed care environments, the risk for health care costs is often shifted to primary care clinics. Teams working in such settings will be subject to pressure from administrators regarding the cost of their services. Until the last decade or two, the culture of health care led professionals to attempt to put aside such pressures; although we would still like to believe that they focus only on patient advocacy, such a view is unrealistic. Assigning services to Mrs. Gomez to help her stay in her home will come at some expense to the professional portion of the team.

The nature of the expense will depend on the type of clinic in which they work. In a public health setting, or a staff-model managed care organization, the expense might be a decreased availability of services to other clients, or incurring the wrath of an administrator for overspending the team's patient care budget. In a private medical practice, the issue may be one of excess time spent for poorly reimbursed services. The team must openly acknowledge these pressures and recognize ways in which such pressures will influence their clinical decision making with Mrs. Gomez.

Case Description: The Hospital

Lucy Gomez is an 85-year-old widowed Hispanic woman who lives alone. One morning her niece stops by to visit Mrs. Gomez and finds her sitting on the floor in the bathroom, unable to get up without extensive help from the niece. She is admitted to University Hospital, where the niece reports that she has fallen five times in the past two weeks. It is not clear if she has sustained a syncopal episode. The acute care geriatrics unit uses an interdisciplinary team approach to patient care. Members of the team include a physician, GNP, SW, OT, and dietitian.

Mrs. Gomez's medical problems include hypertension and diabetes; both of these have been fairly well controlled with medications. According to outpatient records, she has had very mild dementia (MMSE of 22 out of 30) for the past two years, without identified reversible causes. The niece also mentions that she is concerned because her aunt eats poorly, and has lost ten to fifteen pounds in the past three months.

On exam, the patient is obese, in no distress. Skin exam reveals a 4 cm-by-6 cm Stage III ulcer, with poor healing. Mrs. Gomez appears disheveled and dehydrated. She is very deconditioned and cannot stand without full assistance of two people. The remainder of her exam is normal.

She is started on intravenous fluids, and antibiotics for possible occult infection. PT and OT evaluate her and begin daily exercise. Blood tests are performed, as well as a CT scan of the brain; these are noncontributory.

After four days in the hospital, Mrs. Gomez's condition is unchanged. More frustrating to the team is her poor effort and follow-through on exercises and medication intake. The team is also concerned for her safety if she returns home by herself. She tells the discharge planner adamantly that she refuses to have family move in with her because she believes they will steal from her. She refuses nursing home placement, either short term or long term. Despite her dementia, however, she appears to understand her situation, saying, "I know you all are trying to help me and are worried about me and all. I'm worried about falling too. I'd like to have help, but I'm afraid they would steal from me. My niece says I can come live with her, but my house means so much—and I don't really trust her either. I have to go home. I can't stay in this place anymore."

"Power of Place" for the Patient

For most people, few places are as threatening as a hospital. The sounds, smells, and language of the hospital are unlike any they experience in daily life. Although members of the health care team are familiar with hospital technology, such as heart monitors, pulse oximeters, ventilators, and infusion pumps, patients often find these machines alienating and discomforting. Even familiar foods seem to taste different in the hospital.

Even with all of her impairments and her apparent difficulty managing her everyday affairs, Mrs. Gomez retains more control over her life at home than she can hope to have in the hospital. In the hospital, the locus of control is largely external. Mrs. Gomez will, of course, have to sign permission forms for invasive tests and procedures, but otherwise she will be subjected to the routines of hospital life as determined by the staff. Her vital signs will be checked, orderlies will bring her to the X-ray department, and physical therapy will take place on a timetable completely independent of her symptoms or mood. When a team member wished to see Mrs. Gomez in her home, they scheduled an appointment with her; in the outpatient clinic, she scheduled an appointment with them. In the hospital, team members enter her room whenever they have the time to do so. The inequality of the relationship between patient and team is at its maximum in the hospital.

Patients in hospitals may be all too willing in some cases to turn decisions over to the health care team, or more than they would in other settings. In the context of life-threatening illness, or at least the fear of such an illness, patients may prefer to believe in "powerful others" who can cure every disease. They may be aware of their need for intensive and extensive help from "powerful others." Mrs. Gomez's attitude may reflect a belief, conscious or unconscious, that the hospital can fix all of her problems, even without her participation. She may think that her role in the health care team is to be a recipient of the healing services of the professional members, so that she can return home.

Impact of the Locus of Care on Team Goals, Leadership, and Processes

Hospital-based care is characterized by the traditional goals of medicine: the diagnosis and treatment of disease and, to a lesser extent, the relief of suffering. These goals do not appear to fit Mrs. Gomez's case particularly well. Her evaluation has not revealed an undiagnosed acute illness. Once she has received intravenous hydration, she no longer has conditions amenable to intravenous antibiotics or surgery or other acute care interventions. In this setting the team typically takes one of two courses of action: further invasive testing or intervention (e.g., placement of a gastric feeding tube), or expeditious discharge to home or nursing home.

An effective interdisciplinary team could develop alternative strategies to address Mrs. Gomez's dilemma, but they might well feel constrained when operating in the hospital. Of all of the clinical settings discussed in this chapter, the hospital is inherently the most hierarchical and thus may be the most inhospitable to true interdisciplinary teams and innovative problem solving. Given the power of physicians in the traditional hospital setting, other team members may be less willing to use aggressive or confrontational conflict management approaches. How will Mrs. Gomez's team respond if the physician makes a firm declaration: "We certainly cannot allow this patient to return home. We all agree that there is no way that she can care for herself." The facts of the case suggest that the physician is correct in saying that Mrs. Gomez is unlikely to be safe in her home. In the hospital's hierarchical environment, team members' risk-benefit analysis would focus on the risks versus benefits to themselves of contradicting the physician rather than on the risks and benefits to Mrs. Gomez of their decision.

Additional constraints and disapproval may come from other directions. A head nurse complains that Mrs. Gomez is excessively disruptive to patient care on the unit; a specialist talks to colleagues about how the team is failing to be "aggressive enough" in getting Mrs. Gomez to comply with the treatment plan; a utilization manager insists that the team move ahead with a discharge plan for this unreasonable patient. Operating in a manner that is countercultural in the acute care hospital, even an egalitarian interdisciplinary team will feel enormous pressures to conform to institutional norms.

Part of the ethics of place is that the hospital's hierarchical environment tends to place undue ethical demands on the team members who are lower in the hierarchy: nurses, social workers, therapists, and others. Frequently, physicians' opinions ignore the moral sense of others who work with the patient and family. As has been pointed out by the Institute of Medicine's report on medical errors, hospital-based teams must work to develop an "open cockpit" culture of communication in which all participants feel free to speak up for the good of the patient (Kohn, Corrigan, and Donaldson 1999).

In the best scenario, there is little risk of disagreement among team members; the lack of clear benefits from any option available to Mrs. Gomez makes it unlikely that any clinician would be heavily invested in a particular position. JSW say that "[a] medical treatment is ethically mandatory to the extent that it is likely to confer greater benefits than burdens upon the patient" (Jonsen, Siegler, and Winslade 1998, 139). Burck has revised this principle of proportionate care in this manner: "The team's responsibility is to recommend the treatment that is most likely to confer the greatest balance of benefits over burdens upon the patient." Under this principle the professional portion of the team has the same responsibility. Thus, there are ethical reasons, based on patient well-being, for changing the system, so that nonphysician team members feel bold enough to speak up.

But hospital scenarios are often worse. Conflicts flare between nurses and physicians, or family and physicians, precisely about what proportionate care for the patient is. Overt "battles of the advocates" develop. Having a conflict out in the open at least allows it to be addressed more cleanly. In the worst case scenario, fear drives the conflict underground, and it is fought out behind the scenes.

These norms for hospital care remind us that much of what we consider ethics is still closely related to custom. Ethical obligations require the team to challenge these customs. In the case of Mrs. Gomez, each team member is responsible for invoking collaborative and conflict-resolution skills that belong in good teamwork: listening; clarifying others' concerns; keeping the dialogue going when closure would be premature; and humbly but firmly bringing new perspectives and responsibilities to the table. The use of established and effective team processes, even in a hostile environment, are critical to resolving ethical conundrums in the hospital setting.

Interaction of the Patient and Team

Hospital-based teams are at a tremendous disadvantage in dealing with complex patients such as Mrs. Gomez. Most team members will have had little or no prior relationship with Mrs. Gomez and will thus have no shared history or understanding with which to interpret her wishes. Is her intransigence a manifestation of an acute delirium? Does it reflect decreased insight and understanding on the basis of a progressive dementing illness? Or is her response a long-standing coping mechanism, making bad choices at times but sticking to them vigorously and somehow making them work. Unlike the home care team, the hospital has little or no direct data with which to answer these critical questions. Furthermore, the team is unlikely to have time to carefully analyze these questions. In the hospital setting, complex decisions must be made in extremely short periods of time: often in just a few minutes, and at times in a matter of seconds. At best, Mrs. Gomez's statements will be acknowledged and taken at face value; there is too little time to discuss her safety, security, grief, life story, and the meaning of her wishes.

We have already indicated that patients in the hospital may be more willing to turn over their care and decision making to others, especially the hospital team. Some authors compare hospitals to mental institutions and prisons, as "total institutions" or "place[s] of residence where a large number of like situated individuals, cut off from the wider society for an appreciable period of time, together, lead an enclosed, formally administered round of life" (Goffman 1961). In such a setting, desperate and fearful older patients often exchange their independence for the beneficence of nurses and doctors. Latimer describes this behavior as seeking inclusion in "positive medical categories" by "lying low and effacing their distinctiveness as individuals and as social beings" (Latimer 1999). The cost of this behavior, of course, is that the older adult reduces their effectiveness in influencing their own care. Although Mrs. Gomez continues to strongly express her desire to return home, her resistance may buckle in the face of continued negative feedback from the hospital team. The moral dangers here are several and complex. For the team, looking at the options on the ethics continuum, continued negative feedback may be ethically preferable to actual conflict with her: at least this strategy will not result in her complete withdrawal and silence about her treatment preferences.

External Factors

Hospitals operate under a web of local, state, and federal regulations, with increasingly strict oversight of operations, most notably from the Joint Commission on Accreditation of Healthcare Organizations (JCAHO) and Medicare's Office of Inspector General (OIG). Such oversight, as well as fears of litigation, may further constrain the options that the inpatient team considers in working with Mrs. Gomez. Specifically, the team may be subtly influenced to choose a plan that is least likely to violate a regulation. Similarly, discharging Mrs. Gomez to home at least militates against the likelihood of her falling in the hospital or developing a wound infection. While both complications can also develop at home, team members may be falsely comforted by the fact that they would not trigger an institutional morbidity and mortality review. Concern about regulatory oversight or institutional review is a contextual feature that can sneak into decision making almost without notice and contaminate decisions that appear to be solely for the patient's benefit.

At the same time, regulatory bodies create positive opportunities for the geriatric interdisciplinary team. Medicare regulations mandate that patients' advance directives be assessed at the time of admission (the Patient Self-Determination Act). JCAHO assesses a hospital's respect for patient rights, and closely monitors issues such as the use of restraints. Patient-centered geriatric teams can provide invaluable assistance to hospitals struggling to demonstrate their compliance with regulations.

Teams in hospitals must also openly acknowledge the influence of financial issues on their decision-making process. For most elderly patients, hospitals are paid a flat rate on the basis of diagnostic-related groups. Mrs. Gomez can be said to be medically stable at this time, so it is in the interest of the hospital to discharge her as soon as possible. Is this also in Mrs. Gomez's best interest? Will a geriatric team charged with reducing the cost of caring for older adults rationalize pushing Mrs. Gomez out of the hospital as "respect for patient autonomy"?

Ethical analysis of the health care team's responsibility is made difficult by taboos and moralizing pressures. In the hospital setting certain ends, such as the patient's well-being, are favored over that of the clinician and others. In fact, proper ethical reflection requires attention to everybody's good: everybody counts. Usually the patient counts most, but not always. Unless the health care team is clear that it counts, too, self-interest may be hidden behind the dominant acceptable goal, the patient's well-being. Sunshine is the best remedy for moral fuzziness.

Case Description: The Nursing Home

Lucy Gomez is an 85-year-old widowed Hispanic woman who moved to the nursing home two weeks ago, after being discharged from the hospital following a series of falls. The nursing home has been using an interdisciplinary team for Skilled Nursing Facility (SNF) patients who are admitted from the hospital. Members of the team include a GNP, SW, PT, OT, a skin care nurse, and a physiatrist.

According to her niece, until recently Mrs. Gomez was fairly independent in her self-care, although she went out only rarely. She paid a neighbor to pick up her medicines and groceries. Her medical problems include hypertension and diabetes; both of these have been fairly well controlled with medications. She has had very mild dementia (MMSE of 22 out of 30) for the past two years, without identified reversible causes. Mrs. Gomez was admitted to the hospital after falling five times in a two-week period. According to the hospital records, Mrs. Gomez was grossly deconditioned, but no cause was found for her weakness and anorexia.

Since transferring to the nursing home two weeks ago, Mrs. Gomez has made little progress. She has gained only one pound, despite being presented with high-caloric foods. Despite PT and OT twice a day, she has shown little willingness to try to walk and move about. A Stage III ulcer on her left shin is healing very slowly, despite the aides giving her a whirlpool bath every day and careful wound care. Staff nurses are upset because Mrs. Gomez has tried to get up on her own almost every day and on four occasions nearly fell. They have an order from her attending to use a restraint vest to reduce the risk of falls.

When the team meets to review her case, they are concerned about her discharge plans. She has made few gains that justify further SNF care; team members believe she should be moved to the long-term care wing of the nursing home. Mrs. Gomez insists that she wishes to return home, despite her lack of safety and frequent falls. She told the social worker that she refuses to have any family move in with her because she believes they would steal from her. But the team is concerned for her safety if she returns home by herself. Despite her dementia, Mrs. Gomez appears to understand her situation and refuses to remain in the nursing home: "I know you all are trying to help me and are worried about me and all. I'm worried about falling too. I'd like to have help, but I'm afraid they would steal from me. My niece says I can come live with her, but my house means so much—and I don't really trust her either. I have to go home, I can't stay in this place anymore."

"Power of Place" for the Patient

William H. Thomas begins his book *Life Worth Living*, about alternative nursing homes, this way: "The specter of the nursing home haunts the infirm elderly and their families. They know in their hearts that to enter a nursing home is to take an irreversible step down the path toward disability and death" (Thomas 1996, 7). This haunting specter dramatically alters the relationships among patients, families, and health care workers in nursing homes. Patients enter the hospital in the hope that a treatment will cure their disease or at least improve their symptoms. This is not the expectation in long-term care. For long-term patients, residence in a nursing home is evidence of declining health and function. This may be a source of shame for many, frustrated that they can no longer fully care for themselves. For others, the need for a nursing home may generate resentments directed at family who cannot provide necessary assistance or housing.

Families, in turn, often feel shame and guilt at the need for a parent or grandparent to live in a nursing home. They may feel they have betrayed or let down their loved one, triggering other feelings of inadequacy as well. Part of the responsibility of the professionals is to help families understand that feelings of inadequacy are appropriate, but not demeaning. The family simply can no longer handle the situation themselves. In that sense they are not adequate, but being inadequate to their loved one's needs is not a basis for self-judgment. Some handle their guilt by withdrawal, visiting on only rare occasions. Others become demanding of the nursing home staff, alleviating guilt or asserting their sense of responsibility by being "advocates" for the patient, by framing every problem as an infraction, and by demanding the immediate correction of every minor infraction.

What does the nursing home mean for Mrs. Gomez? She is very clear about what it is *not*; it is *not* her home. Bringing in furniture, photos, and other memorabilia from her home might reduce this negative feeling. On the other hand, she might find many conditions unacceptable. She has lived alone since the death of her husband; now she must share a room with one or more other women and take her meals in a dining room with many others. At home she could watch whatever television program she wanted and could keep the volume on the television turned up; in the nursing home, she must watch whatever is on in the dayroom. The food is not the same, the smells are not the same, and the list goes on. We can speculate about what she does not like about the nursing home, but what is really needed is an empathic conversation with her. Someone from the team needs to listen to her discuss these issues and their narrative costs to her.

Impact of Locus of Care on Team Goals, Leadership, and Processes

Staff members in nursing homes are often overworked and undervalued. Nurses report dreading family visits because of the litany of new demands that will greet them. The nursing home team is all too aware of popular prejudices that only second-rate health care professionals would ever consider working in long-term care; they may even have internalized this bias. This is a particularly pernicious ethical aspect of health care at the contextual level. Society's lack of emphasis on the well-being of nursing home residents, like its underemphasis on schools, becomes an attack on the self-esteem of those who serve nursing home residents and perhaps even an attack on their virtue.

In this setting, the power of place can conspire to keep the team from forming effective relationships with patients and families. With limited or poor communication comes greater risk of conflicts and ethical problems. At the same time, other factors provide nursing home teams with unique opportunities for resolving the ethical conundrum posed by Mrs. Gomez.

The goal of the team in a nursing home contrasts with the acute care goals of hospitals and outpatient clinics. Nursing homes are organized as care-giving facilities. The goals of the team here are to prevent disease (rather than diagnose and treat it), to maintain or improve independent function, and to relieve pain and suffering. Services are provided to assist patients with activities of daily living (ADLs). Long-term care facilities thus are an alternative to home rather than to the hospital. The majority of needed services come not from physicians but from nurses or nurse's aides. Rehabilitation specialists such as physical therapists, occupational therapists, speech therapists, and physiatrists play an important role in preserving or enhancing function. Chaplains, social workers, or nursing staff may address spiritual needs. In most cases the attending physician (or the medical director of the nursing home) has the least amount of direct contact with the patients, and provides a comparatively minor component of their care. Thus, the nursing home's focus on personal care of the patient lends itself to balanced, less hierarchical, interdisciplinary teams.

Because Mrs. Gomez's team is focused on her ADLs, it is well positioned to evaluate and enhance her capacity for self-care. The physiatrist and physical therapist provide additional expertise that was not available in the outpatient setting or in the hospital. At the same time, the purpose of this nursing home team is somewhat less clear than that of other teams in this chapter. Is this team charged with maximizing patient function and promoting return to the community? Is it responsible for promoting patient satisfaction and reducing family complaints? Has management charged it with providing preventive care to reduce the risk of avoidable hospital admissions? Has it been assembled to meet the nursing home's regulatory need to have interdisciplinary work groups complete mandated care plans? The answers to these questions are critical to understanding the team's decision-making process in this case.

Interaction of the Patient and Team

Like hospitals, nursing homes can be characterized as one of Goffman's "total institutions." In contrast to the hospital-based team, however, the nursing home team is not forced to make decisions quickly or with insufficient information. This works in the team's favor. Mrs. Gomez can remain in the nursing home without economic pressures mandating a decision and discharge. The team can negotiate with Mrs. Gomez to encourage her to participate in further therapy sessions for a predetermined amount of time to prepare her to return home. While this continues, she receives meals, supportive care, and supervision. At the same time, professional members can patiently develop their relationship with Mrs. Gomez and gain insights into her values, beliefs, and attitudes. The professional members can also attend to other detriments of being in the nursing home experienced by Mrs. Gomez, such as her lack of familiar objects.

Making use of time to resolve this case does not eliminate the risk to the patient. First, Mrs. Gomez could suffer worse malnutrition due to her dislike of the institutional food or her depression about being out of her own home. She could fall and injure herself in the nursing home as easily as she could at home—perhaps even more easily, considering her lack of familiarity with the environment. There is also the risk of asking her to try "just a few more days" and progressively dragging out the stay in the nursing home. While the nursing home team should make use of the time to resolve issues with Mrs. Gomez, it must remain aware of the risks of doing so.

External Factors

Regulations may support effective teaming in long-term care in a way in which they do not support it in the outpatient clinic or the acute inpatient setting. Medicare's requirements for maintaining the minimum data set (MDS) on each patient and the periodic completion of interdisciplinary care plans mandate the use of teams. This environment is familiar with the role of the interdisciplinary team. Of course, in some facilities the interdisciplinary team is resisted in favor of a hierarchical model like that of the hospital, or simply tolerated or accommodated. In other nursing homes, however, such teams may be embraced as critical to the mission of the facility.

Nursing homes, like hospitals, are scrutinized for their respect for patient rights and autonomy. Regulatory bodies include the Health Care Financing Administration (HCFA), state public health authorities, and in some cases the Joint Commission on Accreditation of Healthcare Organizations (JCAHO). This creates an environment in which the nursing home must demonstrate that it has taken steps to assess and honor Mrs. Gomez's personal preferences.

At the same time, the heavily regulated nature of long-term care may lead to risk aversion. This tension will need to be acknowledged openly by the team caring for Mrs. Gomez in the nursing home.

The economics of long-term care pose special challenges for the ethical functioning of teams. During the posthospital component of her care, Medicare's prospective payment system for nursing homes rewards a shorter length of stay and earlier discharge. As with the hospital, the team could be motivated to honor her wishes out of economic interest and not out of respect for her autonomy.

If, however, Mrs. Gomez is receiving custodial long-term care, the economic pressures change completely. In the hospital setting, reimbursement will be the same whether Mrs. Gomez is discharged to her home or to a nursing home. For the outpatient team seeing Mrs. Gomez in her home or in the clinic, a decision to move to a nursing home would have modest financial impact, as the team is paid only for its services and not for where she lives. In contrast, the nursing home's revenues are directly tied to Mrs. Gomez's continued residence in the facility. Although it can certainly be argued that another patient will come to fill her bed if Mrs. Gomez is allowed to return home, the team must recognize that there may be a subtle bias that favors keeping her "safe" in the facility. The employer of the team, the nursing home, has a direct financial interest in the outcome of Mrs. Gomez's case. Keeping her safe appears to be the morally preferable course of action, but it may actually be an example of rationalizing one's actions on the basis of ethics rather than truly choosing the morally preferable course of action.

Finally, the team must recognize that Mrs. Gomez's family will have its own financial concerns about her remaining in the nursing home. Given the out-of-pocket costs of long-term care, some families may act out of economic self-interest to preserve the patient's estate (and their inheritance). In the nursing home setting, advocacy for patient autonomy may cover a range of less altruistic motivations for both team and family and must be guarded against. We must guard against it by stating the financial incentives very clearly.

Conclusion

The discussion of Mrs. Gomez across four different care settings has identified a number of ways in which the environment in which health care professionals work affects the way they understand their ethical responsibility toward patients. Patients are also influenced by locus of care in their own assessments of quality of life and personal preferences. In addition, teams must recognize factors such as team structure and function, decision-making issues, legal and regulatory factors, and financial biases that can influence their deliberations. Human beings are profoundly affected by the power of place, and that power must be acknowledged and given its due in the resolution of any ethical conundrum.

Discussion Questions

The team in the home

1. In the home setting, a team may be subtly biased toward therapeutic nihilism, or at least toward unquestioning acceptance of the patient's position. How can this team avoid both of these biases?

2. How would the issues, including the goals of medicine, raised by this case be different if Mrs. Gomez had moved into this home within the past six months?

3. How would the issues be different if Mrs. Gomez were living in her niece's home?

The team in the outpatient clinic

1. How could team members respond if the physician says, "It's all well and good for you to advocate for the patients' rights, but I'm the one that her niece is going to sue if Mrs. Gomez dies at home!"

2. The mission of this team is not explicitly stated in the case study. How would the analysis of the case change if the primary care team has been formed for each of the following purposes:
    a. to help control clinic costs of providing health care to frail seniors.
    b. to promote patient autonomy and quality of life.
    c. to reduce the incidence of premature morbidity and mortality through the identification and reduction of risk factors.

The hospital-based team

1. How can an interdisciplinary team working in a hospital setting ensure that the patient is active part of the team?

2. What are the risks of the team assuming the role of patient advocate in confrontation with other staff in the hospital? What are the benefits?

3. What processes can a hospital-based team put into place to ensure equal participation among members?

4. Some hospitals have adopted a "hospitalist" model of care in which the physician only takes care of the patient only while they are in the hospital. How might such a model impact team function?

The nursing home team

1. Mrs. Gomez cannot be held as a prisoner in the nursing home. What options does this team have if she announces her plan to go home in a day or two?

2. Although this team has the benefit of time, what is a reasonable time limit for resolving these issues?

3. If Mrs. Gomez continues to have periodic falls despite participating in the team's treatment plan over the course of a year, and still insists she wants to go home anyway, has the team violated her autonomy?

REFERENCES

Burck, R. 1996. Feeding, withholding, and withdrawing: Ethical perspectives, invited review. *Nutrition in Clinical Practice* 11:243–53.

Goffman E. 1961. *Asylums: Essays on the social situation of mental patients and other inmates.* Garden City, N.Y.: Anchor Books.

Hunter, K. M. 1995. "*Narrative,*" listing in Warren T. Reich, ed., *Encyclopedia of bioethics,* 2nd ed. New York: Macmillan.

Jonsen, A., M. Siegler, and W. J. Winslade. 1998. *Clinical Ethics,* 4th ed. New York: McGraw-Hill.

Kohn, L. T., J. M. Corrigan, and M. S. Donaldson. 1999. *To err is human: Building a safer health system.* Washington, D.C.: National Academy Press.

Latimer, J. 1999. The dark at the bottom of the stairs: Performance and participation of hospitalized older people. *Medical Anthropology Quarterly* 13(2):186–213.

Thomas, W. H. 1996. *Life worth living: How someone you love can still enjoy life in a nursing home—The Eden alternative in action.* Acton, Mass.: VanderWyk & Burnham.

Webster's Second New International Dictionary of the English Language Unabridged. 1961. Springfield, Mass.: G & C Merriam.

PART V

Impact of the Organization on Team Care

CHAPTER 14

Ethical Dilemmas of Team Decisions in a Cost-Conscious Environment

Joann Castle, M.A.

Cost-consciousness pervades today's health care environment as health care systems go through a crisis of mergers, bankruptcies, and consolidations. As our economic practices shift in response to the pressures of cost, the ethical responsibility of caring for the old and the very old within the constraints imposed by limited resources will challenge the skills of practitioners involved in their care.

In the shift to more cost-effective strategies, traditional fee-for-service health care has given way to a variety of new approaches intended to reduce costs. These new approaches are collectively referred to as *managed care.* Ironically, while the effects of shrinking health care dollars are being experienced broadly across the health care marketplace, no place is more profoundly affected than the managed care industry itself.

In the effort to forestall financial losses, many provider organizations have developed sophisticated systems to monitor spending. Whether the motivations of the finance monitors are solvency and survival for a nonprofit organization or profits for stockholders, managed care practitioners are often trapped in the middle, finding themselves pushed toward new efficiencies that pose ethical challenges to the care of complex patients.

As the managed care resource pool shrinks, pressures to reduce costs will continue to fall on practitioners. These practitioners are desperately in need of assistance in balancing ethically sound physician-patient relationships and resource constraints. This chapter proposes the thesis that geriatric interdisciplinary team care may be an answer for overburdened practitioners who need support in making sound ethical judgments.

Ethical issues related to cost are not new phenomena. Primary care practitioners have always had to deal with financial issues related to a patient's ability to pay. Early practitioners simply negotiated options directly with patients according to their ability to pay. What has really changed today is the nature of the tension between patient needs and costs, and the clinician's experience of this tension in the process of care management. In managed care, conflicts that promote this tension are even more overt because third-party interests are involved in virtually every aspect of the physician-patient relationship (Fleck and Squier 1997). These third parties have the explicit responsibility to define the practitioner's obligation and to police the interaction between practitioner and patients related to cost. These third parties may include governmental agencies, payers of health benefits, and hospital or health plan administrators who monitor expenditures.

The traditional fee-for-service "piecemeal" model worked well in a period that focused on managing acute illness. But this model consumes resources at a rapid rate. In contrast, the managed care model is based on caring for a defined population of patients. Generally, this model is a better fit for managing chronic disease in elderly persons. In the group practice model, dollars are paid to care providers at a fixed capitation (per patient) rate agreed upon in advance, to cover the cost of care for all patients in the pool. Practitioners are generally retained on contract by a third party and paid by salary. Resource dollars are then "managed" to assure that spending does not exceed the dollars that exist in the pool.

The disbursement of funds from the pool is an ethical matter of distributive justice. Two moral imperatives flow from this model: (1) health care providers and practitioners must achieve fairness in the distribution of scarce resources to the patient population, and (2) practitioners must maintain ethically sound relationships with their patients despite the pressures of cost. Practitioners in the managed care setting often have little training or support in managing dilemmas that flow from complexities involved in achieving these imperatives.

Background

Ethical conflicts related to changes in the economics and financing of health care delivery had become such an issue by 1995 that the Council on Ethical and Judicial Affairs of the American Medical Association (1995) issued a report that unequivocally stated that "physicians, no matter what their plan structure, must remain primarily dedicated to the care of their individual patients." A few years later, Hall and Berenson (1998) noted that "medical ethics and medical economics are increasingly in conflict" and proposed that the situation was so drastic and the economic pressures so unique that a new ethic for managed care is necessary. The authors argued that practitioners need pragmatic ethical guideposts attuned to an era of managed care. Examples of issues they felt would benefit from guidelines were patient loyalty under practice incentives, techniques for communicating resource constraints to patients, and population-based ethics—where the good of the group supersedes the right of any individual patient.

Additional ways to assist practitioners with ethical practice in the "real world" of managed care need to be explored. This paper suggests that the implementation of geriatric interdisciplinary team care is an option that should be considered for providing the necessary support to practitioners. Interdisciplinary teams can expand and improve care approaches for the elderly and produce more ethically appropriate outcomes in the managed care setting.

Interdisciplinary teamwork differs from multidisciplinary practice in that team members engage in collaboration, usually in team meetings. The product of their work will be the result of a synergistic process (Mason et al. 1996). Working together and using an ethical framework, team members may be able to achieve a balance between ethics and cost that would be overwhelming to a single practitioner. The use of teams may well offer a bridge to carry us forward as new care systems unfold.

Team care works well in an atmosphere where colleagues work together and share resources. Managed care has already opened the door to teams, partly due to its collaborative nature and salaried compensation and partly due to the structure of its communication systems. The Bureau of Health Professions (1995) notes that managed care organizations provide an excellent environment for interdisciplinary (team) care. In the setting, "the flow of information and communication modalities . . . bring members of different disciplines together, creating innovative channels of dialogue and emphasizing the value of professional interaction as part of a larger team effort."

Case Description

In the past, we have associated ethics in health care with inpatient end-of-life decisions. As times change, we need to heighten our awareness that the social organization of our care systems and the emphasis on cost containment require vigilance in our day-to-day work in ambulatory care. The following case will demonstrate the struggle of a team to improve its performance on a stage fraught with moral and ethical contradictions related to costs. The experience suggests that the team approach offers much to practitioners and patients, especially those elderly who thrive better with less medical intervention. Yet a primary question remains: In the real world of cost pressures, can team care meet the challenge of cost effectiveness?

The setting for this case is a managed care ambulatory clinic under pressure to reduce costs. The medical center is funded by a capitation agreement with the associated health plan. Thus, the center is at risk for all costs related to the physicians' panels of patients, including inpatient admissions. Keeping patients out of the hospital is of primary concern. As cost monitoring spreads to the ambulatory setting, dilemmas like Mrs. Martin are expected to increase.

Gather Clinical Information

Dr. Johnson is extremely frustrated with Mrs. Martin's unwillingness to cooperate with her plan of care. Although the 69-year-old patient is morbidly obese and has a number of chronic conditions, he is certain that she is competent and that her medical situation is manageable. The patient's diagnoses include chronic obstructive pulmonary disease (COPD) from a history of smoking, congestive heart failure (CHF), diabetes, and arthritis. The patient is on Coumadin for her CHF and recently suffered a spontaneous hip fracture.

Mrs. Martin has had multiple hospital admissions over the past few years. She continues to be uncooperative with her plan of care and refuses to get out of bed even when assisted. After hospitalization for her hip fracture, Mrs. Martin was admitted to a nursing home for physical and occupational therapy. While there, a psychiatrist diagnosed her condition as "passive-aggressive and self-destructive behavior." She was discharged home about two months ago under the supervision of her daughter, who lives nearly. Mrs. Martin's frequent hospitalizations have more often than not resulted from her noncompliance in taking her medications as well as her poor diet.

Dr. Johnson has considered that Mrs. Martin's health is deteriorating because she refuses to help herself. It appears that with her cooperation, most of her hospitalizations could have been avoided. Dr. Johnson has already recommended to the patient that she get another physician. In doing so, he told her honestly that he does not want to be responsible for her health status as she continues in her noncompliance. Despite the doctor's recommendation, Mrs. Martin has made no effort to get another provider. The doctor is all too aware of other patients who would more clearly benefit from his time and attention.

Dr. Johnson is facing an ethical dilemma that managed care providers face on a large scale, often in a hostile environment. What amount of time and resources should be provided to a declining patient who is unwilling to cooperate with the treatment plan? The doctor feels pressured by his inability to be effective with Mrs. Martin and by the processes that hold him responsible for noncompliant patients. He would benefit from the support of his colleagues in resolving this dilemma.

Geriatric interdisciplinary teams offer the promise of more effective care for high-risk geriatric patients. Their collaborative nature also brings more support and satisfaction for practitioners. Team members bring a diversity of skills and perspectives to a complex task and can trade off the burden of care when cases become overwhelming. Core disciplines on the interdisciplinary team include medicine, nursing, social work, and pharmacy. Other disciplines such as physical therapy or geropsychiatry may also interact with a team to support patient needs. There are many characteristics of team care that offer support for practitioners faced with these complex cases. Members provide a cross-section of views, experiences, and cultural backgrounds that bring depth to the patient discussion. Their various perspectives also assure that critical aspects of the case are not missed.

Traditionally, health care disciplines approach their work differently. Physicians are trained to focus on biomedical systems and disease. They approach a diagnosis by ruling out problems and eliminating possibilities. Nurses, on the other hand, are more holistic in their outlook, considering psychosocial needs and focusing on patient preferences and functional abilities. Social workers approach problem solving by ruling in problems and looking at interrelationships. They are specialists in assessing environmental and financial problems. The support of nursing and social work fosters more involvement by the family. Pharmacists bring a wealth of knowledge on drug properties, reactions, and pharmacokinetics. A pharmacist can review medications to identify cost or quality issues, making suggestions for improving the selection of drugs and dosages. A pharmacist can also monitor patient compliance in taking drugs by checking refill records.

Through the team, the burden of care that is so heavy for an individual practitioner will be shared among team members while the situation is brought under control. The whole team shoulders responsibility and accountability for the case. The combination of the team approach and the synergy of members' interdisciplinary interaction open a broad spectrum of new possibilities for complex patients.

In the managed care setting, a team is charged with managing its panel of patients 365 days a year, using a finite resource pool. This team knows that the decisions they make for one patient will affect all patients using the resource pool. Systems update the team on a clinic patient's admissions and emergency room use and allow identification of high-risk patients.

The concept of the interdisciplinary care team is holistic, addressing medical, social and functional needs. If a task is not done by one member, others support and assist. The team meeting is a forum where updates take place and next steps are developed. The model encourages team members to meet targeted deadlines because incomplete actions hold up the whole plan of care. More resources may be used up front, but over time the plan becomes proactive in avoiding excessive costs. While team members report that cost is not an issue in their day-to-day decision making, the judicious use of resources is inherent in the culture, clinical policies, and practices of the medical center as well as the health plan.

Dr. Johnson has been alerted of Mrs. Martin's overuse of resources in a report from the utilization department and has asked the utilization nurse care manager to present the case at today's team meeting. Other members in attendance include the geriatric nurse practitioner who shares patients with the physician, a part-time social worker who is new to the organization, and the pharmacist. Other than the social worker, everyone on the team is familiar with Mrs. Martin because of her frequent hospitalizations.

Dr. Johnson expresses his view that health providers have spent more time on this patient than most others and have had no effect on her health status. He feels that his time could be better spent improving health outcomes for other patients. He questions whether the team is facilitating the patient's inappropriate behavior and suggests that the patient is controlling the practitioners and may be achieving social gain from her interactions with staff, both as an inpatient and as an outpatient.

The utilization nurse reports that she has already checked with the health plan and found that the patient cannot be disenrolled from the plan even though she won't let the providers do anything for her. She also reports that she has taken the initiative to check with the legal department and has found that the clinic is responsible for any medical expenses. At this point, the pharmacist reports that the patient called yesterday requesting a refill of Darvocet. The doctor responds flatly that he will not order any more medications for this patient. She needs to see another physician.

It is not surprising that Dr. Johnson wants to be relieved of responsibility in a situation he is unable to control. The physician's traditional role in the medical model focuses on matters that are amenable to medical treatment. In a one-to-one provider-patient relationship, a patient who is resistant to medical intervention would likely have been lost to the care system except for acute or traumatic events. Additionally, if the physician faced this situation as an individual provider, the broader issues now brought to his attention by the team would probably not have been brought forward.

Evaluate Quality-of-Life Issues

The utilization nurse and the social worker visit the patient while she is in the nursing home to assess her progress. According to nursing home caregivers, the patient appears capable of more functional activity but is unwilling to make the effort. She doesn't seem to display pain or discomfort but just lies in bed all day, watching television. Calls to the patient's home after the nursing home discharge suggest a similar pattern.

It is reported that the patient's daughter comes every day to her home to bring her a meal that is compliant with her diet. A home care nurse has been requested, but the patient, who is home alone during the day, refuses to let her in. Because Mrs. Martin is on Coumadin, she needs regular monitoring of her blood levels. But she refuses to come to the clinic even by prearranged ambulance, an idea the team proposed partly because Medicare would cover the cost. When the ambulance arrived, the patient simply stated that the time was inconvenient. From all appearances, the patient is happy, relaxing in her home and watching television to pass the time in spite of the continued deterioration of her medical condition. Admission to the hospital for crisis intervention is a way of life for her.

Unable to persuade the patient to accept care, the utilization nurse approaches Dr. Johnson, requesting a lab order to have Mrs. Martin's blood drawn at home. Doing so is intended to avoid any possible suggestion that the team has abandoned a homebound patient. But since the patient is no longer homebound but rather chooses not to leave her home, the circumstances no longer meet the Medicare criteria for home care, and as a result the health plan rejects bills for these services, forcing the clinic to absorb the costs. The utilization nurse notes her concern that the clinic is financially at risk for the cost of care, even with the patient's history of noncompliance.

Identify Patient and Family Preferences

Considering the case from a different disciplinary perspective, the social worker urges the team to expand the discussion beyond the clinical issues to the patient's lifestyle and resources. The social worker asks whether there is a guardian and is told that the patient is reluctant to give up control and the family won't force the issue. Mrs. Martin is a survivor on her husband's health policy from a major auto corporation and appears to have sufficient financial resources. There are no advance directives. No one is clear whether the patient has been properly informed of the benefits and risks of her behavior. The social worker suggests a family meeting where issues can be explored and the patient's views and understanding clarified. She also proposes that ethical dimensions of the case should be evaluated, commenting that the patient's right to choose could be more appropriately managed.

Consider Contextual Factors

The growth of managed care and the support of modern technology have brought more formalized structures for monitoring the cost of care. Organizational policies and procedures that influence how practitioners perform their daily care activities are grounded in cost-consciousness. Directives from administration are often based on utilization data and updates from health plans involved in day-to-day operations. As data systems improve the ability to monitor costs, medical practitioners are increasingly pressed to control the use of resources within their patient panels. Pressure on practitioners is sometimes used by administration as a short-term strategy for addressing fiscal shortfalls. Practitioners who are targeted must be especially cautious that these factors do not influence ethical treatment decisions.

Patient noncompliance is a major dilemma for practitioners, who must balance legal and financial responsibilities to the organization while still remaining faithful to their patient's best interest. Ethical dilemmas related to the treatment of noncompliant patients are not new. In the past, noncompliance was often addressed by bedside rationing or avoidance. Today advances in technology produce quick and easy data to monitor care activities. Lack of follow-up may be noted in the data at some later date. The team is duly concerned about possible allegations of abandoning Mrs. Martin. In the face of all these dynamics, Dr. Johnson's frustration is understandable. Removing the patient from his panel to avoid future problems is uppermost on his mind.

Ethical Problems

While justice frames the broader discussion in this case, the search for the etiology of the patient's noncompliant behavior uncovers additional ethical issues. Themes unfold as the team works through the case. Primary among them are autonomy, the patient's right to choose, and fidelity—the requirement that practitioners remain faithful to their patients, pursuing their patients' best interest despite the circumstances.

Ethical dilemmas will be embedded in any system that is motivated by cost. This case suggests that certain characteristics in the design of managed care contribute to ethical contradictions between the needs of patients and the limited resources available for their care. A review of the managed care model reveals characteristics that may present barriers to ethically appropriate care.

First is the physician or medical center's accountability for the cost of their patients' care. This essential principle of managed care thrusts cost considerations to the forefront and, despite the intent of the practitioner or care team, makes cost an integral part of the practitioner-patient relationship. Such accountability may be established voluntarily (e.g., by seeking a contract with an HMO) or involuntarily (e.g., by being told by HCFA that DRG payments must be accepted for Medicare patients).

A second feature of managed care is the provider's opportunity and the obligation to be proactive in care planning. As providers work diligently on the most efficient and cost-effective approach to meeting a patient's needs, it is easy to forget that their perspectives as practitioners may be in conflict with autonomy, the patient's right to self-determination. More simply put, there is a potential for providers to become preoccupied with serving their own or someone else's economic interests, to the exclusion of serving patient needs or desires. This moral dilemma risks abusing the promise that physicians make to be primarily dedicated to their patients.

A third feature—really a manifestation of the first two—is the increased use of the outpatient setting. Treating a patient in the outpatient setting serves to avoid costly hospitalizations. It follows that when the patient is primarily treated in the outpatient setting, the care environment extends beyond the clinic to the patient's home. Often missed, in the practitioner's rush to be efficient, is taking the time necessary to assure the patient and family's understanding and cooperation as partners in the care plan. Practitioners should solicit basic information about the home environment to determine if the care plan is feasible in the home setting. Home visits or family meetings will help practitioners understand the patient's social and cultural milieu and avoid misunderstanding.

A fourth characteristic is the exclusive use of interventions that are proven to be efficient for the patient population at large. Managed care plans tend to cover and promote only treatments for which there is solid evidence of effectiveness. This may be problematic in the treatment of patients with particular conditions where other approaches may be effective. Benefits design is used to exclude inefficient or costly treatments for which there are less costly alternatives. For instance, managed care plans will promote cost-efficient drugs on the formulary and may avoid or shorten hospital stays. Referrals and inpatient services are limited to facilities associated with the provider or where negotiations have resulted in reduced rates for services. While most plans have appeal mechanisms to evaluate patient preferences, providers will often be discouraged and face barriers in proposing a treatment of choice that is not covered by the HMO's benefits.

These overriding principles of managed care are a prescription for efficiency and cost savings. They are also a way of life for managed care practitioners who struggle with the clash of values in the care of their patients. Patients with conditions that are not expected to improve present special dilemmas for practitioners pressured by cost containment. The frail elderly in our population are the most vulnerable with the greatest risk. Caring for the frail elderly with declining conditions is a complex and time-consuming task that takes both a physical and a psychological toll on practitioners who are trained to heal.

Using Ethical Theories to Analyze a Problem

Ethics are a powerful tool for analyzing a case. Using basic ethical principles as a discussion guide can benefit a team. As Mrs. Martin's team revisits her case, the members respond to the social worker's comments, review the ethical principles that apply, and consider their implications.

The dilemma of administering distributive justice for a large population of patients is evident to the team. They realize their obligation to be discretionary in using resources intended for all patients. They will also need to set reasonable limits on the use of time. But they are aware that what they learn in this case will help them in other cases with noncompliant patients.

As the team revisits the case, the members decide that patient autonomy, the patient's right to self-determination, has not been sufficiently addressed. As a result of this discussion, they fully realize how essential it is to clarify the patient's goals before proceeding to develop a plan of care. This realization is a big step forward for the team.

An evaluation of the issues makes it clear that the team has not addressed whether the patient understands her condition or the consequences of her actions. Perhaps the patient wants to be noncompliant but still wants care. Dr. Johnson believes the patient to be competent, and the team knows that with appropriate informed consent, competent patients have a right to refuse treatment. Jonsen, Siegler, and Winslade (1998) tell us that "informed consent is a practical application of autonomy." Steps need to be taken to assure Mrs. Martin's understanding and to involve her in the care plan. Patient participation in care decisions brings a unique piece to the broader picture that is otherwise incomplete.

Poor patient education can be a huge problem when treating a complex patient in the outpatient setting. When the care environment extends to the patient's home, patient education and family-caregiver communication are essential components of the treatment plan. The team also needs knowledge of the patient's home environment so that its plan may complement the setting. The patient and family may need assistance in preparations to carry out the plan. A home visit from a team member whom the patient trusts may be helpful.

As consumers of health care, elderly persons often have little knowledge of their health care contracts, how their physicians are paid, or what ethical conflicts may be faced. They may have insurance that is provided by previous employers, by deceased spouses, or through a plan based upon affordable cost. Health plans themselves do not always provide full disclosure of benefit limits. Additionally, an older patient may be represented by a family or caregivers that have had no role in the patient's choice of a care plan and are uninformed themselves. Time needs to be taken by staff to educate the patient and family on the health plan and benefits.

Treating patients in the outpatient setting is intended to reduce costs, but it also circumvents the risk of iatrogenic illness so prevalent in older adults when treated in an acute care setting. Treating Mrs. Martin in the outpatient setting should be of benefit to both the patient and the provider. Efforts to keep Mrs. Martin out of the hospital were not successful however, partly because of her habitual noncompliance but also because the practitioners were focused on economic interests to the exclusion of the patient's needs and desires. Other factors include gaps in communication and lack of patient-family participation in the care plan. Input from the patient may open other avenues for creating a plan that is integrated with the patient's lifestyle.

Finally, a physician has a responsibility, beyond any obstacles created by policies or service limits, to be faithful to his or her patient. The principle of trust that flows from this covenant between doctor and patient is essential to the healing process. In this case, transferring Mrs. Martin from Dr. Johnson's care to that of another physician could result in interruptions in her care. Furthermore, repeating the experiences with someone new would not be cost effective. Dr. Johnson needs help with this complex case. With the team's support, sharing the care can lighten the burden. The team decides to work on a plan to support Dr. Johnson in continuing the care of Mrs. Martin.

Resolve the Ethical Issues and Create the Plan

Ultimately, the team adopts an action plan to address the ethical issues and to take the pressure off Dr. Johnson. The nurse practitioner has a good relationship with Mrs. Martin and agrees as a first step to contact her at home to assess her understanding and discuss her goals. The social worker will do a psychosocial workup for the team. The utilization nurse proposes to call the patient and ask her to personally pay for continued lab services at her home. This way the monitoring of her blood thinner medication will not be interrupted due to the health plan's refusal to pay. The social worker agrees to stand by for a contact with the patient's daughter to propose a family meeting or a home visit where they can talk with the patient about her desires and alternatives.

In case the plan fails, the team has a backup plan. The utilization nurse will contact the legal department about writing a letter to the patient and family giving them notice that the team is unable to care for her if she does not cooperate. All members of the team agree to document their interactions and the patient's response. The case is ongoing.

Resolve the Ethical Issues and Create the Plan

A number of issues in this case emphasize how, in the managed care setting, the cost of care has become part of the practitioner-patient relationship. In their efforts to be cost efficient, the team lost sight of the broader picture and also lost time by rushing to poorly considered conclusions. They did not listen to the patient's voice or assess her understanding, ignoring her right to autonomy. They simply drew on available resources to get the patient to comply. Attempting to be proactive, they concluded that getting Mrs. Martin into the clinic could solve the problem, and because it was a covered benefit, they sent an ambulance to her home. This plan failed to produce a response. Differences between the staff's and the patient's wishes had not been considered. The team needed an approach that would readjust its focus. The social worker's suggestion that the team consider the ethical aspects of the case was a pivotal point in the discussion.

Implement the Plan (with Special Consideration of Team Issues)

Cost-consciousness pervades this case, interfering with the practitioners' abilities to be effective in the care of Mrs. Martin. Patients like Mrs. Martin take time, a luxury the team does not have. Cost-saving practices imposed by the principles and practices of managed care have led them astray. Their attempt to be proactive caused them to ignore the patient's right to determine her own goals. In an attempt to resolve issues before there was mutual understanding, their plan failed and the patient was repeatedly admitted for costly care. A discussion of the ethical aspects of the case will provide the basis for a reevaluation of their decisions.

As stewards of scarce resources, the team needs to weigh what level of resources Mrs. Martin has a right to. At the most basic level, the team carries a social burden of deciding how much time and resources can be given to her without infringing on the rights of others. Clancy and Brody (1997) propose that the fairest and most defensible principle would be to match treatments with those patients most likely to benefit, and to begin to discourage or to withhold expensive treatments for patients whose chances of benefiting are very slim or nearly zero. Addressing Mrs. Martin's needs may take an inordinate amount of time and result in little benefit. In addition to time, the task is complex. Setting boundaries in a fair and equitable manner is difficult and takes practice. The task requires collective input and careful reflection, a necessity despite the time constraints.

Over time the team may be able to develop guidelines for establishing issues of justice for individual patients. Ideally, their diversity of perspectives and ability to reflect on their work together will result in a synergistic product that is more than the sum of its parts. Further, it is essential that they find a way to share the burden of care for complex and difficult cases. While teams seem to provide the best answer for exploring options and addressing patient quality-of-life issues, they also find themselves limited by time and resources in extensively pursuing all their insights. Teams bring a better outcome, but often the product is cost prohibitive.

The case of Mrs. Martin illustrates many of the ethical dilemmas faced by practitioners in an environment controlled by cost. With all the effort the team has made, the patient remains distressed, the physician annoyed, and the team frustrated with the increasing amount of dollars being spent. Little progress has been made in treating the patient, and she has been hospitalized several times for care more appropriately rendered in the outpatient setting. In this case, the team's tendency to consider cost first and not take the time to develop a comprehensive approach has interfered with an ethically appropriate process. The outcome became exactly what they were trying to prevent.

Through their work together, the team members have moved forward in resolving the conflict between the proactive principle of managed care and the patient's right to autonomy. While they need to be reminded of the importance of considering the patient and family as members of the team, they are making progress in this concept.

There are other aspects to the case over which the team has no control. Considering the intensive use of resources and the likelihood of a poor outcome, Mrs. Martin may not be appropriate for team care—or for managed care. Perhaps the physician is correct that for the benefit of other patients in the pool, Mrs. Martin should be removed from his panel. Faced with legal advice to the contrary, the team continues its work. In the end, the pressures of cost in the managed care design appear to have interfered with maximizing the benefits of team care.

Other contradictions outside the control of teams continue to affect their acceptance in the cost-constrained environment. For example, to survive over time, teams need some means of measuring outcomes to demonstrate their effectiveness. But measuring the value of the team's intervention is complex. One of the problems teams face today is the lack of adequate measures to demonstrate dollar value for time spent in care planning for high-risk elderly patients. If Mrs. Martin stays with the team a long time after the intervention, the center may benefit from the time expended by the team. These savings will be hard to measure. Until more evidence shows that teams are cost effective, team time will be allocated reluctantly if at all. This patient, because of the complexity of her medical condition, may never measurably improve. Improved outcomes in elderly patients with debilitating conditions are especially difficult to demonstrate using conventional measures. Many older patients die during periods of evaluation. Although new patient-centered evaluation methods are being tested (Fischer, Stewart, and Block 1999) at this point in time health care organizations are better at scrutinizing practitioner time and productivity— measures that are easily quantifiable and readily available. Unless teams can demonstrate effectiveness in cost and outcomes, their survival will probably not be easy.

Patients with declining conditions will be a continuing problem not only for providers but also for society at large. Teams bring promise of a new level of accountability and insight to alleviate this burden. Reflective teams working together over time can build on their collective experiences and bring new levels of awareness to resolving ethical issues. In this case, Dr. Johnson in frustration was prepared to abandon or disenroll the patient. As a result of the team's work, he realized that this was ethically and legally inappropriate. As our population ages, practitioners will require more and more support. Teams seem to be the answer.

Conclusion

The team reviewing Mrs. Martin is expending a costly effort addressing ethical issues. At the conclusion of their effort, they will have some opinions about the time spent and the appropriateness of the resources expended on this patient instead of other patients, with the likelihood of more positive outcomes. Individual cases can best be resolved when practitioners who know the patients take their medical histories and conditions into account (Clancy and Brody 1997). No one is more equipped than the team to make decisions about allocation of resources for patients in their care. Their experiences may or may not be successful with this patient, but it will provide a new level of learning that can benefit their future work. Most specifically, the team has learned of a need to be more systematic and thorough in developing care plans that are ethically appropriate. In doing so, they will improve their product.

As practitioners, this team is convinced that the team concept is a valid and ethically superior method to address the multiple and complex needs of older adults. The team members also appreciate the camaraderie and the shared learning experiences that help them grow as professionals. They believe that they provide better geriatric care as a unit than they could as individual practitioners. Their views of justice are developing and maturing through their teamwork. They have been reminded of their patients' right to autonomy and its conflict with their efforts to be proactive. They understand and can remind each other that all these principles must be balanced in practice.

In retrospect, the team's performance in this case was effectively cost conscious but the pressures of cost interfered with the members' ability to resolve the dilemma of the patient's noncompliance effectively. While health care works on alternatives to bottom-line decision making, teams demonstrate characteristics that help us assure ethically appropriate consideration for elderly patients with declining conditions and potential adverse outcomes. Because of their inherent contradictions, however, practices related to cost containment can be expected to continue to function as barriers to the expansion of team care as a practice. These inhibiting factors will probably prevent teams from gaining widespread prominence in the current period.

Ultimately, new care systems will evolve to meet our economic mandates. It is our task to assure that efforts are made to keep them ethically appropriate to the needs of older patients. In the meantime, until doors open to new options, teams offer a transitional means of support for overburdened practitioners. Working together in the care of the elderly, teams can learn from their experiences and apply what they have learned with new patients. Interdisciplinary team care is a model for continual improvement.

Discussion Questions

1. What are some essential differences in this case between care provided by the team and care provided by a single practitioner, from the perspective of (a) the practitioner? (b) the health provider? (c) the patient?

2. There is a suggestion that Mrs. Martin is not an appropriate patient for team care—or managed care. Should there be a screening process to identify patients appropriate for team care? If so, what criteria should be used to determine appropriateness?

3. Should Mrs. Martin be removed from Dr. Johnson's panel? If so, what ethical and legal issues are involved?

4. Suggest a guideline for practitioners to evaluate whether they are serving their own or their patient's best interest.

5. What can practitioners do if a patient wishes to be noncompliant but still wants care?

6. In a fixed-income environment like managed care, how can decisions best be made about the allocation of resources when a patient's condition is not expected to improve?

7. The case in the chapter is ongoing. What do you think the outcome will be?

REFERENCES

Bureau of Health Professions. 1995. Health resources and services administration. Interdisciplinary education. In Susan Klein, ed., *A national agenda for geriatric education: White papers.* Vol. 1, Administrative Document.

Clancy, C., and H. Brody. 1997. Managed care: Jekyll or Hyde? In J. Glaser, and Hamel, R., eds., *Three realms of managed care: Societal, institutional, and individual.* Kansas City, Mo.: Sheed and Ward.

Council on Ethical and Judicial Affairs, American Medical Association. 1995. Ethical issues in managed care. *JAMA*. 273:300–35.

Fischer, D., A. L. Stewart, D. Block, et al. 1999. Capturing the patient's view of change as a clinical outcome measure. *JAMA*. 282(12):1157–62.

Fleck, L., and H. Squier. 1997. Facing the ethical challenges of managed care. In J. Glaser, and R. Hamel, eds., *Three realms of managed care: Societal, institutional, and individual.* Kansas City, Mo.: Sheed and Ward.

Hall, M. A., and R. A. Berenson. 1998. Ethical practice in managed care: A dose of realism. *Annals of Internal Medicine* 128(5):395–402.

Jonsen, A. R., M. Siegler, and W. J. Winslade. 1998. *Clinical ethics,* 4th ed. New York: McGraw-Hill.

Mason, R., S. Moore, C. Sciulli, N. Wadsworth, and P. Whitehouse. *Great Lakes GITT, Characteristics of multidisciplinary teams, interdisciplinary teams and interdisciplinary learning teams.* Unpublished work.

CHAPTER 15

Duly Compensated or Compromised? Multiple Providers and Cross-Institutional Decision Making

Kathryn Hyer, Dr.P.A., M.P.P.,
Lori A. Roscoe, Ph.D., and
Bruce Robinson, M.D., M.P.H.

The modern health care landscape is characterized by competing service providers, multiple reimbursement mechanisms, and complex organizational arrangements and reporting relationships. The complexity in the environment influences the roles that particular facilities play in the provision of care and the roles that individual health care professionals play within institutional hierarchies. For example, nursing homes that historically provided custodial care now also serve as subacute care facilities for recovery and rehabilitation. New roles—such as geriatric nurse practitioner and director of palliative care—have emerged as health care facilities struggle to address the needs of an aging population in cost effective ways.

Health care professionals are increasingly employed and compensated in ways that are often not openly disclosed or discussed. When clinicians are paid on a modified fee-for-service formula based on actual services delivered, there are incentives to improve revenue by providing more service than might be necessary. Increasingly, individual earnings are aligned with the larger corporate structure's goals to increase profitability. In managed care especially, but not exclusively, bonuses may be tied to clinicians' ability to control patient costs and increase the profitability of the corporation. At the same time, providers may feel conflict between their professional and service mission to patients and their new accountability for profitability. While there is a general unwillingness to openly discuss compensation, especially individual compensation, incentives established by employers may have important implications for patient care.

Despite possible ethical conflicts, few clinicians or organizations fully disclose the structure of compensation packages, and even fewer have created mechanisms or norms that allow for the open discussion and consideration of possible conflicts as a result of shifting organizational hierarchies and reimbursement structures. Yet in the new complex world of for-profit health care, these are essential considerations for patients, families, fellow clinicians, and the organizations that employ these professional staff members. Because of the regulatory environment as well as the patient population served, long-term care facilities may be particular sites of conflicting loyalties and ethics. This chapter explores how financial incentives influence interactions between and among clinicians jointly caring for the same elderly client but receiving compensation from competing multiple sources.

Impact on Nursing Homes

Nursing homes are highly regulated institutions and are suspect providers of quality care. Inspections of facilities by teams of state surveyors are scheduled annually, but under recent Medicare rules inspections must now begin at night or on weekends to ensure that regulators monitor the quality of care at "off-hours." Suspicion about quality of care has increased federal spending on state survey and certification efforts and heightened tensions between regulators and providers. Finally, HCFA maintains a web-based list of all facilities, entitled "Nursing Home Compare," that reports facility-level findings by state from each state's survey. While such interaction may be meant as an aid for families, it further increases providers' fears of the survey process.

Reimbursements for nursing home services have also been squeezed in recent years, especially since the Balanced Budget Act of 1997, when nursing homes were forced into prospective payment for services. One result is plummeting revenue and decreased value of for-profit nursing home companies. Florida estimates that 23 percent of total nursing home beds in the state are in facilities that have filed for Chapter 11 bankruptcy protection. Nursing homes are also a target of lawsuits across the nation. Again, Florida is a leader, with its facilities three times more likely to be sued and the average $278,000 settlement more than twice as high as the national average. In this climate, nursing home administrators worry about keeping their facilities solvent and their jobs intact. Balancing smaller budgets, maximizing reimbursement for services, and complying with federal and state regulations to avoid monetary fines in the increasingly hostile survey process are tasks that are paramount to survival. In addition, the image of the long-term care facility in the public record and the professional community must be maintained to insure goodwill and client referrals.

Geriatric Care Teams

Adapting to changes in roles and responsibilities as well as responding effectively to economic pressures and environmental uncertainties may be especially difficult for members of geriatric care teams. Members of multidisciplinary care teams are charged not only with representing their respective professions and the patients in their care but also with responsibility for the effectiveness of the services they provide and often the viability and competitiveness of the facilities in which they practice. In some instances health care professionals may practice in particular facilities but be partially compensated by federally funded programs with different goals (i.e., to reduce costs and limit hospital admissions). Team members who play multiple roles may also have multiple and sometimes competing loyalties—to their professions, their facilities or institutions, and to the signer of their paychecks, as well as to the patients and families in their care. The norms and priorities that prevail at a particular point in time depend on the nature of the decisions to be made, the respect of the team members for one another, the tolerance of the team to fully discuss disagreements, and the conflicts that surface during the course of team interactions.

Members of geriatric care teams are also challenged by the complexities inherent in their patient population. While many clinical interactions are straightforward and require only cursory introspection about the ethical consequences of decisions, the care of residents of long-term care facilities rarely presents such easy choices. For example, clinicians treating frail adults must weigh comorbidities and probable drug interactions against a treatment's effect on function and quality of life. The average nursing home resident has been described as an 85-year-old cognitively impaired widow, involuntarily admitted to a nursing home directly from the hospital (Kane 1990). Such residents may arrive with little or no documentation about their preferences for treatment, and without family members or caregivers familiar with their values or willing to act as surrogate decision makers should the need arise. Impaired cognitive ability and depression, common among those who reside in long-term care facilities, may also cloud the ethical parameters of decision making. Thus, geriatric care teams generally shoulder the enormous responsibility of making life-and-death decisions for residents who lack either decision-making capacity, responsive surrogate decision makers, or clear advance directives.

Although hospitals and nursing homes are required by law to offer patients an opportunity to complete an advance directive upon admission, many patients decline to do so; even when an advance directive is completed by a patient, it often fails to accompany the patient when the care setting changes. Long-term care facilities have few incentives to create the structured process for clarifying and documenting residents' treatment preferences if initial offers are refused, yet such documentation can provide much-needed guidance for future decisions.

Not only are advance directives and other medical documentation frequently misplaced when the setting of care changes from the hospital to a long-term care facility, but relationships with primary care providers are also displaced. Few community care physicians follow their patients into the nursing home setting. Nursing home physicians regularly examine residents, but these cursory examinations offer only limited opportunities to develop rapport with the patient and gain knowledge of treatment preferences. As cognition deteriorates, patients' preferences and ability to understand the risks and benefits of treatment choices are even more difficult to ascertain.

Despite sometimes-limited opportunities for physician interaction, patients who become permanent nursing home residents often do interact with nurses, aides, social services staff, activity directors, and therapists—all of whom may be in a position to ascertain the treatment preferences and concerns of residents through informal and unstructured conversations. Ironically, many of these staff members are not empowered to represent the voice of the patient when important clinical decisions need to be made and deference is paid to physician expertise and authority.

The case presented below highlights some of the conflicting loyalties and ethical dilemmas that surface in the emerging world of multiple employers, subcontracts, and varied sources of compensation for health care professionals engaged in the care of residents of long-term care facilities. The physician's multiple sources of compensation complicate not only relationships with patients but also relationships with other members of the health care team.

Case Description

In June 1997 Theresa Lyons, an 81-year-old widow, was admitted to Sunnyside Nursing Home, in a large metropolitan area of Florida, from a local hospital after a bout of malnutrition, dehydration, and anemia. The hospital record stated that she had deteriorated mentally due to multi-infarct dementia and was unable and uninterested in meeting her nutritional needs. Mrs. Lyons did not object to placement in the nursing home. She had no known children or family and no advance directives or other documentation about her treatment preferences upon her transfer to Sunnyside.

Mrs. Lyons had limited income but was admitted as a self-pay patient and converted to Medicaid within two months of admission as her finances dwindled. For forty years she had worked as a waitress before retiring at the age of 60. In 1985 she and her husband moved to Florida, where they lived on a modest pension from his company and a small Social Security check she received. Mr. Lyons died in 1993, and his pension stopped immediately upon his death. After her husband's death, Mrs. Lyons moved to a smaller apartment in another neighborhood and was unable to maintain relationships with old friends because she did not drive.

Even though her decisional capacity was in question upon admission to the long-term care facility, no efforts were made at adjudication of competence or appointment of a guardian. In addition to a minimum filing fee of $300, there was a long waiting list for public guardians; the court also discouraged the routine appointment of guardians unless the patient's life was imminently at stake. As she had no primary physician who would follow her care in the nursing home, and no other physicians accepted new patients at Sunnyside, the medical director of the facility became her primary care physician.

Mrs. Lyons was a slight, frail woman barely 60 inches tall and weighing 90 pounds at admission. She was quiet and did not voluntarily participate in activities, although she did not object to being included and seemed to enjoy the change of scene and companionship. In February 1998, seven months after her admission, the social services director at Sunnyside recommended that Mrs. Lyons be considered for a new Medicare replacement program run by a for-profit managed care company that had a contract with Sunnyside. The program was a capitated plan that aimed to reduce emergency department visits and hospitalizations by providing additional medical services on-site delivered by a geriatric nurse practitioner (GNP). The GNP was employed by the Medicare replacement program but worked at Sunnyside and other participating facilities to provide services to the patients enrolled in the program. Physicians were also employed by the program to oversee the medical care of enrolled patients.

As part of the contract, the enrollment procedure required the social services director to screen all residents living in the facility to determine whether they were acceptable candidates for the program and to protect them from undue pressure to join. The social services director used two criteria to screen potential members: the resident was expected to live in the facility on a permanent basis, and the resident was assigned to a physician under contract with the Medicare program so that changing physicians would not be required. Mrs. Lyons satisfied both selection criteria; she was expected to be a long-term resident and the medical director, Mrs. Lyons's physician, was one of the contracted managed care physicians participating in the Medicare replacement program. In February 1998 Mrs. Lyons was deemed eligible to participate, and the membership coordinator for the Medicare replacement program contacted her to explain the program. The social services director was present for the interview as required by the Medicare replacement program and Sunnyside. Mrs. Lyons smiled during the interview and agreed to enroll, happily signing the papers. The Social Services director verified that Mrs. Lyons voluntarily agreed to enter the managed care program, and two months later, on April 1, 1998, Mrs. Lyons became a member of the program.

Sunnyside was eager to increase the number of residents participating in the Medicare replacement program. The more residents who were enrolled in the program, the more time the GNP allocated to Sunnyside, and all Sunnyside patients and staff benefited. The GNP served as a resource to the other nurses at the facility because in addition to monitoring her assigned residents, she was available to confer with physicians and other staff about the care of all patients. The medical director, recognizing the value of the GNP as a highly skilled clinical provider who visited the residents more frequently than required by Medicare, encouraged his patients' participation in the program and was very supportive of the GNP assigned to his patients. He also benefited financially in two ways: he received additional income from the Medicare replacement program for enrolling patients, and a GNP visit to his patients could substitute for his required Medicare visit.

On admission to the managed care program, the GNP assigned to Sunnyside conducted a history and physical with Mrs. Lyons as part of an initial comprehensive assessment. As a standard part of the initial interview, the GNP talked about advance directives, but Mrs. Lyons was unable to participate fully in the discussion. When asked if she had family or friends who could help her, Mrs. Lyons shook her head and said, "no one." The GNP's notes also indicated that Mrs. Lyons scored a 20/30 on the MMSE and that she was oriented to person and place but had 0 out of 3 in recall. She did note, however, that Mrs. Lyons seemed able to describe her current symptoms and did not seem depressed as she smiled and talked with the GNP.

Mrs. Lyons weighed 85 pounds, and the GNP noted the drop of five pounds since her arrival at the facility. When asked about her weight, Mrs. Lyons said that she was always small and never ate much. She said she ate "some of the food," but that the food served was "cold and not very good." The GNP told Mrs. Lyons that it was important that she continue to eat and, pointing to a resident with a feeding tube, reminded her that eating was a significant part of her life in the nursing home. When Mrs. Lyons looked at the resident with the feeding tube, she seemed to grow fearful, shook her head forcefully back and forth, and cried "No, no." The GNP, concerned about Mrs. Lyons's weight loss, noted in the chart that her body mass index was less than 19, which placed her at risk for malnourishment. She also ordered a dietary consult and requested that Mrs. Lyons be offered small calorie-rich snacks during recreational activities.

In July 1998 Mrs. Lyons had a seizure and was unwilling to eat even though she could swallow. After a neurological consult, the physician determined that Mrs. Lyons had had a minor stroke. Nine days later the GNP's note read "dysphagia, weight loss, mouth drooping to the right, taking 50 percent of her meals by mouth." In consultation with the dietitian, the GNP ordered high-calorie shakes thinned with liquid and noted that Mrs. Lyons would need encouragement from the staff to drink the shakes and eat the puddings that were to be offered throughout the day.

On August 27, during a routine examination by her physician, Mrs. Lyons weighed 71 pounds but was alert, smiling, and eating small portions. The staff complained that it took a long time for her to finish her meals; because of the dysphagia, even thinned liquid supplements were difficult for her to swallow. The physician corroborated the GNP's orders to continue to push fluids. The physician noted in her chart that her rapid weight loss continued to be of concern, that a feeding tube might need to be considered, and that her lack of capacity made it unlikely that she could make decisions about her medical care. Five days later Mrs. Lyons weighed 69 pounds. The GNP and director of nursing at Sunnyside talked briefly and agreed that she was unable to eat or drink sufficient quantities to maintain an adequate nutritional status.

Throughout the course of Mrs. Lyons's stay at Sunnyside, but particularly after her enrollment in the Medicare replacement program, she had seldom been the focus of the geriatric care team's concern. The team usually consisted of the physician, the nurse assigned to the patient, the director of nursing, a dietitian, and at times a social worker. The care of patients in the capitated program was overseen by the GNP, who was responsible for calling the team together as necessary to evaluate the care plans of enrolled patients. Anticipating the need to hospitalize Mrs. Lyons even though she participated in a plan whose primary goal was to keep patients out of the hospital, the GNP called a meeting of the medical director, the director of nursing, and the dietitian. The director of nursing invited the administrator of Sunnyside to attend because this patient's significant weight loss would surely trigger her record to be reviewed in the upcoming state survey. Recognizing the likelihood of Mrs. Lyons as the focus of a state survey, the nursing director wanted to be certain that everyone participated in the discussion.

At the hastily called team meeting, the director of nursing and the medical director agreed that Mrs. Lyons's decisional competence was questionable and argued that it was unlikely that she would understand the life-and-death significance of refusing a feeding tube at this point in her care. The GNP stated her belief that Mrs. Lyons did not want a feeding tube and that discussion about treatment preferences had occurred prior to her most recent stroke. The GNP made a side comment to the director of nursing that Mrs. Lyons's competence had not been an issue when she agreed to enter the managed care program, that was not shared with the team. The director of nursing advised the team that she understood the importance of maintaining adequate oral intake and was concerned about the record review during the upcoming state survey. But a series of articles on tube feeding in dementia patients suggested that such interventions rarely improved survival or maintained quality of life, and that such clinical findings should be incorporated into protocols for patient care (Callahan et al. 1999; Finucane, Christmas, and Travis 1999; McCann 1999). The GNP offered that the Medicare replacement program would like to bring the case to the ethics committee of the local university for a fuller discussion and assistance in working through the issues to be resolved.

The meeting concluded when the administrator of Sunnyside stated that she was unwilling to expose the facility to possible legal or regulatory action or to negative publicity "for starving an old lady." Nor would an ethics consultation help, since the Labor Day holiday and the beginning of the semester would certainly delay any decision for a few weeks. The administrator reminded the team that weight loss of more than 5 percent of body weight was classified as a sentinel event under the unintended-weight-loss protocol instituted by the federal government's nursing home regulatory group. The upcoming annual survey was due, and Mrs. Lyons's record would certainly be reviewed. After reading the record, the administrator worried that the facility had not adequately documented the constant offering of nutritious snacks. She also questioned the dietitian about how she had documented that the food served Mrs. Lyons was warm and appealing. "These surveyors can always say we haven't accommodated the patient's needs enough," she sighed. At the end of the meeting, the administrator stated that the scrutiny of the surveyors' reviews would be mitigated if the home were aggressive about putting in the feeding tube. "I'm not risking citations because we aren't being aggressive, nor am I testifying in court that Mrs. Lyons was capable of making the decision to reject a feeding tube," she declared.

The next day Mrs. Lyons was admitted to the hospital with dehydration. Her primary physician from Sunnyside and another hospital surgeon agreed to insert a percutaneous endoscopic gastrostomy (PEG) tube on the basis of medical necessity. They noted her inability to make decisions and indicated that no advance directives were in her record. Mrs. Lyons tried to remove the feeding tube when she regained consciousness and seemed very distressed by its presence. To prevent her from being able to remove the feeding tube, Mrs. Lyons was fitted with "geri-mitts," a mittenlike restraint that uses Velcro to immobilize the patient's thumb, making it difficult to grasp items. Mrs. Lyons was also fitted with a "belly band," a wide cloth placed over the feeding tube and around her waist to hold the tube in place.

On readmission to the nursing home two days later, Mrs. Lyons continued to try to remove the tube and needed to be restrained to avoid doing so. When the GNP visited Mrs. Lyons after her return from the hospital, she was very troubled. She complained to her supervisors at the Medicare replacement program that her professional judgment was not appreciated. Mrs. Lyons was clearly uncomfortable with the tube and her restraints. The GNP was distressed by her inability to change a decision that she viewed as not clinically sound and as a defensive move to avoid citations or litigation. Further, the nursing home's administrator, a person whose agenda of care, the GNP believed, was philosophically opposed to the Medicare replacement's model of care, had driven the decision. The GNP requested reassignment to another facility and a different physician since she believed her credibility had been compromised. She stated that she did not believe the physician was supportive of her philosophy of care, and she could not understand how he had chosen his medical director role over his role as primary care physician.

After the tube was placed in Mrs. Lyons, the GNP had demanded that her employer find another nurse practitioner to practice in the facility. She stated that she was troubled by the emergency nature of the decision making, her inability to change a decision she felt violated her own ethical standards, her patient's wishes, and the precepts of the Medicare replacement program that employed her. She claimed she could not continue working in a facility where the administrator usurped the team process and undermined the decisions of the staff who knew the patient best. The nursing director and staff were dismayed that the GNP would no longer be part of their protocols and demanded to know who would provide that skilled service. The medical director, also upset at the reassignment request of the GNP he respected and valued, worried about the quality of care at Sunnyside as well as his reputation. In seeking to avoid another situation like that of Mrs. Lyons, the administrator agreed to establish an ethics committee with outside consultants at the facility.

Mrs. Lyons remained on the feeding tube with no more complications for three months. On December 5 she died in the nursing home of aspiration pneumonia.

Case Analysis

The case of Mrs. Lyons highlights how caring and competent providers are subtly influenced by unacknowledged conflicts of interest and competing loyalties to the multiple systems for which they work. Using the Jonsen, Siegler, and Winslade (1998) template for ethical analysis, we will first review the facts of the case in the following four areas: gather clinical information, identify patient and family preferences, evaluate quality-of-life issues and consider contextual features. The major ethical conflicts in this case arose over the patient's ability to state preferences and the interpretation of contextual factors, especially the financial, economic, and institutional interests of the individual clinicians and the organizations they represented.

Gather Clinical Information

There was little disagreement about the medical indications. A woman with obvious limits in cognitive capacity and no acceptable surrogate decision maker experienced the loss of ability to eat and drink. Already dehydrated and malnourished, the woman would die with no intervention.

Identify Patient and Family Preferences

Clinicians recognize that patients have the right to forgo life-sustaining treatment, including artificial nutrition and hydration; but for many nursing home residents, questions about their competence to make such decisions are fraught with justifiable concern. The GNP was the individual who spoke directly with the patient about the use of artificial nutrition and hydration. She believed that Mrs. Lyons did not want a feeding tube and that she was quite clear about her decision. This discussion, however, required cautious judgement in interpreting Mrs. Lyons's responses and her capacity to understand what was presented to her. Mrs. Lyons's mental status score at the time of the advanced directive discussion was low and clearly called into question her capacity to make decisions. Furthermore, judgments by cognitively compromised people are extraordinarily open to reflecting the views of the interviewer. At a minimum decisions of demented people require careful documentation and corroboration by other members of the care team.

In this case Mrs. Lyons's questionable capacity empowered the administrator to act in such a way as to avoid negative publicity and possible fines based on surveyors' citations. The administrator's decision to intervene, combined with the medical director's judgment that imminent action was required to prevent further decline, trumped the GNP's conviction that a feeding tube went against the patient's treatment preferences and the opinion of the director of nursing that such intervention might not be medically appropriate for dementia patients.

Evaluate Quality-of-Life Issues

The director of nursing raised the issue about quality of life and the prognosis for the patient when she reported that the professional medical journal articles on tube feeding in dementia patients questioned the value of feeding tubes (Callahan et al. 1999; Finucane, Christmas, and Travis 1999; McCann 1999). In response, the medical director reminded the team that the patient could certainly have the tube removed if her swallow function returned. But the unspoken consensus was that Mrs. Lyons would continue tube feeding until her death. As the literature suggests, patients with dementia have a poor prognosis and the tube does not improve quality of life. In fact, the GNP's position in the team meeting was that the tube interfered with Mrs. Lyons's quality of life and that Mrs. Lyons should be offered palliative care and allowed to die.

Consider Contextual Factors

The crux of this case was the potential financial and organizational affiliations that present conflicts of interest and called into question the motives of the clinicians and administrators involved in the care of Mrs. Lyons.

Physicians and nurse practitioners who receive substantial financial benefit by representing both a nursing home and a managed care program are apt to be influenced by these financial entities in making decisions about patient care. In this case both the physician/medical director and the GNP may have received financial benefit when Mrs. Lyons agreed to participate in the program, but the potential patient care benefits to Mrs. Lyons seemed to outweigh any conflict of interest. Still, as medical director of Sunnyside, the physician had yet another conflict—he received about 40 percent of his annual income from the nursing home. Mark Hall (1999) argues that "while capitation or other financial incentives—such as bonuses or withholds—directed to physicians are permissible, they are not however, ethically ideal since they create a financial conflict of interest between the patient's best medical interest and the physician's economic interest" (111).

While the physician might retrospectively have preferred to remove himself from the dual role of patient primary care physician and medical director of the facility, the reality was that few community physicians were willing to take Medicaid clients. Transferring Mrs. Lyons at the time the conflict appeared would have left her with a physician who knew her even less well. Besides, the medical director agreed that the decision to insert the tube was reasonable because she was unable to eat or drink sufficiently to maintain adequate nutritional status. Aggressive care is part of the socialization of physicians, he reasoned, but he recognized that the GNP was far more supportive of palliative care because of her socialization in nursing (see also Chapter 8). Finally, he also worried that in the increasingly litigious nursing home environment, his license and reputation would be jeopardized by a decision not to put in a feeding tube.

The GNP in this case was directly employed by the managed care organization, but she worked in the nursing home facility and thus had an obligation to represent the program, the facility and the interests of her patients. She was rewarded financially for increasing the patient census on her caseload and in the Sunnyside nursing home. Thus, she had incentives to please the nursing home and certainly to be careful about whistleblowing and making waves. Furthermore, the program routinely analyzed costs of care for enrolled patients assigned to each GNP and reported the data regionally, which influenced both her bonus and her promotion. Certainly this GNP was concerned about the overall financial stability of the program, and putting people in hospitals was not only against the program's philosophy but also not in her financial interest. In the end, however, the GNP was so distraught over the decision to insert the tube that she withdrew from that facility.

The administrator in this case had a compelling need to protect the facility from litigation and adverse regulatory action. These responsibilities weighed heavily and caused him to play a heavy-handed role in a matter of clinical judgment. While the administrator did not want to force a person to have a feeding tube without sufficient documentation, a decision to let someone die from malnourishment would have been tantamount to inviting a surveyor's wrath. Recognizing that the records would be scrutinized, the administrator did not want to jeopardize the reputation of the facility and did not trust that the records would demonstrate sufficient effort.

The director of nursing had compelling clinical evidence to offer about the efficacy of tube feeding, but ultimately she deferred to both the medical director and the administrator, particularly since she did not have a long history with the patient. Moreover, the patient record troubled her as well, and she worried that the surveyors or lawyers would find something more that the staff should have done to help the woman gain weight. She also recognized that she could never adequately document the number of attempts made by overburdened nurse aides to encourage Mrs. Lyons to take small sips of booster shakes.

The reality was that the home had a tremendous turnover in nurse aides and that tubes made it easier to feed demented residents with poor swallow reflexes.

Faced with compelling arguments for both options (tube placement or not), providers searching for an acceptable solution could not easily resist the influence of professional culture, administrative systems, and personal bias. The seemingly precipitous intervention of the administrator and the willingness of the medical director to agree compromised years of working relationships. The intervention failed because it defied the clinicians' sense of justice. They were thwarted in their ability to arrive at a moral standard because real discourse was not permitted. What is needed in resolving ethical dilemmas is an approach to discuss difficult cases and a decision-making process that allows for dissension and disagreement but ultimately for coordinated action in the service of both good patient care and respectful professional relationships.

Discussion

Practical discourse, an approach in communicative ethics, is a "procedure for testing the validity of norms that are being proposed" (Habermas 1990). Jürgen Habermas and communicative ethics argue that ethical norms are developed through an individual's interaction with society and that the societal norm is what people use as a community standard. But the societal norms can be realized only through discourse. Habermas states that "real conflicts . . . in which actors consider it incumbent upon them to reach a consensual means of regulating some controversial matter . . . create a process in which particular values are ultimately discarded as being not susceptible to consensus" (1990, 103). As Moody (1992) notes, "the value of a communicative ethic is to find commonly agreed upon ways of negotiating differences when we fail to agree in binding principles and rules" (13). Communicative ethics requires a mutuality of understanding and a noncoercive discussion that honors and respects patient autonomy and preferences for treatment and permits a full discussion of team members' norms and values. Habermas's practical discourse recognizes that clinicians can reach consensus about a plan of action while simultaneously acknowledging the inherent conflicts in their multiple roles and arriving at a community-derived standard.

Clinicians in this process have a responsibility to acknowledge and articulate their own values, biases, and observations while at the same time attempting to understand the opinions of others involved in each case. A difficult environment does not absolve practitioners of the responsibility to make ethical decisions, and difficult cases demand disclosure of conflicts of interest and an even more complete airing of competing ideas before the group can proceed. The communicative ethics of Habermas is summarized by Seyla Benhabib (1992, 30–31) as a six-step approach to the establishment of the norms of universal moral respect and egalitarian reciprocity. Once there is a disagreement around a moral judgment, Benhabib claims:

- A "reasonable agreement" must be arrived at under conditions that correspond to our idea of a fair debate.
- These rules of fair debate can be formulated as the "universal-pragmatic" presuppositions of argumentative speech, which can be stated as a set of procedural rules.
- These rules reflect the moral ideal that we ought to respect each other as beings whose standpoint is worthy of equal consideration (the principle of universal moral respect).
- Whenever possible, social practices embodying the discursive ideal (the principle of egalitarian reciprocity), which allow each participant to express their own point of view, should be developed and put in practice.

Benhabib (1992, 37) emphasizes the moral importance of the process to discuss disputes because "not that everybody could or would agree to the same set of principles, but that these principles have been adopted as a result of a procedure, whether of moral reasoning or of public debate, which we are ready to deem 'reasonable and fair.' It is not the result of the process of moral judgment alone that counts but the process for the attainment of such judgment." Thus, the process Benhabib describes allows justice to be served. In this case a team meeting must enable the group to arrive at a moral standard for the participants, including the patient, and develop the consensual position.

While not all decisions require elaborate decision-making processes, those that have implications for policy and those in which important values and goals come into conflict merit a more formal process for reaching consensus. The Woodstock Theological Center (1999) has proposed a straightforward decision-making process that was specially formulated for addressing and preventing ethical dilemmas in managed health care organizations. Briefly, the steps involved are (1) assemble facts and describe the problem; (2) identify the stakeholders affected by the decision; (3) identify the interests, values, and preferred outcomes of each stakeholder; (4) evaluate priorities; (5) brainstorm possible solutions or courses of action; (6) make the decision; (7) communicate the decision; and (8) monitor, learn, and make adjustments for future decisions. All decisions that clinicians and administrators make should reflect careful attention not only to ethical principles but also to "the needs, values and goals of the many stakeholders affected by the decision" (25). Thus, we review the case of Mrs. Lyons briefly highlighting the preventive ethics approach of teams using the Habermas standard of practical discourse.

Assemble Facts

The ethical dilemmas in this case did not unfold quickly. Rather, they played themselves out over multiple months and multiple decisions. While there were not many conflicts over the facts, if Mrs. Lyons had been the subject of a case review earlier, the significant weight loss would have been noticed and addressed more systematically by the care team. More documentation of feeding efforts would have been possible, and routine discussions would have also allowed others to ask Mrs. Lyons about her desire to have a feeding tube. Weight loss and a notation in the chart that read "at risk for a feeding tube" might have prompted the nursing home to request a guardian who could represent Mrs. Lyons's best interests without some of the competing claims for loyalty.

Identify the Stakeholders

Along with more regular team meetings, all key stakeholders in the care of Mrs. Lyons should have been more clearly identified. By discussing the case earlier and in less heated conditions, the values, interests and preferences of the players would have been easier to identify. A fuller discussion of the state surveyors' process could have prompted better record keeping by the GNP, floor nurses, social service staff, and dietary staff. The administrator might have felt better able to defend the case during the review of the surveyors.

Identify the Interests, Values, and Preferred Outcomes of Each Stakeholder

The multiorganizational conflicts that arose around the proper care of Mrs. Lyon show why managed care organizations and nursing homes should be explicit about their contracts. Details about the incentives for each party, the physician, the GNP, and the nursing home should be explicit. It is apparent from this case that nursing homes must also create a process for reaching decisions that are both ethically justified and consistent with the institutional mission, philosophy, policies, and procedures. Decision-making processes that build consensus by permitting open communication from all members of the care team may best render decisions that are acceptable to all and in the best interests of the patient.

Discuss Fully and Openly

The next three steps—(4) evaluate priorities, (5) brainstorm possible solutions or courses of action, and (6) make the decisions—involve a collaborative decision-making process that honors the individuals who comprise the team providing care to Mrs. Lyons. While the team might develop a clear sense of its values with practice and more explicit discussions, this case would have benefited from an effective clinical ethics consultation.

Discussion Questions

1. At what level of an integrated delivery system should decisions involving conflicts between delivery obligations and business goals be made? By whom and by what process should they be made?

2. Which if any organization should have provided the organizational ethics resource in Mrs. Lyons's case? What would you recommend when setting up a clinical ethics team?

REFERENCES

Benhabib, S. 1992. *Situating the self: Gender, community and postmodernism in contemporary ethics.* New York: Routledge, Chapman and Hall.

Callahan, C. M., K. M. Haag, N. N. Buchanan, and R. Nisi. 1999. Decision-making for percutaneous endoscopic gastrostomy among older adults in a community setting. *Journal of the American Geriatric Society* 47:1105–9.

Finucane, T. E., C. Christmas, and K. Travis. 1999. Tube feeding in patients with advanced dementia: A review of the evidence. *Journal of the American Medical Association* 282: 1365–70.

Habermas, J. 1990. *Moral consciousness and communicative action.* Cambridge, Mass.: MIT Press.

Hall, M. A. 1999. Referral practices under capitation: Commentary. In K. Gervais, ed., *Ethical challenges in managed care: A casebook.* Washington, D.C.: Georgetown University Press.

Jonsen, A. R., M. Siegler, and W. J. Winslade. 1998. *Clinical ethics.* 4th ed. New York: McGraw-Hill.

Kane, R. 1990. *Everyday ethics: Resolving dilemmas in nursing home life.* New York: Springer.

McCann, R. 1999. Lack of evidence about tube feeding: Food for thought. *Journal of the American Medical Association* 282:1380–81.

Moody, H. R. 1992. *Ethics in an aging society.* Baltimore: Johns Hopkins University Press.

Woodstock Theological Center. 1999. *Ethical issues in managed care organizations.* Washington, D.C.: Georgetown University Press.

CHAPTER 16

Transitions from Setting to Setting along the Care Continuum: The Case for Megateams

Judith L. Howe, Ph.D., Jeremy Boal, M.D.,
Kirsten Ek, B.A., and Christine K. Cassel, M.D.

Older adults often move from setting to setting along the care continuum, generally because of changes in health status. This pattern presents special challenges to health care professionals because of the diversity of settings, ranging from institutional, community, and home settings, and the increased numbers of providers involved.

Transitions for older patients occur under many guises and may involve many steps. It is not an unusual scenario, for example, for an older adult in a home-based care setting to require an emergency room visit—a transition in care in itself. The emergency room may only be the beginning step of a mazelike process of care, in which the client is shuffled between settings within the admitting institution or to one or more different institutions entirely. The journey may not necessarily end with the client back in his or her original setting. Over the course of this process, the typical older patient will encounter numerous different health care providers, many of whom have never met each other, operating in a variety of settings. There is a greater chance of role confusion and blurring, miscommunication, and general confusion about who does what. In worst-case scenarios, these transitions occur with little continuity of care between settings.

Teamwork in caregiving is already inherently complex, particularly when personal values come into play that may not always contribute to the best interest of the client. Team members from different professional or cultural backgrounds may bring different expectations and ways of communicating. Leadership may be poorly defined. Family members may or may not feel part of the team and in some cases may act in opposition to it. These issues become more complicated, with a greater chance of poor outcomes and miscommunications, when the older client is in transition and encountering not one but several teams, resulting in confusion and a flawed care plan. Consistency among the various teams in prioritizing the patient's overall needs often becomes an elusive goal.

Ethical issues also arise during these transitions. Care providers must often weigh issues of patient autonomy against their own ideas of the patient's best interest. They may disagree and not know it. Ethics committees, where they exist, are typically housed in one institution, not spanning several of them. Different clinical settings and providers with different ways of operating and communicating complicate the issues. Financial incentives for discharge, insufficient information exchange between settings, and inadequate follow-up exacerbate ethical dilemmas, hampering clarification of values and consensus building.

One model of care, the Program of All-Inclusive Care for the Elderly (PACE), has had increasing success by working not only to eliminate the multiple teams that patients encounter during transitions but also to eliminate many of the transitions themselves (Chin Hansen 1999). PACE was developed as a demonstration project at On Lok Senior Health Services, in San Francisco's Chinatown, in the 1970s and 1980s. It was designed to offer older patients continuity of care provided by a single health care team.

The elderly persons served by PACE all have chronic impairments severe enough to make them nursing home eligible, but the majority wish to continue living at home. The average PACE client is 80 years old and depends on outside help for at least three activities of daily living, and two-thirds are cognitively impaired through dementia or depression (Chin Hansen 1999). The majority are women and members of minority groups, and most are from low-income brackets (Eng et al. 1997).

To help these clients avoid or delay nursing home placement and promote their expressed wish for autonomy, an interdisciplinary megateam of care providers, ranging from eight to twenty-three members, provides adult day care services, in-home visits, and inpatient services as needed. Rather than drifting through emergency room visits and uncoordinated transitions in care settings as the patients in the cases in this chapter do, PACE patients are monitored extensively by the team. PACE team members provide care exclusively for PACE participants, meeting as often as daily to discuss cases and treatment plans.

The team ordinarily consists of a center coordinator, a social worker, a nurse, a home care aid, and a physician, as well as recreational, occupational, and physical therapists. Pharmacists, dietitians, chaplains, and transport technicians may also be involved (Zimmerman, Pemberton, and Thomas 1998). The team physician or nurse practitioner serves as the client's primary care provider, handling inpatient services as well. He or she may seek services from other health care specialists for the client if necessary (Eng et al. 1997).

Here we present three cases that demonstrate the complexities, contributions, and ethical pitfalls of teamwork in caring for older clients who are in transition. The problems raised by the cases suggest the need for megateams such as PACE that span all settings along the continuum of care.

Case Description: Mrs. Rodriguez

Mrs. Rodriguez, a 79-year-old widow with a history of diabetes mellitus, breast cancer, poor vision, and gait instability, lived in a senior housing facility in the inner city. When she was diagnosed with a recurrence of her breast cancer, the cancer was found to be widely metastatic. She was advised by her primary care physician that there was no hope of cure. She continued to live in the senior housing facility. Soon thereafter her health began to decline.

Three months after being diagnosed with the recurrence, Mrs. Rodriguez fell at home. She was taken to the emergency room by her pastor and was subsequently hospitalized at an academic medical center with a fractured arm. Due to Mrs. Rodriguez's decline in functional status, the medical center's inpatient social worker recommended that Mrs. Rodriguez be placed in a nursing home. The patient and her pastor were strongly opposed to nursing home placement. A nurse who had become quite close to Mrs. Rodriguez during her inpatient stay also tried to advocate on Mrs. Rodriguez's behalf against nursing home placement in heated discussions with the inpatient social worker, but she was unsuccessful in her efforts. Based on the evaluation of the medical center's inpatient social worker, the social worker at Mrs. Rodriguez's senior housing facility steadfastly refused to allow Mrs. Rodriguez to return to her home, citing liability restrictions of the housing facility.

Against her wishes, Mrs. Rodriguez was sent to a nursing home to convalesce while the pastor continued efforts to get her adequate home attendant services so that she could be returned to the senior housing facility. Medicare personnel would approve only nine hours of home attendant service, however, and neither the staff of the nursing home nor the senior housing social worker would accept this as adequate for her care.

An interdisciplinary meeting was held at the nursing home. The senior housing social worker, the pastor, and the nursing home's geriatrician attended. The pastor continued to press for discharge to the senior housing facility in keeping with the patient's wishes, while the housing facility's social worker reluctantly continued to deny permission. It was noted at this meeting that Mrs. Rodriguez had become much more withdrawn and depressed at the nursing home. At the end of this meeting, the nursing home's geriatrician promised to push Medicare for a round-the-clock home attendant care for the patient, which the senior facility social worker agreed would be adequate for her return. Mrs. Rodriguez also signed a health care proxy form naming her pastor as proxy. She was approved for twenty-four-hour home attendant care, then was transferred to the senior housing facility. There she died in her sleep four days later.

Case Analysis

Identify Patient and Family Preferences

The patient wished to be returned to her apartment in senior housing. At first glance she appeared to have the capacity to make her own decisions, but a

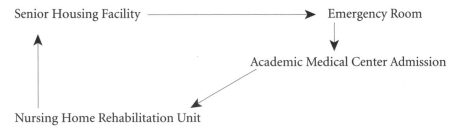

FIGURE 16.1 Case of Mrs. Rodriguez: Transitions in clinical settings

clear assessment of her decision-making capacity was not carried out. The nurse's notes indicate that Mrs. Rodriguez was "alert and oriented x 3." But her alertness and orientation did not necessarily reflect her capacity, unless assessed at various times throughout the day. Elderly patients especially may have fluctuating levels of capacity during the day—they may be lucid and retain capacity at certain times but not at others, as with "sundowner" syndrome commonly seen in nursing homes. For Mrs. Rodriguez to have evidenced capacity, her ability to understand her situation, weigh the benefits, burdens, and risks of options, appreciate the consequences of decisions, and make and communicate decisions would have had to remain consistent. If this ability waxed and waned throughout the day, her capacity was impaired. According to Jonsen, Siegler, and Winslade, "The expression of preferences in such a state should not be considered determinative, unless there is consistency in the preferences expressed during periods of clarity" (1998, 63).

The patient was allowed to sign a health proxy form, but this alone does not indicate that she had capacity. Capacity is decision specific, and a lower level of capacity is needed to appoint a proxy than to make many health care decisions. In this case, it was not made clear that the patient had the capacity to do both, although this might in fact have been the case.

Mrs. Rodriguez's case was made difficult by this lack of clear assessment. The foremost ethical conflict here was the conflict between autonomy and beneficence: the desire to respect the patient's wishes and right to self-determination balanced with the desire for health professionals to act in what they perceive to be the patient's best interest. Here several of Mrs. Rodriguez's health care providers emphasized finding the optimal care setting for the preservation of her life, giving the issue of beneficence more primacy than the stated desire of both Mrs. Rodriguez and her confidants to have her back in her own home. Mrs. Rodriguez was kept out of her home until four days before her death—which might have been avoided had an explicit assessment of her capacity been made and communicated to the entire team. A better compromise between autonomy and beneficence might also have been worked out had a round-the-clock home attendant care been readily available.

Evaluate Quality-of-Life Issues

Mrs. Rodriguez was unable to return to normal life in the senior housing facility and required a round-the-clock care; but she still desired this option over life in a nursing home. As previously noted, it was not made clear whether Mrs. Rodriguez appreciated the consequences of her stated wish.

Consider Contextual Factors

Team Composition. Team composition in this case was blurry. There were several care providers, but it is not clear that there was a functioning team at all. Certainly the provision of care was not coordinated. The health care providers at the hospital, including the hospital's inpatient nurse and social worker, did not play an active role once the patient mad the transition beyond the hospital doors. Yet the inpatient social worker's evaluation of the patient had such primacy that it continued to directly affect the patient by forming the basis on which Mrs. Rodriguez was prevented from returning home.

The patient might better have been served had members of the hospital involved in Mrs. Rodriguez's care—or at the very least the inpatient social worker—stayed involved in the case until its resolution. It is not known, however, what other burdens these providers faced and whether continuing involvement was even a possibility given other time and staffing constraints at the hospital. The interdisciplinary meeting involving professionals from the nursing home and senior housing facility as well as the patient's confidants was an attempt on the part of these providers to function as a single team. In fact this meeting did serve to accomplish the patient's goal, albeit too late to be of benefit to her.

Team Management. Even if all the various health professionals involved in this case are regarded as functioning as a single megateam, a lack of clear team management still obscured what should have been the central role of the patient in being able to make her own choices about living arrangements. Without the needed combination of awareness of the importance of patient autonomy and the power to return her to her apartment, several members of the team appear to have operated under the assumption that the patient lacked decisional capacity. A case manager was badly needed here, whether it be the patient's primary care provider, someone from the hospital who had the patient's trust, such as the inpatient nurse, or any of the other professionals involved in Mrs. Rodriguez's care, preferably one upstream in the transition process.

The Role of Family or Confidants on the Team. The pastor tried to follow the patient's wishes but was powerless to convince the senior housing social worker. In Mrs. Rodriguez's case, the role of confidants on the team and the level of decision-making involvement that should have been afforded the pastor was another central team issue.

Collegiality. Another facet of team dynamics that can complicate decision making is the desire of colleagues to respect each other's decisions. For a team to function effectively, team members must behave toward each other in a manner consistent with how they behave toward the patient—ideally, by respecting autonomy. A premium is placed on colleagues respecting each other's autonomy and decision-making capacity: just as patients with capacity must be permitted to make poor choices, health care professionals may feel that their team colleagues should be permitted to make poor choices. (This aspect of professional autonomy is also illustrated in the chapters in this book that discuss how teams make decisions and resolve conflicts.) Thus team members' desire not to affect the group dynamic of a team adversely may prevent them from confronting each other when they encounter what appear to be poor judgment calls. This may have been the case with the senior housing facility social worker, who appeared to the other team members to lack sufficient knowledge about the importance of respecting patient autonomy. Other members of the team, had they felt comfortable educating the social worker in this regard, might have been able to convince her that transfer back to the adult home was indeed appropriate. When team members do not know each other very well, which is often the case with multi-institutional teamwork, there is a greater reluctance to disagree with a colleague.

Legal Implications. Teams' effectiveness can be compromised by influences entirely outside their control. One example is the senior housing social worker's refusal to permit Mrs. Rodriguez's reentry into the housing facility. Her hands were in fact tied by her duty to heed the regulations of the facility. Here it could be argued that the senior housing social worker—or those who initially determined the housing's policies—violated Mrs. Rodriguez's right to autonomy. This argument must be weighed against the legal liability of the housing facility should Mrs. Rodriguez have an accident upon her return or cause accidental injury to others through fire or other means. An ethical dilemma arising during Mrs. Rodriguez's transitions is whether persons living in a housing facility have less right to autonomy than persons living in a private home (i.e., a conflict between patient autonomy and housing facility liabilities).

From the point of view of clients who need long-term care most likely for the rest of their lives but wish to live at home as long as possible, as Mrs. Rodriguez did, a single agency responsible for providing all care and assuming complete accountability is preferable to the patient being shuffled from setting to setting. A model of care like PACE might have avoided unnecessary hospitalizations and prevented this particular ethical dilemma from arising.

Allocation of Resources. Another contextual feature of this case was Medicare's unwillingness to provide more hours of daily home attendant care, making what could have been a logical team compromise—for Mrs. Rodriguez to remain at home with extended home attendance—an impossibility. Medicare personnel, presumably for cost-control reasons, blocked the way for this compromise by approving only nine hours of daily home care. Medicare regulations and personnel played an important role in this case, yet no Medicare representatives were part of the team. Managed care administration may very often play a central role in a team's decisions without actually being a physical part of the team. This situation can engender frustration from care providers, patients, and family members alike. Here again a megateam model is instructive, where those parties responsible for making cost decisions are actively involved in the team decision-making process for each patient. The case that follows discusses how the PACE model accomplishes this goal.

Case Description: Mr. Stokes

Mr. Stokes, an ethnic West Indian in his late eighties, lived with his wife in a four-story walk-up building in Harlem. Mr. Stokes had become bed-bound and nonverbal due to a series of devastating strokes. His wife was becoming increasingly overwhelmed with the responsibility of caring for him. At length, Mr. Stokes was enrolled in a hospice program that provided him with four hours of home attendant services per day as well as his prescription medications. Hospice was the only way for him to obtain these services, as Medicare was his only insurance. He was also referred to a program that provided physician home visits since he was unable to get transportation to outpatient facilities.

It was clear to Dr. Richards, on his first visit to Mr. Stokes's apartment, that Mr. Stokes needed more services than were available through the hospice program. Mr. Stokes was developing skin breakdown in multiple areas, and his wife was showing signs of caregiver burnout and depression. Dr. Richards suggested nursing home placement for Mr. Stokes as the best option. The wife was adamant that Mr. Stokes remain at home. Dr. Richards asked the hospice nurse to make more frequent visits and left orders for aggressive wound care and an air mattress.

The nurse found herself increasingly frustrated that the wife insisted on keeping Mr. Stokes home, and felt strongly that the patient was suffering unduly from the wife's inability to carry out care in her absence. She complained frequently to the hospice social worker, who himself felt that Dr. Richards had adequately assessed the situation and left appropriate orders for care. Neither the social worker nor Dr. Richards realized that the order for an air mattress had not been carried out; nor were they fully aware of the nurse's suspicions that Mrs. Stokes was beginning to drink heavily on occasion.

Several months later Mr. Stokes was brought to an inner-city emergency room after his wife called 911 seeking help. Her husband's ulcers had become much worse, despite her and the nurse's attempts at care, and they were now foul smelling and extensive in size. Mrs. Stokes was overwhelmed and exhausted. Mr. Stokes was admitted to the hospital. A hospital nurse explained to Mrs. Stokes the importance of placing a feeding tube to help Mr. Stokes keep up his strength. The resident treating the patient, however, seemed not to be concerned with carrying out the tube placement when Mrs. Stokes questioned him about it.

Dr. Richards was not informed of this hospital admission until the increasingly distraught Mrs. Stokes called him to get his opinion about placement of the feeding tube. Dr. Richards, on learning of Mr. Stokes' clinical deterioration, again attempted to persuade Mrs. Stokes to allow her husband to be placed in a nursing home, even temporarily, to address his wound status and to give Mrs. Stokes a brief relief. Mrs. Stokes insisted that her husband return home.

Dr. Richards made repeated attempts to get the hospice program to provide more home attendant hours for Mr. Stokes—all to no avail. He also entered a protracted battle with the hospice administration to get it to authorize placement of the air mattress. The administration insisted that the mattress was too expensive and that care of the decubiti was not covered by the hospice benefit since this was not Mr. Stokes's "terminal diagnosis."

Not long thereafter, Mr. and Mrs. Stokes reappeared at a different emergency room, this time at the academic medical center where Dr. Richards worked. The hospice nurse brought them to the hospital—against the wishes of Mrs. Stokes—when during a home visit she found Mrs. Stokes extremely distressed and Mr. Stokes in worsening health. Mrs. Stokes claimed not to be a regular drinker, but she had had a substantial number of drinks that day, to the point where her gait was affected. Mr. Stokes was admitted to the geriatric care unit with a diagnosis of multiple infected decubitus ulcers. His wife begged Dr.

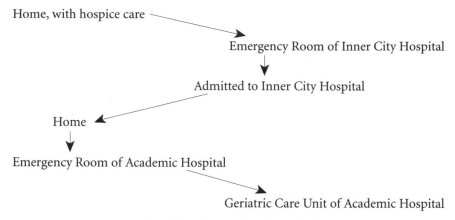

FIGURE 16.2 Case of Mrs. Stokes: Transitions in clinical settings

Richards and the other hospital staff not to transfer him to a nursing home. Dr. Richards recommended that Mr. Stokes be transferred instead to the palliative care cluster within the hospital. Before resolution of this issue, Mr. Stokes died.

Case Analysis
Identify Patient and Family Preferences

The patient's wishes were not known. He was nonverbal and could not answer even simple yes-no questions. Mr. Stokes did not have decisional capacity but had previously assigned his wife proxy. His wife did not know his own prior wishes but wanted him to remain at home. She was unwilling to consider nursing home placement, yet was under extreme stress and might have been developing a drinking problem.

The important value of respecting the proxy's decisions existed in tension with the responsibility of the health care providers to ensure that Mr. Stokes was getting reasonable and adequate care. Care providers may override potentially life-threatening decisions made by a surrogate who herself appears to be losing decisional capacity. Similarly, if a patient is clearly feeling pain or other distress that cannot be relieved adequately at home, one could make a moral case that his suffering requires overriding the wife's stated wishes and provides a justification for the social worker to engage adult protective services.

In this case we have neither of these situations. Mrs. Stokes was not definitely an alcoholic and could not definitively be determined to have inadequate decisional capacity herself, which would have compromised her role as proxy. It also does not appear that Mr. Stokes was suffering, although there is no way to determine what he was experiencing as a result of his progressive skin breakdown. A common ethical pitfall is the tendency to assume that patients or their proxies—especially elderly ones—who reject health professionals' recommendations, or make what appear to be unwise choices, by definition lack capacity.

Additionally, there were no life-saving measures appropriate for his situation. It is particularly difficult for care providers to resolve the conflict between patient autonomy and beneficence when the providers are not doing everything possible to preserve life. When dealing with palliative care patients unable to communicate their wishes, the conflict is especially thorny. In this case, Dr. Richards, the home care nurse, and the hospice social worker had to balance their duty to place Mr. Stokes in the optimal setting for care (e.g., a nursing home) with a desire to respect Mrs. Stokes's wishes. In doing so they also had to struggle with the larger moral issue of whether it was wrong to allow Mr. Stokes to fester in his decaying flesh when they did not know whether this was what he would have wanted. Here, because it was impossible to speculate on Mr. Stokes's preferences, the team members never resolved the issue of whether to allow Mrs. Stokes's wishes to take precedence.

Evaluate Quality-of-Life Issues

The apparent results of the inadequate care Mr. Stokes received included multiple decubitus ulcers and inadequate hygiene. It is important to distinguish pain—a physiological response of the body—from suffering—an assault on the personhood. It can be argued that in this case one or both were being experienced by patient and wife. While the wounds were offensive to the care providers, they might not finally have caused pain to Mr. Stokes; on the other hand, not having Mr. Stokes at home might cause him or his wife suffering. It could be argued that respect for the family's choices overrode the need to adequately treat the decubitus ulcers and keep the patient in an institution.

Mr. Stokes had a degenerative and incurable set of illnesses that would lead to his death. Therefore, the goals of care in this case were palliative. There was no absolute value in this case, which engendered disagreements among the various team members about where the priorities should lie.

When care of a patient involves providers at multiple settings, the goal of operating in the patient's best interest may take on many different meanings depending on the setting. The various care providers may share little more in common with each other than the client, and they may never reach consensus on how to resolve the ethical conflicts.

Consider Contextual Factors

Multiple Settings. Deciphering team composition during such transitions can be puzzling for both patients and the professionals involved in their care. Here it is not clear whether there were several teams operating, or—in name only—one megateam. In Mr. Stokes's case, the hospice physician, the hospice home nurse, the hospice social worker, and the hospice administrators (who make cost-control decisions) seemed to act without coordination with the hospitals involved in Mr. Stokes's care. The emergency room staff at the inner city hospital contacted neither the hospice nor the academic center staff, something an already exhausted and overwhelmed Mrs. Stokes was left to do on her own.

Even the hospice personnel, ostensibly a team, did not function well together. Dr. Richards, although himself employed by the hospice program, found his orders for care not followed through due to hospice administrative restrictions. The hospice nurse's oft-expressed opinion that the patient care was compromised appeared not to make its intended impact on the hospice social worker or on Dr. Richards. It appears there were multiple providers for Mr. Stokes but no definitive teams. They did not meet or have an established liaison to coordinate care.

Team Management. From the point of view of Mrs. Stokes and the various health care professionals alike, the lack of a defined team framework meant leadership of the case was also ill defined. Dr. Richards found his orders for care stymied by hospice administration. The hospice administration found its decisions on appropriate management of Mr. Stokes's care challenged by Dr. Richards. The inner city emergency room nurse's advice to insert a feeding tube was undermined by the treating resident and questioned by Mrs. Stokes. Without a clear coordinator for Mr. Stokes's case, continuity of care was markedly diminished, and the result was several unnecessary transitions.

In the PACE model, by contrast, a client encounters a team that is accustomed to working collaboratively and that shares the common goal of avoiding duplication and fragmentation of services. Poor care management, common among chronically ill elders wishing to remain at home, is avoided, thereby preventing many unnecessary hospitalizations and exacerbations of illness.

The Role of the Family on the Team. Mrs. Stokes was in no position—no matter how willing she was—to successfully fill the role of care coordinator herself. She might have seen herself as the main coordinator of her husband's care by her status as proxy and by virtue of time devoted to his care and her intimacy with him, but she was clearly distressed by the day-to-day responsibilities of keeping him at home. Alternatively, she might have seen Dr. Richards filling the role of coordinator, as she at times sought his advice. But she was in conflict with the main advice he provided—to have her husband placed in a nursing home. She had far more frequent contact with the hospice nurse than with the doctor, and might view the nurse—who did make a transition decision in bringing Mr. Stokes to the academic center emergency room—as the leading care provider. Ultimately Mrs. Stokes appeared disenfranchised from the teamwork altogether. From her perspective, she was dealing with several transitions for her husband, and no one person was in charge of coordinating his care.

Decision making such as that employed in the PACE model would have better served Mrs. Stokes and her husband. Here the megateam designates a central coordinator rather than different teams in different settings making a haphazard collection of decisions. Family members and participants are extensively involved in care issues but are not left to coordinate care themselves from multiple sources.

Communication. Lack of continuity of communication among the various parties can also deepen conflicts in caring for a patient. Care of patients with complex advanced disease necessitates close communication between the team members involved, or ideally the existence of a single cohesive megateam. In this case the hospice nurse's unilateral decision to bring Mr. Stokes to the emergency room might have been the right thing to do. Mrs. Stokes at that point was at the end of her rope and unable to make such a decision. It appears that her resistance was not with intermittent hospitalization but rather with long-term institutionalization. But if the hospice home care team had made a treatment plan that involved allowing intermittent hospitalization at the wife's request, it could have been communicated to Mrs. Stokes and to the academic hospital staff who would be admitting Mr. Stokes, to ensure that the goals of care were understood and that any inadequacies in the care he was receiving at home were understood. Because Mr. Stokes was twice brought to emergency rooms without the knowledge of his physician, the receiving physicians were unable to ascertain whether he had a do not resuscitate (DNR) order or any other advance directives. This is another kind of ethical responsibility of the health care system, but it is also largely a teamwork issue. Those involved in the care of complex patients have some responsibility to make the system work for the patients, however frustrating it may be. A good example is the patient orders for life-sustaining treatment forms (POLST) that are now in wide use in the state of Oregon, which successfully communicate advanced directives throughout the different levels of the health care system.

Trust. Trust was another important team issue operating in this case. Dr. Richards repeatedly pointed out that he didn't "trust" the hospice administration, which he had only recently begun working with, to provide adequate care for Mr. Stokes. A cohesive care environment is unlikely to exist when there is lack of trust and familiarity between caregivers, whether they are working on the same team or on separate teams involved in patient transition. It is difficult to build a level of trust among team members when the teams do not work together on a regular basis.

Justice and Reimbursement. A hospice has an ethical responsibility to provide optimal care in the face of its own financial constraints. In this case the hospice administration justified not placing the expensive air mattress in the family home and not authorizing more than four hours of a hospice attendant's services per day by invoking cost considerations. Additional hospice services were clearly in the best interest of the patient and would also have better allowed Mrs. Stokes's preference for home care to be respected, but if authorized they might have been at the expense of other patients or the financial stability of the hospice itself. The hospice's medical director had planned to review the case as Dr. Richards had requested but was unable to do so before Mr. Stokes's death. Resource allocation considerations often raise difficult ethical issues and may be worse when the patient is served by more than one institution.

Finally, in many cases team conflicts are driven by the implications of organizations having different reimbursement structures. In this case the hospice administration set limits on the amount of care it could reasonably provide Mr. Stokes, given its financial considerations, which put its team of care providers in direct conflict with Dr. Richards, the home nurse, and Mrs. Stokes. Were all Mr. Stokes's care providers operating under the same set of financial constraints, a compromise position might have been more readily negotiable. Patient "dumping," although not an issue in this case, can be an unfortunate result of different reimbursement structures for different organizations. Victims obviously lose continuity of care priorities altogether as they are shuffled between settings and teams.

A better model such as PACE can obviate some of these resource allocation problems. PACE receives capitated payments from Medicaid, Medicare, and limited private-pay sources for each client, which it then pools. Although the program bears full risk for all costs incurred for each client regardless of the duration and complexity of the client's participation, it does not face service-by-service restrictions and has complete flexibility in designing long-term care plans. Preventive and rehabilitative care is emphasized, and the team makes all allocation decisions. There is no incentive for cost shifting or "dumping" the patient to another outside facility; conversely, there is no incentive to keep the patient in an endless cycle of transitions simply because a payment is received each time the patient appears at the emergency room.

Under traditional fee-for-service programs, cost shifting between Medicare and Medicaid is rampant. Medicaid insufficiently covers simple acute services, such as fever management, while Medicare will not cover hospital stays of less than three days. Bennett (1997) describes the resulting cost shifting thus: "Therefore, rather than receive care in their own environment, patients with simple febrile illnesses must endure $400 ambulance trips to the hospital; $500 emergency room evaluations; and $3,000 four-day hospital stays—all paid for by Medicare."

Patients needing more extensive care services are similarly ill served by the traditional fee-for-service system and are often transferred to subacute care units to maximize Medicare payments. Bennett (1997) describes the situation: "Under the prospective payment system in effect in the United States (except in Maryland), hospitals are paid based on the patient's diagnosis at discharge. Under this system, the shorter the hospital stay, the greater the profit from the admission. . . . The result is the rapid movement of patients out of the hospital into a skilled nursing unit largely because of reimbursement considerations."

PACE participants have lower overall utilization rates of hospital and nursing home services than the healthier general Medicare population. This translates into fewer transitions for PACE clients than they would otherwise have encountered in a traditional system of care. Although both PACE participants and general Medicare populations average 2,400 hospital days / 1000 / annum, PACE clients are a much more frail, nursing-home-eligible population and would be expected to have higher utilization rates (Baskins 1997).

Case Description: Mrs. Hodges

Mrs. Hodges is a 104-year-old woman who presented to an academic medical center emergency room with respiratory distress. She was diagnosed with pneumonia and subsequent respiratory failure and hospitalized. During the course of her four-month hospitalization she was intubated repeatedly, developed acute renal failure and many deep decubitus ulcers, and spent the majority of her time in a nearly comatose state. All during the hospitalization, the patient's 80-year-old daughter, Sandra—an Ivy League–educated professor—demanded that everything be done to keep her mother alive.

Sandra often disagreed with the hospital care team—nurses, a medical resident, and the attending geriatrician—who were uncomfortable with the aggressive care they were asked to deliver. It was clear to the team that Mrs. Hodges was not going to progress much in terms of her functional status. Nurses in particular voiced concerns on many occasions that the patient was being "tortured" by being forced to receive such aggressive care, given her very advanced age and terrible functional status. Sandra refused to consider a more palliative approach to her mother's care, which left many persons on the hospital team feeling frustrated and angry with her. The resident and several nurses had conversations with Sandra, during which they expressed their discomfort. Sandra never wavered in her demands.

At Sandra's request, a hospital-based speech pathologist was brought in to assess Mrs. Hodges's communication status. It was determined that the patient was able to mumble a few words but unable to express her wishes or preferences. Sandra took this as evidence that her wishes as proxy were to be followed.

Mrs. Hodges's clinical condition eventually stabilized. She remained relatively nonverbal, ventilator dependent, and covered in decubiti, but her pulmonary and kidney function improved enough that transfer to a subacute facility was warranted. The medical resident and nurses thought Mrs. Hodges was appropriate for a regular nursing home floor. The attending geriatrician concurred, explaining to Sandra the team's position. Sandra refused such a move, fearing that aggressive care would be discontinued. She became irate, mentioning that she was in touch with her lawyer.

Ultimately the hospital department's senior doctor became involved. He called an interdisciplinary meeting so a variety of other options could be discussed. He, the attending geriatrician, a nurse practitioner, and a nurse from

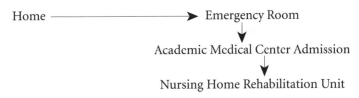

Home ⟶ Emergency Room
↓
Academic Medical Center Admission
↓
Nursing Home Rehabilitation Unit

FIGURE 16.3 Case of Mr. Hodges: Transitions in clinical settings

the nursing home floor were in attendance. Sandra brought the speech pathologist, with whom she had become quite close. A compromise was suggested by the speech pathologist whereby Mrs. Hodges would be transferred to an affiliated rehabilitation unit rather than to the nursing home. The attending geriatrician—who was also affiliated with the rehabilitation unit—voiced strong disagreement with this plan, since Mrs. Hodges was unable to follow commands or participate in physical therapy. The speech therapist then disclosed that she had learned in conversation with Sandra that Mrs. Hodges had been cognitively intact and revered in the family for her wit right up until the night of her hospitalization, so the daughter therefore did not feel that aggressive care and rehabilitative efforts were futile. It was agreed that Mrs. Hodges would continue to receive aggressive care while on the rehabilitation unit, as well as the continued services of the hospital-based speech pathologist, whose services Sandra would pay for out-of-pocket.

On receiving the patient, the nurses and the physical therapist at the rehabilitation unit initially also felt Mrs. Hodges was an inappropriate candidate for rehabilitation and found caring for her very frustrating. Moreover, they found the daughter a very difficult and demanding person. The speech pathologist and the now-supportive attending geriatrician were still involved in Mrs. Hodges's care, however, and were able to explain to them why rehabilitative efforts were meaningful to the family.

Six weeks into her treatment on the rehabilitation unit, Mrs. Hodges was able to open her eyes, sit up with assistance, and speak coherently on occasion. She continued to receive very aggressive medical care at the request of the daughter. Her decubiti healed, and she began to be weaned from her feeding tube as she took in more nutrients orally. At this writing, Mrs. Hodges remains on the rehabilitation unit with preparations beginning for her return home.

Case Analysis
Identify Patient and Family Preferences

The patient's preferences are not known. The patient's daughter, the designated proxy, insisted that her mother receive aggressive life-saving care at all times. She demanded the transfer of her mother from the hospital to the rehabilitation unit against the advice of the hospital medical team.

The care goal was not clearly palliative. The daughter, when asked to consider palliative options and sign a DNR order for her mother, refused on the grounds that her mother had no diagnosed terminal illness. Because the patient had designated her daughter as proxy, the daughter had to be viewed as representing what Mrs. Hodges would have wanted in the way of autonomy. But it should be noted that the team was under no obligation to provide what it believed to be ineffective treatment, even in the face of proxy or patient demands.

As seen in Mr. Stokes's case in this chapter and in Chapter 5, ethical dilemmas may arise when teams question the appropriateness of a proxy's wishes. In Mrs. Hodges's case, the team wished to avoid prolonging the suffering of a very frail, very old woman with numerous incapacitating illnesses, while the proxy wished to preserve life at all costs.

Here the mental competency of the proxy was beyond doubt—the daughter in no way appeared unable to handle the responsibilities she had been assigned. Nor could it be definitively argued that the decisions of the daughter were not in the best interest of the patient. Rather, there was a conflict between the values of the daughter and those of the medical team members treating Mrs. Hodges, and no clear imperative favoring either side, although the additional facts made available by the speech pathologist helped the decision-making process.

Evaluate Quality-of-Life Issues

The hospital and rehabilitation unit nurses, the medical resident, the attending geriatrician, and the physical therapist participating in the care of Mrs. Hodges felt as though they were "torturing" her. The ethical stumbling block behind their reluctance to treat—that doing everything medically necessary to preserve life seemed to prolong suffering needlessly—is all too common and difficult to resolve. Here the conflict was exacerbated not only by the patient's poor prognosis but also by her very old age. None of the team members explicitly stated why they felt caring for her was different from caring for other critically ill patients, but treating a critically ill patient at 104 years old may seem more futile to team members than treating a 70- or 80-year-old. Whether limits should be set based on the patient's age, functional status, or poor prognosis for recovery becomes a particularly poignant dilemma when family members place clear value on preserving life.

Providers must be careful not to let bias—such as ageism—color their decision making; on the other hand, the burdens of treating a 104-year-old patient may legitimately seem to outweigh its potential benefits. According to the principle of proportionality, "no . . . absolute duty exists: preservation of life is an obligation that binds only when life can be judged more a benefit than a burden by and for the patient" (Jonsen, Siegler, and Winslade 1998, 139–40). This case brings up the best interest standard and discussion of medical futility, which Jonsen, Siegler, and Winslade also discuss: "Physicians have no obligation to perform actions beyond or contradictory to the goals of medicine, even when requested to do so. . . . It is our opinion that patient preferences, as important as they are, do not impose an obligation on physicians to act contrary to their best medical judgment" (94–95). In Mrs. Hodges's case, the patient preferences were unknown; therefore the surrogate's decisions had to promote the "best interests" of the patient (i.e., a quality of life that a "reasonable" person would choose) (87, 112). The daughter's demands seemed to be justified by that fact that Mrs. Hodges, after six weeks of the aggressive rehabilitation treatment, not only stabilized but also even improved.

Consider Contextual Factors

Team Composition. Here, the team composition was more clear-cut than in the cases previously discussed and may be viewed as a single megateam. An interdisciplinary meeting was held with representative care providers, who remained in open negotiation with a very assertive family member whose advocacy of the patient clashed with their judgment. The speech pathologist and attending geriatrician remained involved with the patient throughout the transition and her subsequent care in the rehabilitation unit. Their continued involvement successfully bridged the two settings and created a single team where there might otherwise have been two separate ones.

The Role of Family. In this case, most of the multi-institutional care providers were in agreement about the goals and appropriateness of care for the patient but were in conflict with a proxy. The daughter was very well informed about her importance as proxy in decision making and played an important role as a team member. She was not open to discussion about anything other than the most aggressive, life-saving approach. At issue was the degree to which a family member should coordinate care, and whether the other members of the team were willing to accept the family member in this role.

Communication. A team is more likely to benefit the patient most by maintaining close communication between members and by coming to a reasonable compromise—where possible—with the health care proxy. In this case the various team members did collaborate with one another and presented one unified voice to the daughter. The team's agreement about the goals of care helped facilitate an open discussion with the proxy on transitioning the patient to a less-aggressive care plan. The speech pathologist, meanwhile, was able to get to the root of the daughter's reluctance to give up aggressive care and thereby suggest a compromise palatable to all parties involved.

Team Conflict. The frustration among health care providers that this kind of case generates could have led the various teams or team members to act against each other. Here the frustration of the family member led to the involvement of the senior physician, who until that time had not been involved in the care of Mrs. Hodges. Because of Sandra's persistence in going above their heads to a more senior physician, both the hospital and the rehabilitation staff felt they had been bullied into acquiescing to unreasonable demands on the part of the proxy leadership. The interdisciplinary meeting and the continued involvement of team members through the transition instead helped stop resentment from all sides, led to a better patient outcome, and may have avoided a lawsuit.

In the PACE model of care, family members and participants are extensively involved in care issues but do not coordinate care themselves from multiple sources. In Mrs. Hodges's case, as with PACE, a single interdisciplinary team across two settings provided integrated care. Both team and ethical dilemmas can best be mitigated by a single, fully accountable, ongoing care team, particularly one that involves but does not solely rely on family or the patients themselves to coordinate care services. In addition, the megateam can present a unified voice to the proxy, a particularly important point when the proxy's demands seem inappropriate to the care providers. Here the successful patient outcome was owed in large part to the fact that one member worked closely with the family member, ascertained the source of conflict, and brought the issue out on the table for the team to discuss until a suitable compromise could be reached.

Conclusion

All three of the cases presented here would have been better handled with a model of care that allowed patient transitions to be bridged by a unifying team. The cases raise many of the obstacles to good care that elderly patients encounter as they move through the health care system from setting to setting. For the health care providers who treat these patients—however briefly, before the patient is moved to a new setting—the ethical and team problems raised are common and often frustrating. For those professionals who strive to ensure continuity of care for their clients, the goal can be compromised or lost completely in the face of numerous transitions.

In all of the cases in this chapter, problems in leadership, communication, and trust could have been avoided had the same team members worked together to provide care regardless of site. Ethical issues too are easier to resolve when teams are well defined and members are comfortable working together. Family members played an important, if ill-defined, role in all three cases and would have been better served if they were clearly involved as members of a permanent, ongoing care team. Additionally, in at least two of the cases, the ideal resolution for all involved would have been for the patient to stay at home with caring family members and significant home attendance.

A desire for autonomy on the part of patients and family members was deeply felt in all three cases presented here. This goal is best served by a team familiar with each other and with the client. When multiple transitions occur, patient autonomy, along with continuity of care, is compromised. The frail elderly, very often the victims of multiple transitions, are also often the people least equipped to deal with them. A reduction in the number of transitions for frail patients in the last years of life is another benefit of megateam models.

Discussion Questions
Small groups

1. Identify the "team" members (all persons involved in care of the patient). In any given case, was more than one team operating? Were the patient and family members legitimately part of the team(s), or were they disenfranchised instead?

2. Could any of the transitions have been avoided through better coordination of care?

3. Are there other ethical issues not explicitly addressed in the analysis?

4. As a megateam, create a better-coordinated care plan for one of these patients at the point of the patient's first transition, including provisions for disagreements among team members on ethical issues related to the case, or team leadership.

Entire class

1. What transitional or ethical dilemmas occur in more than one of these three cases?

REFERENCES

Baskins, Judith Pinner, R.N., B.S.N. 1997. Testimony before the House Ways and Means Committee, on Health Medicare and Medicaid Dual Eligibility. April 29.

Bennett, Richard G., M.D. 1997. Prepared testimony before the Senate Aging Committee. April 29.

Chin Hansen, J. 1999. Practical issues for delivering integrated services in a changing environment: The PACE model. *Generations* 23(2):22–28.

Eng, C., J. Pedulla, G. P. Eleazer, et al. 1997 Program of all-inclusive care for the elderly (PACE): An innovative model of integrated geriatric care and financing. *Journal of the American Geriatrics Society* 45(2):223–32.

Jonsen, A. R., M. Siegler, and W. J. Winslade. 1998. *Clinical ethics: A practical guide to ethical decisions in clinical medicine,* 4th ed. New York: McGraw-Hill.

Zimmerman, Y. A., D. A. Pemberton, and L. Thomas. 1988. Factors contributing to care management and decision making in the PACE model. Report submitted to the HCFA under contract No. HCFA 500-910027. Cambridge, Mass.: Abt Associates.

CHAPTER 17

Emerging Ethical Issues in Geriatric Team Care

Peter J. Whitehouse, M.D., Ph.D.

Geriatric team care is an evolving form of clinical service in a rapidly changing health care environment. First I will briefly consider social forces that are influencing both team care and bioethics as a discipline. I then survey emerging ethical issues, with a focus on aging individuals who perceive that their health is not optimal and label themselves as ill. (I refer to these individuals not as clients, patients, or even consumers but rather as ill older persons. Illness recognizes a broader notion of health and well being than just the absence of disease, as it refers both to the subjective experience of the individual and the relationship of individual health to that of the community.) I go on to consider larger and larger social units, moving from the ill person to his or her family and from the individual provider to the health team, finishing with a discussion about how cultural and environmental issues affect organizations providing care (Morris 1998).

The geriatric team is a critical social unit in this analysis. It is composed of a small number of individuals trying to assist an often similarly sized patient and family caregiver group. Thus, it often serves as a bridge for individuals to large organizational and community units. Unlike other, more practically oriented chapters, in this chapter I attempt to place teamwork in its broader political and cultural context.

At all levels of social organization, changes are occurring in our understanding of the components of each particular level. For example, the concept of being a healthy person, let alone being an ill person, is being reexamined by critics of modernity (Gergen 2000). Personhood is being explored with attention to the post-Enlightenment fascination with the intellectual side of human nature rather than the affective, and to the postmodern concern with our perhaps illusionary sense of a unified self. Families are continuing to evolve from nuclear families (or other traditional forms) into different forms of care relationships. This evolution is occurring in different ways in different countries based on existing kinship systems. Increasing cultural diversity within national and local health care systems will contribute to more complex networks of informal care and challenges to provider teams.

The organization of work is being reexamined in various sectors of social life including health care systems. Academic health systems that train most geriatric team members have been notoriously poor at improving their organizational processes (Ludmerer 1999). Information systems are a critical part of organization life, yet the use of such technology to support clinical care and education has been limited. In the emerging digital age, distribution of information in society will link even more closely to the distribution of power. Information systems create great opportunities for new and powerful virtual organizations and distance learning. But fundamental issues lie ahead in terms of the distribution of knowledge among the haves and have-nots (the so-called digital divide) both within our country and worldwide.

Like information technology, biotechnology is advancing rapidly. We are living in an era of unprecedented change in the ecological footprint of the human species on the planet (Potter and Whitehouse 1998). First, too many people burden the biosphere. Second, partly as a result of our attempts to control population, in the future we will have large numbers of older people compared to younger individuals. Finally, this past millennium has seen the human race create technology that has wrought considerable havoc on the ecosystems of our planet. Our arrogance (through neglect or, worse, malignant attempts to dominate nature) will have severe consequences (Orr 1994; Potter 1971, 1988). New efforts to achieve greater wisdom and humility will be necessary in order to ensure the survival of the human race and other life on this planet. The evolution of values underlying health care systems will play an important role in redefining not only rights but also duties as well as our responsibilities to each other and to other life-forms. Too often our health care systems are unhealthy for both ill persons and providers as well as sources of expensive pollution and maladaptive behaviors, such as dependence on medical technology. Geriatric teams have the potential to be agents for change in the underlying values of our health care systems in these tumultuous times.

Biomedical ethics, as it has evolved over the last thirty years, stands at a focal point of the creation of knowledge and exploration of human values in health care. Bioethics as a movement and interdisciplinary endeavor has enhanced the discourse surrounding value issues in clinical consultation. Moreover, new generations of students have been educated to examine the complex cultural and social factors affecting health. Positive direction can also be seen, as ethicists begin to attend to the moral issues that arise as new organizations for health care emerge. Discussions among geriatric team members and with patients and families may serve as a model for addressing ethical issues creatively in practical care situations.

Despite these significant contributions to the health care field, questions can be raised concerning the role of bioethics in the future. Will it become a voice for change or part of the establishment? What role will it play in the distribution of knowledge and power in health care systems? Bioethics is becoming increasingly professionalized and incorporated into the main body of medicine (Jonsen 1998). Biomedical ethics as a field has limited the scope of its activities focusing excessively on the implications of medical technological advances. The presumption seems to be that if we just have enough intelligent bioethicists, we will be able to address the fundamental issues raised by cloning human beings and destroying entire species, within our current rational philosophical tradition. The expectation appears to be that we will fine-tune the technology with limits here and there but basically continue our march of everlasting progress toward some scientifically defined utopia.

Critical views of these so-called standard medical bioethics approaches are growing (McKenny 1997; Jonsen 1998). Feminist philosophers have raised concerns about the role of women in the power structure of care systems. The health of women has been relatively neglected compared to men—in the undertreatment of cardiovascular disease for example. The ethics of caring needs to balance the curative approaches that are so often the focus of traditional medicine. Communicative or discourse ethics, along with casuistry, emphasizes the importance of fostering dialogue about the particulars of individual cases (Post, Ripich, and Whitehouse 1994). Richard Rorty (1989) and other neopragmatists suggest that the analytical foundational philosophy upon which much standard bioethics has here to fore been built, has been less than satisfactory. Many ethicists have been engaged in the stories of the ill individuals whom they attempt to assist. This experience is a rich source of narrative. Narrative ethics will likely evolve as a more potent force for change as we listen carefully to the stories of ill persons. Martha Nussbaum argues eloquently that stories, including those from the classics and from history, best capture the full complexity of ethical issues playing out in our lives (Nussbaum 1992).

The most important criticism of bioethics, however, comes from those who emphasize its ignored historical roots as a global environmental ethic. As Van Rensselaer Potter has taught us, bioethics should encourage broader discussion about the relationship between biology and values (Potter 1971, 1988). Human health and even species viability are dependent on our environment. We have neglected the ecosystem's role in health as we have focused on mapping the genes of our species. Gene therapy offers much promise, but more immediate and long-lasting improvements in the health of individuals and populations can come from respecting the environment.

One of the essential features of human beings is their ability to learn and to use this knowledge to anticipate future events. This feature places a special responsibility on them as stewards not only of the biosphere but also of the noosphere—the world of ideas. Our contributions to global knowledge are enormous in terms of the amount of detailed information. We are driven by curiosity and should continue research at all levels of intellectual endeavor relevant to health. But we should also focus on integrating information into knowledge and making wise social decisions based on data that is not always comprehensive enough to answer our questions (Fineberg et al. 1995).

Individual Ill Persons

A considerable amount of discussion about ethics in the American health care system focuses on individual rights. A reexamination of the dominance of autonomy and rights is under way in our culture and in bioethics as well (Jonsen 1998). We celebrate, for example, preserving independence for older individuals with functional impairment, but we do not give enough recognition to our fundamental interdependence, not only among ourselves as members of society but also in relationship to other elements in our environment. The very principles of teamwork illustrate the interdependence that health care professionals should recognize in their own process of care management.

Cognitive impairment is frequent in the elderly, whether it is due to delirium, dementia, cerebral vascular accident, or other causes. These conditions create new dependencies and also new concerns about the effects of disease on personhood. As mentioned earlier, the self is being reexamined in terms of its essential rationality. Since the Enlightenment, the use of our rational faculties to solve social and environmental problems has dominated the modern agenda. Science and technology drive change in our health care system and its costs. We believe that if we could just "think smarter," we could solve ethical dilemmas and societal issues such as maldistribution of resources. We must, however, also recognize the nonrational aspects of ourselves relating to our motivations and values—for example, spiritual and religious beliefs—that are being viewed as more important to aspects of good health (Larson, Sawyers, and McCullough 1998).

The examination of self is also occurring in the context of reexamining the fundamental concepts of health and disease (Aronowitz 1998; Jobst, Shostak, and Whitehouse 1999; Whitehouse, Maurer, and Ballenger 2000). Health involves broad psychosocial and even spiritual well-being rather than merely the absence of disease. The illnesses that are common in older people are chronic. Chronic disease, for which the clinician's intention is caring rather than curing, raises issues of who is responsible for what aspects of an individual's health and function. At a conceptual level, who defines health—the professions (especially physicians) or other elements in society (Morris 1998)? At the microlevel of the bedside or the office examining table, who is in control of establishing individual goals for health—the ill person, or the health care provider? Once again, teams should illustrate the importance of collaborative goal setting. A critical issue for the future of teams is how to incorporate patients and families affected by chronic disease into the decision-making process.

A related fundamental change in our global society is the reorganization and redistribution of knowledge, for example, of health information (Goodman 1998). The senior baby boomers of today will interact with physicians and others in the health care system in different ways than their parents (Friedland and Summer 1999). They will have greater access to medical information through a variety of sources, including the World Wide Web, and will be more prepared to work collaboratively with health care teams. Shifts will also occur in the distribution of knowledge, power, and influence among providers. The bio-psychosocial model will continue to challenge the medical model, especially in regard to chronic disease.

The creation of new knowledge, at least in science, depends heavily on the engagement of the research "subject." This is the word that we have used in the past to characterized ill people who agree to consent to our experimental attempts to help either them or other affected members of society. The process of negotiating participation (we should call individuals participants or partners and not subjects) is called informed consent. In the process of seeking informed consent, the experimenter needs to provide the potential partner with information relevant to making the decision about whether to participate in research. At a social level, has science tried to convince us that major breakthroughs are just around the corner with a degree of irresponsibility that is excessive? Gene therapy illustrates the power of promises that do not achieve many results and the dangers of misleading research participants. Would a truly informed consent reveal more of the complexities and ambiguities of the scientific process? Should scientists allow potential partners (who are also taxpayers who pay for scientific work) a more intimate glimpse of the processes of normal science as well as the unpredictable changes in methods and focus that have been called paradigm shifts? It is to be hoped that a more knowledgeable populace would participate more actively in the research endeavor as long as scientists work to maintain trust.

Thus, the individual ill older person coming for clinical care into a health care system or into an academic center to participate in research should play an increasingly important role in the future of geriatric care. Professionals bring their knowledge and skills to the collaborative endeavor that characterizes good teamwork and good team care.

Family

Older patients are members of families who may be more or less available to participate in care. The changes in family structure that we have already observed will continue and grow as a challenge for geriatric practitioners (Friedland and Summer 1999). The average age of ill persons, as well as their caregiving relatives, will increase. We will be dealing with clinical and community situations in which multiple frail individuals interact with one another. More changes in family structure will take place: for example, because of the ravages of drug abuse and AIDS, older individuals who have survived will be raising younger children. Thus, more grandmothers and other friends and relatives who are not the biological parents will care for children. Moreover, other ties, such as living in proximity with one another rather than with blood relatives, may define long-term "kinship" relationships.

The amount of elder abuse will depend on many factors, including the economic climate. As the number of older people increases and the number of younger individuals working to support them decreases, there will be even more issues around these so-called dependency ratios.

Elder abuse is but one reason for our society to renew opportunities for intergenerational discourse. In the United States and Western Europe, the opportunities for children and grandparents to share the stories of their lives have been decreasing because of changes in mobility and family life. We need to create new opportunities for communication and learning to occur among individuals of different ages, not only to directly benefit those individuals but also to support the negotiation of the mutual social dependencies that exist among generations. Older individuals will be retiring later, volunteering more, and, one hopes, becoming increasingly concerned about the future of the planet. In general, more older individuals who are relatively wealthy and educated will be supported by fewer younger individuals who are more likely to be poor and struggling. Thus, we need to invest more in education and in the health of children in order to support the long-term survival of the human species. In Cleveland, for example, we are starting the first public intergenerational school (Whitehouse et al. 2000). We hope that it will represent a novel and effective organizational form to promote health and environmental education involving young, middle-aged, and aged persons. Clearly, how we provide opportunities for communities to form will be key (hopefully, including opportunities for learning). We may also need to explicitly provide training opportunities for individuals to participate in the life of the different communities in which they live and work.

As we try to assist individuals and families in thinking about their moral values in relation to health, the diversity of their voices will increasingly need to be recognized. The range of cultural backgrounds of the individuals and families who come to clinics in the United States is already amazing and challenging. Good doctors and other health care providers have always needed to be anthropologists, and the need is even greater now, as they try to understand the context of the illness of the person based on knowledge of that particular individual's social background (Cohen 1998; Sacks 1995). Physicians and other health care providers need to be as knowledgeable about cultural concepts of disease as they are about modern genetics and technologies. A so-called bio-cultural perspective, which blends biological knowledge of disease with broader social perspectives, will be increasingly necessary (Morris 1998).

Health Care Providers

The roles of various health care providers will continue to evolve in our health care system. More than two hundred "allied" health disciplines currently exist, including not only the dominant ones of medicine, nursing, and social work but also the disciplines of various types of laboratory technicians, therapists, and assistants to providers. A redistribution of workload is occurring as a function of the cost and value added of particular disciplinary approaches. Health care systems will likely hire the least expensive employee to accomplish a particular task, barring evidence that a higher-level person is required. The role of the physician continues to be reexamined in different care settings in part because of cost. Nurses continue to struggle to define just what a nurse is, as the number of nursing degrees proliferates. Attracting young people to social work careers is increasingly a challenge as a result of the relatively low wages. Classroom teachers, often the first nonfamily individuals who teach about lifelong health, are underpaid as well.

Probably the greatest force at work in our health care system is the increasing number of women entering the system in positions of power—for example, as physicians and managers. Their different attitudes toward caring and family life will likely become a positive influence on the dominant values in the health care system.

A fundamental question associated with the redistribution of knowledge discussed earlier relates to the role of professionals in society. Whether it be with nurses, social workers, doctors, lawyers, or others professionals, society is renegotiating social contracts (Ludmerer 1999). Discussions about the autonomy and accountability of individual professionals abound. One issue is whether to permit professionals to continue to have as much control over the entrance, training, and discipline of members of the professions as they have had. Another relates to whether health professionals are to be dominant over managers of the bureaucracy or vice versa. Clearly, health system administrators seem to have the upper hand as efforts to control costs dominate organizational behavior. But this reevaluation of the role of professionals and the control of knowledge is not just about the accumulation of more information and data, but about social values as well (for example, the so-called knowledge-value revolution [Sakaiya 1991]). What new knowledge do we need? How can we learn to use better the knowledge we already have and to what particular individual and global ends?

Teams

In the future, individual health care providers will undoubtedly continue to be brought together in groups to help ill persons and their communities. Teamwork will remain essential, recognizing that one particular individual in a system is not adequate alone to care for a particular problem. Training for teamwork, such as that offered by the Geriatric Interdisciplinary Team Training (GITT) grant, will likely increase in importance. Teaching individuals to work effectively in teams and to avoid the problems of single disciplinary or personal domination of leadership will be important. Teams will need to demonstrate their added value, as they are not necessarily the cheapest or most efficient model for providing all types of care. The very need for teams, however, provides a lesson for the professions. Perhaps each individual profession can train new members in skills that are more congruent with social needs—for example, better understanding of cultural diversity. We should be sure to develop teams to meet the needs of ill persons and not the needs of doctors, nurses, social workers, or other professionals.

One model of team developed in Cleveland as part of the GITT process is geriatric interdisciplinary *learning* teams (Wadsworth et al. 1998). These self-organizing groups attend to the process of learning together in order to improve care through outcome-oriented educational activities. Learning is an essential part of the continuous quality-improvement process in which we should all be engaged.

Unfortunately, health care systems are changing so quickly that certain issues that are not immediately on the forefront of the health executives' minds are ignored. The appropriate use of teams and, even more broadly, the appropriate methods of care for geriatric patients are not usually given adequate attention. This neglect is in part related to unclarity about what the goals of care ought to be for older individuals, particularly those who are frail and near the end of life.

Organizations

Teams are themselves small groups or organizations, but they exist in larger organizations and communities. The evolution of our health care system as a whole will affect the environment for team care. For example, capitated managed care systems are now a dominant but still evolving force for change. Such organizations contribute new ethical demands for team practice (Hall and Berenson 1998). The roles of nonprofit and for-profit organizations in providing care needs further study. As hospitals (mostly nonprofit) and nursing homes (mostly for-profit) merge to form integrated health systems, they should be assessed for their effectiveness.

Teams are subject to many forces at work within the health care system, such as the demand for economic efficiency. Such pressures may limit critical team activities, such as time for discussion among team members and with the ill person. Different attitudes toward health itself and health care interventions may be required before the value of teams is given appropriate recognition. Teams are "low tech" in an environment where much of the excitement and expense comes from the introduction of new but inadequately tested technology. Relationship-based care is at the heart of good team care.

Some technology will clearly influence team care. Teams will interface more directly with computers, using them for communication and storage of information as well as assessment of data. The idea of virtual teams will continue to develop—some teams may interact as much electronically as in person. These teams will take on different forms, with different roles for information systems and human providers. One can even imagine an artificially intelligent computer becoming an intelligent member of a team (Whitehouse et al. 1999). Ideally, the use of information systems will make care more efficient, although issues of confidentiality will intensify (Goodman 1998). Moreover, issues of accountability become more salient when decision making is distributed.

The continued evolution of health insurance will play an important role in how teams are perceived and employed in the health care system. The United States has not yet developed the social will to provide a minimal-benefit package for everyone in the nation. Medicaid, our current most comprehensive form of public insurance, is provided only for ill persons who are labeled as poor. Many citizens become eligible by virtue of health care costs creating family impoverishment.

We can hope that discussion about improving national health insurance will include consideration of long-term care. A fundamental restructuring is required to integrate acute and chronic care. A variety of national demonstration models are available, from SHMOs (social health maintenance organizations) to PACE (Programs of All-Inclusive Care for the Elderly). The National Chronic Care Consortium is an organizational umbrella for development of these model systems. One issue for the future will be to avoid the dominance of the medical model and to allow biopsychosocial and public health models to achieve more prominence. Such integrated models will provide new opportunities for teamwork, as well as create new potential value conflicts, as ill persons move through new systems of care.

Ultimately, health care systems need to be coordinated with public housing efforts and other social services for the elderly, including transportation. Much of the impact of chronic disease on the elderly has to do not with the structure of the health care system but with the organization of society in general. For example, urban sprawl has contributed to access problems for the elderly who depend on public transportation (Orr 1994).

All health care organizations exist within a larger society. They compete for attention and resources and try to deliver a product that will receive continued societal support. Social forces play a fundamental role in creating and modifying conceptions of health. There is no single cultural view of health, but public spaces provide opportunities for ongoing discussion about what health is, how much we should pay to insure it, for what population, and to what extent.

The growing public interest in complementary and alternative medicine (CAM) represents one critical point of interface between the traditional, dominant Western allopathic form of medicine and other more diverse health beliefs and methods of care (Jobst, Shostak, and Whitehouse 1999). The fact that the American public visits alternative providers more than their primary care doctors and spends over $20 billion out of pocket annually suggests the magnitude of interest in different forms of health care (Whitehouse and Edwards 2000).

Although many academics reject CAM as unscientific, there is some evidence for the efficacy of some aspects of certain practices. It is not the scientific issues that need to be attended to, however, but the broad cultural critique offered by CAM. Western allopathic medicine has exalted the randomized controlled trial as the gold standard and has considered the placebo a necessary uninteresting comparator in that process. In fact, placebos represent the power of human beings to heal themselves. The epistemology of medicine needs to be reexamined. Certainly, the randomized controlled trial has a critical place in the development of new knowledge. But it is not the only source of information we need in order to change our health care system and its goals. A focus on individual-centered care, personal responsibility for health, community models of health, prevention, and elaborated conceptions of human health in the context of the environment are aspects of CAM approaches that should be understood better and integrated into our allopathic approaches.

Thus, the very concept of disease and its meaning needs to be reexamined (Whitehouse, Maurer, and Ballenger 2000). Diseases are more than biological entities. Health is more than the absence of disease. Depression has been called a disease of meaning. Depression may relate to imbalances of chemicals in the brain, such as serotonin and noradrenalin. But it can also be, at the same time, a response to the stresses and strains of modern life. Diseases also can be viewed as manifestations of health in that they are a part of the mind and body's response to changes in the environment (Jobst, Shostak, and Whitehouse 1999). Another way to reexamine disease is from the perspective of metaphor. George Annas (1995) suggests that in our concepts of disease and medical practice, we replace military and market metaphors with ecological metaphors.

One of the fundamental difficulties of medicine is defining the boundaries of life and death. In a time of overpopulation, medicine still focuses considerable attention on improving the reproductive capabilities of individuals and enabling the survival of premature infants, many of whom will require enormous social resources through their lives. At the end of life, medicine has an even greater difficulty (Cassel et al. 1997). In broad conceptions of health that include the biosphere, death is a normal part of maintaining the "health" of the entire process of evolution. As long as medicine sees death as an enemy to be conquered, we will not be able to formulate the broader conceptions of health necessary to produce sustainable medicine, or sustainable human life on the planet.

Finally, perhaps the most important long-term issue for team members involved in care of older patients to attend to is that of environmental health. We will continue to damage our health and that of future generations if we do not limit air, water, and other pollution. In their personal and professional lives, team members should participate in the democratic processes that may lead to better care for older individuals. We should also participate in the broader ethical discussion about care for all people and other life-forms in the context of ensuring the survivability of the human and other species.

Conclusion

This chapter is different from others in this book, as its charge was to address *emerging* ethical issues. Geriatric team care will be affected by broad social trends that will modify society's ways of providing health care to its individual members. The discipline of bioethics has improved the level of discourse about fundamental value issues in clinical care and increasingly in the organization of health systems. The focus in this chapter has been a critical view of current models of health care and their impact on older patients and clients. I have suggested that bioethics has an opportunity to play an increasingly important role in future debates, but it needs a more expansive vision of the relationships between biomedicine and human values. If geriatric teams are allowed to thrive, they have the potential to bring the discourse about individual clinical ethical issues, as well as health care delivery, to new levels. Teams are places where the values of medicine, nursing, social work, and other health care professions can interact creatively. Sincere, open discourse can occur in an atmosphere of shared responsibilities and authority both among the professionals and with clients and families.

Discussion Questions

1. Geriatric teamwork can be expensive and time-consuming. Suppose a curriculum is developed to train health care professionals that could accomplish all the goals of a physician–nurse–social worker team in more efficient and effective ways. What are the advantages and disadvantages of teams compared with solo providers?

2. The advantage of information systems in fostering the creation of rich knowledge bases as well as improved communication between team members seems apparent. But the introduction of these systems into health care has been slow. What methods could improve the use of information technology in supporting team care?

3. The focus of geriatric team care is frequently said to be the family, particularly in cases where an older individual has cognitive impairment. Geriatric teams should also be concerned about community health and environmental health, as they impact on the quality of life of their clients. Consider the ethical issues that might arise when conflicts occur between the needs, wants, and desires of the client, his or her family, and the community.

REFERENCES

Annas, G. 1995. Reframing the debate on health care reform by replacing our metaphors. *New England Journal of Medicine* 322:744–47.

Aronowitz, R. 1998. *Making sense of illness: Science, society, and disease.* Cambridge: Cambridge University Press.

Cassel, C., R. Burt, M. Campbell, R. Kleigman, M. Loscalzo, J. Lynn, N. MacDonald, W. Manning, R. Payne, G. Thibault, T. Varner, and Institute of Medicine Committee on Care at the End of Life. 1997. *Approaching death: Improving care at the end of life.* Washington, D.C.: National Academy Press.

Cohen, L. 1998. *No aging in India: Alzheimer's the bad family, and other modern things.* Berkeley: University of California Press.

Friedland, R., and L. Summer, in collaboration with the Expert Working Group. 1999. *Demography is not destiny.* Washington, D.C.: National Academy on an Aging Society: A Polity Institute of The Gerontological Society of America.

Gergen, K. 2000. *The saturated self: Dilemmas of identity in contemporary life.* New York: Basic Books.

Goodman, K. 1998. *Ethics, computing, and medicine: Informatics and the transformation of health care.* Cambridge: Cambridge University Press.

Hall, M., and R. Berenson. 1998. Ethical practice in managed care: A dose of realism. *Annals of Internal Medicine* 128(5):395–402.

Jobst, K., D. Shostak, and P. Whitehouse. 1999. Diseases of meaning: Manifestations of health, and metaphor. *Journal of Alternative and Complementary Medicine: Research on Paradigm, Practice, and Policy* 5(6):495–502.

Jonsen, A. 1998. *The birth of bioethics.* Oxford: Oxford University Press.

Larson, D. J., J. P. Sawyers, and L. B. McCullough, eds. 1997. *Scientific research on spirituality and health: A consensus report based on the scientific progress in spirituality conferences.* Rockville, Md.: National Institute for Health care Research.

Ludmerer, K. 1999. *Time to heal: American medical education from the turn of the century to the era of managed care.* New York: Oxford University Press.

McKenny, G. 1997. *To relieve the human condition: Bioethics, technology, and the body.* Albany: State University of New York Press.

Morris, D. 1998. *Illness and culture in the postmodern age.* Berkeley: University of California Press.

Nussbaum, M. 1992. *Love's Knowledge: Essays on philosophy and literature.* Oxford: Oxford University Press.

Orr, D. 1994. *Earth in Mind: On education, environment, and the human prospect.* Washington, D.C.: Island Press.

Post, S., D. Ripich, and P. Whitehouse. 1994. Discourse ethics: Research, dementia, and communication. *Alzheimer Disease and Associated Disorders Journal* 8(4):58–65.

Potter, V. 1971. *Bioethics, bridge to the future.* Englewood Cliffs, N.J.: Prentice-Hall.

———. 1988. *Global bioethics: Building on the Leopold legacy.* East Lansing: Michigan State University Press.

Potter, V. and P. Whitehouse. 1998. Deep and global bioethics for a livable third millennium. *Scientist* 12:1:9.

Rorty, R. 1989. *Contingency, irony, and solidarity.* Cambridge: Cambridge University Press.

Sacks, O. 1995. *An anthropologist on Mars: Seven paradoxical tales.* New York: Knopf.

Sakaiya, T. 1991. *The Knowledge-value revolution or a history of the future.* New York: Kodansha America.

Wadsworth, N., J. Castle, S. Moore, J. Rose, M. Tupper, N. Whitelaw, P. Whitehouse, and J. Wisniewski. 1998. Interdisciplinary geriatric learning teams: A model for "next generation" interdisciplinary teamwork. Paper presented at Twentieth Annual Interdisciplinary Health Care Team Conference, Williamsburg, Va.

Whitehouse, P. J., and T. I. Edwards. 2000. Complementary and alternative medicine. In Jeremy Sugarman, ed., *20 common problems: Ethics in Primary Care.* New York: McGraw-Hill.

Whitehouse, P. J., K. Maurer, and J. F. Ballenger. 2000. *Concepts of Alzheimer disease: Biological, clinical, and cultural perspectives.* Baltimore, Md.: Johns Hopkins University Press.

Whitehouse, P. J., E. Bendezu, S. FallCreek, and C. Whitehouse. 2000. Intergenerational community schools: A new practice for a new time. *Educational Gerontologist* 26:761–70.

Whitehouse, P. J., N. S. Wadsworth, P. Fioritto, J. Bendis, and C. Manling. 1999. Technology support for geriatric interdisciplinary health care. Paper presented at the Twenty-first Annual Interdisciplinary Health Care Team Conference, Louisville, Ky.

Compiled by Chandhana Paka, B.A.(c)

Activities of daily living (ADLs): Functional self-care tasks that may include feeding and eating, dressing, grooming, hygiene, bathing and showering, toileting, sexual expression, and transfers.

Adherence: The extent to which a patient continues or follows an agreed-upon method of treatment under limited clinical supervision; often called compliance.

Adult protective services: Government agencies involved in the identification and treatment of elders who are at risk of being abused.

Advance directive: A legally and ethically binding statement of health care wishes made by a capacitated person, to be honored after capacity has lapsed. The two types are a living will, a list of instructions about treatments that the individual does or does not want, usually at the end of life; and a health care proxy, the appointment of an individual with the authority to make health care decisions on behalf of the incapacitated person.

Antipaternalism: The belief that (strong) paternalistic intervention cannot be justified because it violates individual rights and unduly restricts free choice.

Authority: The power to influence or command thought, opinion, or behavior. The word *authority* (the right and power to command) originates from the word for a creator of a work of art or craft, having the power to make decisions about it.

Autonomy: The human capacity for self-determination, the respect for which recognizes the person as the ultimate source of value. Individual preferences for action are based on values, preferences, and choices, voluntarily and without controlling interference, and from personal limitations that prevent meaningful choice such as inadequate understanding.

Bedside rationing: Patient-by-patient decisions to provide or withhold beneficial care in order to allocate limited medical resources. See also *Health care rationing*

Beneficence: An ethical principle that refers to the moral obligation to act for the benefit of others, to further their important and legitimate interests.

Benefit-burden analysis: Evaluation of the likely positive and negative consequences of a therapeutic option in terms of the patient's medical condition, prognosis, care goals, values, and wishes.

Biocultural perspective: The interface of knowledge of biological disease processes with broader social perspectives.

Bioethics: The study of ethical issues in the health care professions, health care organizations, and biomedical and behavioral research with animal and human subjects. See also *Biomedical ethics; Clinical ethics; Medical ethics*

Biomedical ethics: A movement and interdisciplinary endeavor that has enhanced the discourse surrounding value issues in clinical consultation and generally limits its scope of activities to focus on the implications of medical technological advances. See also *Bioethics; Clinical ethics; Medical ethics*

Capitation: A fixed amount of payment per patient, per year, per pay period (generally one month) that each patient requires regardless of the volume or cost of services.

Capitation agreement: See *Capitation*

Caregiving: The act of providing assistance or care to a family member, friend, or client, enabling the care recipient to maintain an optimal level of independence. See also *Formal caregivers; Informal caregivers*

Clinical ethics: An interdisciplinary activity that identifies, analyzes, and resolves ethical problems that arise in the care of patients. Its major thrust is to work for outcomes that best serve the interests and welfare of individual patients and their families. See also *Biomedical ethics; Clinical ethics; Medical ethics*

Communicative ethics: Ethical theories holding that ethical values are grounded in discourse. Social norms, policies and actions, and guiding principles are generated in a process of reasonable deliberation in a public forum open to equal and public participation; also called discourse ethics.

Competence: The *legal* presumption that a person has the requisite cognitive ability to negotiate certain *legal* tasks, such as entering into a contract or executing a will. Incompetence is thus a determination made only by a court that an individual lacks this ability and must be deprived of the opportunity to do certain things.

Complementary and alternative medicine (CAM): Health practices used for prevention and treatment of disease that are not paid for by an integral part of the dominant health care system but are used by patients to supplement their health care.

Compliance: See *Adherence*

Confidential information: A statutorily protected right, afforded to specifically designated health professionals, to nondisclosure of information gathered during consultation with a patient. In clinical ethics confidentiality concerns the obligation of clinicians and health care organization to protect medical information from unauthorized access. See also *Clinical ethics*

Consequentialist ethics: Ethical theories holding that certain actions are right or wrong according to the balance of their good and bad consequences.

Contextual features: Information from a case focusing on the particular concerns of family members, clinicians, institutional issues, costs, questions of research, and the like.

Continuing care retirement community: A facility that provides independent living arrangements and medical care within a single setting.

Coping: The process though which an individual can achieve psychological adjustment to stressors.

Cost control: The methods used to help decrease the level of health care expenditure.

Culture: The sum of beliefs, practices, habits, likes, dislikes, norms, customs, rituals, and so on, that are learned from other individuals and society at large.

Decisional capacity: The ability of an individual to understand his or her medical situation, weigh the benefits, burdens, and risks of therapeutic options, apply a set of values, arrive at a decision that is consistent over time, and communicate that decision. The patient without capacity (incapacitated) requires health care decisions to be made on his or her behalf. This clinical rather than legal determination is specific to the particular decision under consideration.

Decision-specific capacity: The patient's ability to understand a specific health care decision, implying that individuals have gradations of capacity along a continuum of cognitive ability to make some but not all health decisions.

Decision theory: An analytical approach to understanding how people weigh alternatives in a given situation.

Deontological ethics: Ethical theories that hold that some inherent feature of an action, other than or in addition to its consequences, makes that action right or wrong.

Dependency: Physical or cognitive impairments and disabilities that lead an older person to require increasing levels of caregiver assistance for psychological, physical, and economic support. See also *Caregiving*

Depression: A mood disorder that involves symptoms of sadness, discouragement, and feelings of hopelessness, as well as loss of appetite, difficulty sleeping, and loss of energy. Depression can be a transient state or a long-term, chronic problem.

Diagnostic-related group: A Medicare payment plan under which a hospital receives a lump sum payment based on the discharge diagnosis, without regard to actual quantity or cost of treatment provided.

Discourse ethics: See *Communicative ethics*

Distributive justice: An equitable distribution of social benefits and burdens, in which resource allocation varies according to different levels of need or merit given the circumstances.

DRG: See *Diagnostic-related group*

Elder abuse: Harmful behavior directed toward older persons by family members or professional caregivers that causes physical, psychological, or economic injury; also called elder mistreatment or maltreatment.

Elder maltreatment/mistreatment: See *Elder abuse*

Ethical dilemma: A situation where two or more competing values are important and in conflict, yet one must be chosen.

Ethical team communication: Team communication that is open about issues and authority, clarifies areas of conflict and dispute, and collaborates in the development of a plan of care that meets the needs of the patient and incorporates the unique contributions and strengths of all the members of the team.

Ethics: The study of human values, moral concepts, and systems of morality.

Ethics committee: A committee organized within or across an institution to deal with patient-specific and institution-wide ethical dilemmas. A committee may perform a variety of activities, including review of ethical and other values involved in individual patient care decisions, clinical and organizational policy advisement and review, counseling and support to caregivers, clinical consultation and case review, and staff education.

Fee-for-service payment system (FFS): A traditional medical payment system in which payment is based on office visits, procedures performed, and hospitalization. In FFS, physician income is proportional to the billing generated by services rendered to patients.

FFS: See *Fee-for-service*

Fidelity: The relationship between a professional and a patient in which special obligations exist, such as truth telling, preserving confidence, and securing patient consent before treatment.

Formal caregivers: A professional or semiprofessional who is paid to provide caregiving services for an elderly person in any of a variety of settings.

Game theory: A form of decision theory and a branch of applied mathematics fashioned to analyze certain situations in which there is an interplay between parties that may have similar, opposed, or mixed interests. In typical decision making, each of the "players" has a goal, and the game is resolved as a result of the players' decisions. A solution to the game prescribes the decisions the players should make and describes the game's appropriate outcome.

Geriatric assessment: An evaluation of medical problems and relevant comorbidity, functional status, psychological status, social support network and activities, economic needs, and environmental considerations for an older adult, generally made by a clinical professional.

Geriatric health care team: A small number of people with complementary skills who are committed to a common goal of providing care for older clients, performance goals, and a clinical approach for which they hold themselves mutually accountable. See also *Interdisciplinary health care team; Multidisciplinary health care team*

Geriatric interdisciplinary learning team: A self-organizing group of health professionals who participate in the learning process together to improve care through cycles of outcome-oriented educational activities.

Goal of medicine: Any of a variety of goals that are proposed as the appropriate focus of a particular patient's medical care, including: promotion of health and prevention of disease; relief of symptoms, pain, and suffering; cure of disease; preventing untimely death; improvement of functional status or maintenance of compromised status; education and counseling of patients and family regarding condition and prognosis; and avoiding harm to the patient in the course of care. To the extent that the goal of medicine varies, the patient care plan may also vary.

Health: In the World Health Organization's definition, "a state of complete physical, mental, and social well-being and not merely the absence of disease or infirmity." Medical care aims to restore, promote, or preserve health.

Health care ethics: The part of bioethics that is focused on the delivery of health care, on patient obligations and rights, and on the ethics of the providing professions, including medicine, nursing, and dentistry. See also *Bioethics*

Health care rationing: The attempt to allocate scarce medical resources equitably among members of a population (i.e., in ways that reflect fair decision-making processes and fair distribution of benefits and burdens).

Health maintenance organization (HMO): A prepaid health plan that delivers comprehensive care to members through designated providers, has a fixed monthly payment for health care services, and requires members to be in a plan for a specified period of time.

Horizontal responsibilities: Responsibilities of members of a health care team toward one another, shaped by their personal values, professional training, and organizational standards of conduct.

Iatrogenic illness: Any illness that results from a diagnostic procedure or therapeutic intervention and is not a natural consequence of the patient's disease; it may include illness resulting from an environmental event (e.g., a fall), underdiagnosis, undertreatment, or negligence.

Identity: A person's sense of self, incorporating various physical, psychological, and social characteristics, and continuity of the self over time.

Impaired decision making: See *Mental capacity*

Individual ethics: The study of the balance and proper relationships among various dimensions (spiritual, mental, physical, emotional, etc.) of a single individual, and the rights and duties that exist between separate individuals.

Individual practice association (IPA): A managed care plan that contracts directly with physicians in independent practice, or with one or more associations of physicians in independent practice, or with one or more multispecialty group practices. The plan is predominantly organized around solo-single practices.

Informal caregivers: A family member or close friend who cares for an individual, either in the caregiver's home or in the individual's home, generally without being paid.

Informed consent: A patient's agreement to undergo a treatment or procedure, in a situation in which the information needed to understand the decision is fully disclosed, and the patient comprehends all disclosed information and acts voluntarily.

Institutional ethics: The study of issues that support the health, vigor, balance, and equity of an institution's key systems and structures, enabling the institution to accomplish its mission while attending to the rights and duties of the individuals. Also, an analysis of the ethical obligations of an institution as health care provider, as distinguished from those of the individual clinician.

Instrumental activities of daily living (IDALs): Specific tasks performed for the maintenance of health, including cooking, functional communication, and financial management tasks.

Interdisciplinary health care team: A functioning unit, composed of individuals with varying specialized training, including patient and family caregivers who coordinate activities that provide services to a client or group of clients and have important input into the care plan for the patient. The team as decision maker acts not just once, at the inception of the process, but in a continuing way. See also *Geriatric health care team; Multidisciplinary health care team*

Long-term care: The assistance provided to a client over an extended period due to chronic illness or disability, either at home or in an institution. Long-term care generally involves a change either in the level of support or in the place of living.

Managed care: A system of organizing health care services in which the responsibility for both the payment and the delivery of care rests within a single organization.

Medical authoritarianism: The traditional medical paradigm in which physicians believed that they knew what was best for the patient and acted accordingly. The focus was traditionally paternalistic and emphasized cure and the preservation of life over quality of life. See also *Paternalism*

Medical ethics: A branch of bioethics that is generally aimed at examining the moral obligations of physicians in patient care, organizational management, and health policy. See also *Bioethics; Biomedical ethics; Clinical ethics*

Mental capacity: The availability of information-processing resources to perform a cognitive task; often construed as being either present or absent. See also *Decision-specific capacity*

Moral fiduciary: The common obligation of members of a health care team to make the protection and promotion of the patient's health-related interests and the integrity of the surrogate decision-making process the primary concerns.

Multidisciplinary health care team: A group of professionals from multiple disciplines in which each provides vital information toward decision making about a patient's care; in general, however, only one person makes the treatment decisions. See also *Geriatric health care team; Interdisciplinary health care team*

Narrative ethics: The study of ethical dilemmas using a model for determining appropriate moral decision making in which reasoning is performed through analogy to stories (narratives), including clinical case descriptions.

Neglect: The failure to provide goods or services that are necessary for optimal function or for avoiding harm.

Noncompliance: See *Adherence*

PACE: See *Program of All-Inclusive Care for the Elderly*

Palliative care: A type of care emphasizing the reduction of pain, symptom management, and the enhancement of quality of life for dying patients and their families. While not limited to end-of-life care, it is a central concept of hospice services.

Paternalism: The intentional limitation of one person's autonomy by another through actions justified exclusively by the goal of helping that person.

Patient Self-Determination Act (PSDA): A Federal law that requires health care facilities to ask if patients have advanced directives to govern their treatment and that encourages the use of advance directives.

PPO: See *Preferred provider organization*

Preferred provider organization (PPO): An organization in which an insurer contracts with a limited number of physicians and hospitals who agree to care for patients, usually on a discounted fee-for-service basis with utilization review.

Preventive ethics: A model for ethical decision making that emphasizes developing skills and practices for recognizing the potential ethical conflicts in their early stages and promotes decisions and actions to prevent occurrence of full-blown conflict.

Primary care: First-contact care, usually typified by the responsibility for coordination, continuity, and comprehensiveness of that care.

Principle of proportionate care: A clinician's responsibility to recommend treatment that is most likely to confer on a patient the greatest balance of benefits over burdens.

Program of All-Inclusive Care for the Elderly (PACE): A program in which Medicare and Medicaid funding is integrated into one stream, payment to providers is capitated, all health care services—including physician, day health, home health, hospital, and skilled nursing facility (SNF) care—are directly provided by and coordinated through case management, by interdisciplinary teams.

Quality of health care: The extent to which a health service increases the likelihood of desired health outcomes and is consistent with current professional knowledge.

Quality of life (QOL): A subjective evaluation of either life in general or its individual components, such as social, occupational, or financial functioning. Quality of life involves four dimensions: psychological well-being, which describes the individual's emotional state (lack of anxiety or depression); behavioral competence, which consists of physical health, cognition, and functional competence; the environment, which comprises the physical attributes of the surrounding environment; and perceived quality of life, which is one's subjective life satisfaction.

Rationing: See *Health care rationing*

Reflective equilibrium: The goal to match, prune, and adjust considered judgments so that they may coincide and are rendered coherent with the premises of theory.

Responsibility: From the Latin root *respondere,* meaning "to answer an accusation, to answer for, to be answerable to" liability for the consequences of one's actions and accountability to someone for those consequences in a moral or legal sense.

Restrictive gatekeeping: A system in which the money available to physicians to provide care for patients is connected to the physician's proficiency in limiting tests, treatments, and consultations for the patients.

Self-neglect: Failure by an older adult to provide adequate personal care, care of the home or surroundings, or access for him- or herself such that the failure poses a threat to the older adult.

Shared authority: Joint responsibility for an outcome, whether the decision making is explicit or not.

SHMO: See *Social health maintenance organization*

Social health maintenance organization (SHMO): A program that links Medicare primary and acute care services with limited long-term care into a single benefit package to provide care, generally for older adults.

Societal ethics: The study of ethical issues dealing primarily with the key systems and structures of society (i.e., its city, state, country, political, economic, legal, and educational structures) aimed at reaching the overall and long-term goodness of a society.

Stress: Initially, the rate of wear and tear on the body; at present, the difference between the demands placed on an individual and his or her potential capacity to meet those demands.

Surrogate decision making: The rendering of judgments by a surrogate decision maker. The preferred, decision-making standard is the substituted judgment standard, under which the surrogate makes the decision that is as close as possible to the patient's known preferences and beliefs. The secondary standards, the best interests standard, is used when the patient's preferences and beliefs are not known. It aims to protectg the patient's health and mental status (which can include allowing the patient to die).

Utilitarianism: See *Consequentialist ethics*

Vertical responsibilities: Responsibilities of members of a health care team to both the patient and organizational or contextual levels within which the team works.